EATING DISORDERS
A REFERENCE
SOURCEBOOK

EATING DISORDERS
A REFERENCE
SOURCEBOOK

Raymond Lemberg, Ph.D., Editor
with
Leigh Cohn

Revised Edition of
Controlling Eating Disorders with Facts, Advice, and Resources

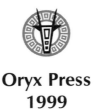

Oryx Press
1999

© 1999 by The Oryx Press
4041 North Central at Indian School Road
Phoenix, Arizona 85012-3397

Published simultaneously in Canada

Printed and Bound in the United States of America

∞ The paper used in this publication meets the minimum requirements of American National Standard for Information Science—Permanence of Paper for Printed Library Materials, ANSI Z39.48, 1984.

Library of Congress Cataloging-in-Publication Data

Eating disorders: a reference sourcebook / Raymond Lemberg,
    consulting editor, with Leigh Cohn.
      p.   cm.
    Includes bibliographical references and index.
    ISBN 1-57356-156-8 (alk. paper)
    1. Eating disorders—Diagnosis.   2. Eating disorders—Social
aspects.   3. Eating disorders—Treatment.   I. Lemberg,
Raymond.
II. Cohn, Leigh.
RC552.E18E2815   1999
616.85'26—dc21   98-48506
                                                          CIP

Contents

Preface

by Ray Lemberg, Ph.D.

The field of eating disorders, although still in its infancy, has evolved into a sophisticated, multifaceted, multidisciplinary area of research and treatment. Much more is understood about the eating disorders: bulimia nervosa, anorexia nervosa, and binge eating disorder (or what some call compulsive overeating). Obesity is not an eating disorder, per se, but is sometimes a consequence of disordered eating.

This volume has been written for varied audiences: the college or graduate student doing research on eating disorders, the professional who treats these problems, and the individual or family looking for self-help. Readers searching for additional information should read older, but significant, works, including Hilda Bruch's *The Golden Cage,* 1978, and Minuchin, Rosman, and Baker's *Psychosomatic Families: Anorexia Nervosa in Context*, 1978. An invaluable reference for the professional is Garner and Garfinkel's *Handbook of Treatment for Eating Disorders*, 2nd edition, 1997.

Eating Disorders: A Reference Sourcebook is an excellent, and perhaps one of a kind, volume with new viewpoints on treating eating disorders and a resource for the latest information available in print, audiovisual, and electronic media, as well as treatment centers throughout the United States.

This current edition is well-grounded in research and is authored by acclaimed investigators and clinicians on the cutting edge of eating disorders treatment. The latest in physiological issues and medical dangers are presented, along with a recognition of sociocultural influences primarily affecting women in Western societies. There are numerous chapters representing exciting developments in the field, including those on preventing eating disorders, the influence of culture and media, the effects of childhood trauma, and such therapeutic approaches as Narrative Therapy, Brief Therapy, and Drama/Expressive Therapies. Individuals with eating disorder behavior are becoming more understood as *people* with unique conflicts, histories, motives, and competencies.

The chapters in this book are meant to stand alone and therefore may be overlapping. They are organized into the following sections: 1. Understanding Eating Disorders: Symptoms and Causes; 2. Physiological and Medical Issues; 3. Sociocultural Issues and Subgroups Affected by Eating Disorders; 4. Dieting and the Obesitites; and 5. Current Treatment Approaches. These chapters are followed by Part 6, Facilities and Selected Resources, listing treatment centers, nonprofit organizations, and sources for other information. In addition, a glossary defining terms used in the eating-disorders field follows this Preface.

UNDERSTANDING EATING DISORDERS

One way to understand the development of eating disorders is to recognize that there are *predisposing factors*, i.e., those that create risk for the individual; *precipitating factors*, i.e., those that trigger the onset of the eating-disordered behavior; and *perpetuating factors*, i.e., those that "stamp in" an eating-disordered identity or a "stance" that is taken toward others through disordered eating that serves many purposes including the development of emotional separation in order to create a sense of self.

Predisposing factors include problems with sociocultural pressures, particularly for young women to be thin; hereditary factors; family upbringing; and mastering developmental milestones. Dieting itself is one of the key forerunners for the development of eating disorders. In bulimia, with few exceptions, periods of *prolonged* dieting precede the onset of binge-purge behavior.

Precipitating factors commonly seen at the onset of an eating disorder involve the emotional and biological upset of puberty; childhood and early adult trauma (particularly sexual abuse); and the developmental stress of forming a sense of self and individuating from family of origin.

Perpetuating factors include embracing an "anorexic (or bulimic) stance" toward parents or spouse in order to create a separate identity. Those who are seen as "chronic cases" seem to have established an eating disorder identity that is based on the resignation that one cannot break free from the chains of the eating disorder and/or on the fear that giving up one's identity will result in loss of close relationships, feelings of being special, and, essentially, the loss of an entire way of life.

WHEN TO SEEK HELP

The *severity* and *duration* of problematic eating behaviors are key indicators of whether an individual needs to seek help. Questions to ask about the severity of the eating problem include whether there has been a dramatic or rapid weight loss (greater than or equal to 15 percent of usual body weight or 10 pounds or more in a one-month period of time), or frequent binge behavior—two or more times a week—accompanied by out-of-control feelings of guilt and the compulsion to "undo" the effects of overeating by vomiting, exercise, or unhealthy dieting practices.

The degree of severity of an eating problem needs to be gauged by a person's psychological state and physical health risks. Serious depression, with loss of motivation, sleep disturbance, and suicidal thoughts, requires treatment. Dizziness, poor concentration, muscle spasms, and fatigue are all medical signs suggestive of the possibility of electrolyte imbalance and an increased risk for serious heart problems and even heart failure.

Even milder forms of emotional problems require attention if the problem continues for a length of time. As a general "rule of thumb," if emotional problems continue for three months or more, professional help should be considered.

There are other important considerations in recognizing whether an eating problem is of serious proportions. An individual with a true eating disorder becomes caught in a self-perpetuating vicious cycle in which attempts at trying to control eating through willpower result in increased guilt, overeating, obsession about weight loss, and, in bulimia, alternating cycles of starvation and out-of-control eating.

A final consideration in determining if an eating problem is serious is whether the eating behavior has become "bound up" in relationship issues, often involving the family system. There are few emotional problems or symptoms that occur in isolation. Often family conflict produces and promotes symptoms, and/or symptoms become the focus for family concern, ultimately resulting in power struggles and damage to interpersonal relationships. In these cases, outside professional intervention is usually indicated and can be very helpful.

FACILITIES LISTED IN THIS BOOK

The listings in Part 6 "Facilities and Selected Resources" are programs found in U.S. hospitals, residential treatment facilities, and other inpatient facilities. Information was compiled from questionnaires mailed between February and August 1998 and some telephone contact. Each entry provides, at a minimum, name of facility, address, telephone number, and type of eating disorder treated. Most entries list other information including name of contact person; fax, e-mail, and Web site addresses; type(s) of treatment offered; setting; population treated; type(s) of programs; number of patients program can treat; and what kind of follow-up care is offered, if any. The directory is arranged geographically by state and city.

Please note: The listings in Part 6 are by no means comprehensive, and readers should consult their physicians, local hospitals, medical schools, state medical and psychological associations, and national eating disorders associations for further suggestions. Readers should also carefully check any eating disorder program before enrolling. Type of treatments available, staff, reputation of facility, price, and setting should all be investigated. A listing in this book does not imply endorsement by The Oryx Press, the editors, or any contributor to this book.

SELECTED RESOURCES

Following the directory of facilities in Part 6 are bibliographies of books, major periodicals, Web sites, and video resources. In addition, this section lists names and addresses of nonprofit eating disorders organizations. These organizations offer a wealth of helpful material as well as providing support groups, referral lists, and professional training, research, and conferences.

INDEX

A name index of facilities listed in Part 6 follows the facilities directory. The book concludes with a comprehensive subject index covering the essays in parts 1–5.

Contributors

■ **Ray Lemberg, Ph.D., C.E.D.S.,** is editor of the revised and expanded edition of *Eating Disorders: A Reference Sourcebook.* Dr. Lemberg is a clinical psychologist and director of Psychological Pathways, a multidisciplinary group practice in Scottsdale, Mesa, and Prescott, Arizona. He is associate editor for *Eating Disorders: The Journal of Treatment and Prevention* and past Executive Vice-President of Willow Creek Hospital and Treatment Center in Scottsdale, a specialty hospital for the treatment of eating disorders. He has served as a consultant to various eating disorders programs and coauthored numerous professional articles, including "Fat Is Not a Feeling: Use of Reframing Techniques in the Treatment of Anorexia Nervosa and Bulimia"; "An Intensive Group Process-Retreat Model for Treatment of Bulimia"; "The Impact of Pregnancy on Eating Disorder Symptoms"; "Understanding Eating Disorders: A Guide for Family and Friends"; and "What Works in the Inpatient Treatment of Anorexia Nervosa and Bulimia: The Patient's Point of View."

■ **Sharon Alger**, **M.D.,** author of "Obesity: Causes and Management," is an associate professor at Albany Medical College. Dr. Alger is a Diplomat of The American Academy of Family Physicians and President of the Fellows Committee of the American Society for Clinical Nutrition. She is the author of numerous articles on obesity and nutrition.

■ **Arnold E. Andersen, M.D.,** is professor of psychiatry at the University of Iowa College of Medicine. His career in eating disorders began with research of endocrine functioning in anorexia nervosa while at the National Institutes of Health. He developed and coordinated programs at Johns Hopkins Hospital for 16 years prior to joining the University of Iowa, where he has developed a spectrum of care for eating-disordered patients. He has written the book, "Practical Comprehensive Treatment of Eating Disorders," and edited, "Males with Eating Disorders." He has also published more than 100 papers and chapters. Dr. Andersen is a founding member of the Academy of Eating Disorders and a senior editor of *Eating Disorders: The Journal of Treatment and Prevention.*

■ **Vicki L. Berkus**, **M.D., Ph.D.,** is a psychiatrist at Sierra Tucson. She heads the Eating Disorder Program which deals with anorexics, bulimics, and compulsive overeaters. Professional interests include looking at acupuncture and Revia as alternate forms of dealing with cravings for the compulsive overeaters as well as looking at experiential issues involved with treating patients with eating disorders.

She is currently a member of the International Association of Eating Disorders Professionals and the Academy of Eating Disorders.

■ **Carol Bloom, C.S.W.,** is a faculty member of the Women's Therapy Centre Institute in New York City, a training institute for the practice of feminist relational psychotherapy. She is coauthor of *Eating Problems: A Feminist Psychoanalytic Treatment Model* and author of "Bulimia: A Feminist Understanding," in *Fed Up and Hungry.* She is in private practice in New York City.

■ **Linda Bock, M.D.,** is associate professor of psychiatry at St. Louis University, Department of Psychiatry and Residency Training Director for Division of Child and Adolescent Psychiatry. Dr. Bock is well known for her work in the field of eating disorders.

■ **Thomas F. Cash, Ph.D.,** is professor of psychology at Old Dominion University in Norfolk, Virginia. A clinical and research psychologist for over 25 years, his professional works largely pertain to the psychology of physical appearance, including four books and over 125 scientific publications and most recent book, *The Body Image Workbook* (New Harbinger, 1997).

■ **Carolyn J. Cavanaugh, Ph.D.,** earned her B.A. in Psychology at Duke University and her Ph.D. in Clinical Psychology at Arizona State University. She completed her predoctoral clinical internship at the University of Wisconsin Medical School, where she worked in the Eating Disorders Treatment Center. Her research and clinical interests are in Eating Disorders, Childhood Obesity, and Health Psychology. She currently teaches in the Department of Psychology at Arizona State University and works at Psychological Pathways in Scottsdale, Arizona.

■ **Irene Chatoor, M.D.,** is vice chair of the department of psychiatry and director of the Infant Psychiatry and Eating Disorders Program at the Children's National Medical Center in Washington, DC, and professor of psychiatry and behavioral sciences and associate professor of pediatrics at George Washington University School of Medicine and Health Sciences. She is board-certified in pediatrics by the American Board of Pediatrics and in psychiatry and child psychiatry by the American Board of Psychiatry and Neurology. She has served as a consultant, reviewer, and workshop presenter, and has published numerous papers, chapter, and articles in the field.

■ **Marjorie Crago, Ph.D.,** is a research specialist in the Arizona Prevention Center at the University of Arizona College of Medicine. She has participated in a number of eating disorder research projects focusing on such topics as risk factors, prevention, sex roles, substance abuse, athleticism, prevalence in different ethnic groups, and treatment.

■ **Cindy Davis, Ph.D.,** is a lecturer in the Department of Social Work at the University of New South Wales in Sydney, Australia. Dr. Davis has done extensive research on eating disorders in both the United States and in Asia. Dr. Davis is the author of several publications on the role of culture and eating disorders. She has worked in the U.S., Asia, and Australia.

■ **Kathy Jo Dennison, R.N., C.N.P.I.S., C.A.C.S., C.N.D.A.I., C.N.F.C.S.,** is a Professional Interventionist specializing in eating disorders and chemical dependency interventions. In addition to clinical interventions and extensive experience with the treatment process, she is in demand as a professional speaker at both national and international addiction conferences as well as in the academic arena. Ms. Dennison also serves as Director of Nursing at Sierra Tuscon Treatment Center.

■ **Alexandra O. Eliot, Ph.D., L.I.C.S.W.,** is an adjunct assistant professor at the Simmons School of Social Work, in Boston, Massachusetts, where she teaches social policy and is a graduate faculty advisor. She was formerly instructor in psychiatry at the Harvard Medical School, chief social worker in the Division of Adolescent/Young Adult Medicine, and cofounder of the outpatient Eating Disorders Clinic at Boston Children's Hospital. She maintains a private practice in Belmont, Massachusetts

■ **Nancy Ellis-Ordway, A.C.S.W.,** worked for several years with the Anorexia/Bulimia Treatment and Education Center (ABTEC) at St. John's Mercy Medical Center in St. Louis, Missouri. She also authored "The Impact of Family Dynamics on Anorexia: A Transactional View of Treatment" in The Addiction Process: Effective Social Work Approaches. She is currently in private practice in Montgomery, Alabama.

■ **Andrea Gitter, M.A., A.D.T.R.,** is a faculty member of the Women's Therapy Centre Institute in New York City, a training institute for the practice of feminist relational psychotherapy. She is coauthor of *Eating Problems: A Feminist Psychoanalytic Treatment Model.* She is in private practice in Manhattan and Belle Harbor, Queens.

■ **Elliot M. Goldner, M.D., F.R.C.P.,** is the director of the Eating Disorder Program at St. Paul's Hospital in Vancouver, and is an Associate Professor of Psychiatry at the University of British Columbia.

■ **Susan Gutwill, M.S., C.S.W.,** is a faculty member of the Women's Therapy Centre Institute in New York City, a training institute for the practice of feminist relational psychotherapy. She is coauthor of *Eating Problems: A Feminist Psychoanalytic Treatment Model.* She is in private practice in Highland Park, New Jersey.

■ **Adele M. Holman, D.S.W.,** is a family therapist in Englewood, New Jersey who specializes in treating eating disorders. She is an Executive Board member of The American Anorexia Bulimia Association. She is the author of *Family Assessment: Tools for Understanding and Intervention.* She is also a family mediator and an accredited consultant of the Academy of Family Mediators.

■ **Donna (Meredy) Humphreys, B.S.,** is a chemist by trade, but a writer at heart. She was a regular columnist and contributor to her college newspaper. She is the author of "Inside the Shell," an article that appeared in "Food for Thought," a newsletter dealing with eating disorder issues. She has also contributed several other features to this newsletter.

■ **Annika Kahm, B.S.,** has more than 15 years experience as the director of nutrition at the Wilkins Center for Eating Disorders in Greenwich, Connecticut. Ms. Kahm is also a board member of the American Anorexia/Bulimia Association in New York and a member of the Academy for Eating Disorders.

■ **Melanie Katzman, Ph.D.,** is a clinical psychologist and assistant professor at the New York Hospital Cornell Medical Center in New York. She is a senior lecturer at the University of London's Institute of Psychiatry, where she coordinates an outpatient eating disorders treatment service. She is the coauthor and coeditor of several books on eating disorders, along with multiple articles. She has worked in the U.S., Asia, and Europe.

■ **Matthew Keene, M.D.,** is the founder and director of Feeding Your Feelings, a multidisciplinary team of health care professionals dedicated to the management of compulsive overeating through the development of human potential. He graduated with honors from Georgetown University School of Medicine and received his psychiatric residency training at the Cleveland Clinic Foundation. He is a board-certified physician with the American Board of Psychiatry and Neurology and practices in Phoenix, Arizona.

■ **Barbara P. Kinoy, Ph.D.,** is former director of professional development, staff therapist, and supervisor of the Wilkins Center for Eating Disorders in Greenwich, Connecticut. She is the editor/author of *When Will We Laugh Again: Living and Dealing with Anorexia and Bulimia,* and editor of *Eating Disorders: New Directions in Treatment and Recovery.*

▪ **Laura Kogel, A.C.S.W.,** is a faculty member of the Women's Therapy Centre Institute in New York City, a training institute for the practice of feminist relational psychotherapy. She is coauthor of *Eating Problems: A Feminist Psychoanalytic Treatment Model.* She is in private practice in New York City.

▪ **Debra Landau-West, M.S., R.D.,** is a dietitian in private practice specializing in eating disorders in Scottsdale, Arizona, for 19 years. She has consulted for several eating disorder treatment programs, with a focus toward program development and management of nutrition therapy. She has also lectured at several national conferences on eating disorders.

▪ **Cappi Lang, Ph.D.,** maintains private practices in art therapy and Rubenfeld synergy in both Phoenix and Prescott, Arizona. She received a masters degree in the Expressive Art Therapies from Pratt Institute in New York and a Ph.D. in Human Development from Arizona State University. She is a certified counselor and a supervisor for both art therapy and Rubenfeld synergy. She currently teaches counseling and art therapy at Prescott College.

▪ **Michael D. Levine, Ph.D.,** is professor of psychology at Kenyon College, Gambier, Ohio, and President, Board of Directors, Eating Disorders Awareness & Prevention, Inc. He has written extensively in the area of prevention.

▪ **Stephen P. Madigan, M.S.W., Ph.D.,** is the director of training at Yaletown Family Therapy in Vancouver, and co-director of training for the Toronto Narrative Therapy Project. He is a founding member of the Vancouver Anti-anorexia League.

▪ **Margo Maine, Ph.D.,** is a clinical psychologist, lecturer, consultant, and writer who has specialized in the treatment of eating disorders for the past 16 years. She serves as the director of the Eating Disorder Program at the Institute of Living in Hartford, Connecticut, and as coordinator of the Women's Connection at the Institute of Living, a system of services specifically devoted to women. Dr. Maine is an assistant clinical professor at the University of Connecticut, Department of Psychiatry and an adjunct faculty member at the University of Hartford, Graduate Institute of Professional Psychology. Dr. Maine is the author of *Father Hunger: Daughters and Food,* published by Gurze Books. Her second book, *Body Wars,* is scheduled for publication in 1998. She has written numerous articles related to the prevention and treatment of eating disorders and

is a senior editor of "Eating Disorders: The Journal of Treatment and Prevention."

▪ **Bonnie Marx, R.N., M.S.N.,** is a counselor in private practice in Phoenix, Arizona. Ms. Marx has done extensive work in designing treatment and training programs for the lay and professional communities in the area of compulsive eating behaviors. She is also a co-creator of the Life Management Program, a psychoeducational treatment program for people with long-term problems with weight.

▪ **Barbara McFarland, Ph.D.,** is the founder of the Eating Disorders Recovery Center and the Brief Therapy Center. Dr. McFarland has worked with eating disorder clients and their families for the past 18 years. She has written numerous articles and books on eating disorders, such as "Swords Into Plowshares," *The Family Therapy Networker.* May/June 1997; "Solution Focused Brief Therapy and Eating Disorders," *Solutions: The Newsletter of the Brief Therapy Network.* Vol. 1, #2, August 1994; *Shame and Body Image,* 1990, Health Communications; *Feeding the Empty Heart,* 1988, Hazelden; *Abstinence in Action,* 1986, Hazelden; *A Practical Guide to Solution Focused Work with Clients,* 1995; and *My Mother Was Right: How Today's Women Reconcile with Their Mothers,* 1997.

▪ **Diane W. Mickley, M.D., F.A.C.P.,** is founder and director of the Wilkins Center for Eating Disorders in Greenwich, Connecticut. She is past president of the American Anorexia/Bulimia Association and a founding member of the Academy for Eating Disorders. She is a research associate in the Department of Psychiatry at the Yale University School of Medicine and served on the McKnight Federal Task Force on Eating Disorders. She was a reviewer for the American Psychiatric Associations Practice Guidelines for Eating Disorders and has contributed numerous publications on the medical treatment of eating disorders.

▪ **James E. Mitchell, M.D.,** is Chairman, Department of Neuroscience, University of North Dakota, and President and Scientific Director, The Neuropsychiatric Research Institute, Fargo, North Dakota.

▪ **Erika S. Neuberg, Ph.D.,** is in practice with Psychological Pathways in Scottsdale, Arizona, and has served as staff psychologist of the Southwest Bariatric Nutrition Center. She has done extensive research and therapy with women with eating disorders, and has designed a pregnancy adjustment group for the prevention of maternal and child pathology.

▪ **Bonnie Pelch, A.C.S.W., L.C.S.W.,** is a private practitioner in St. Louis, Missouri. She specializes in the treatment of adolescents/young adults and their families/spouses. She has provided group and medical professional training in the field of family therapy of eating-disordered families at St. John's Mercy Medical Center and St. Luke's Hospital (now Unity Health Care) in St. Louis.

■ **Carol B. Peterson, Ph.D.,** is a senior research scientist in the Eating Disorders Research Program, University of Minnesota, Minneapolis.

■ **Jeanne Phillips, M.A., C.E.D.C.,** is in private practice with Psychological Pathways in Scottsdale, AZ, specializing in women's issues, anorexia nervosa, bulimia, and compulsive overeating. She was founder and director for 13 years of SHED (Self Help for Eating Disorders), Phoenix's first eating disorders support group which provided support for individuals with either anorexia nervosa or bulimia. She is a Certified Eating Disorders Counselor and frequent speaker to the lay and professional communities and has co-authored several articles on eating disorders.

■ **Donald S. Robertson, M.D., M.Sc.,** is the author of *The Snowbird Diet,* a program for staying slim with gourmet dining. He has also published articles in a number of journals, including the *American Journal of Clinical Nutrition, Arizona Medicine, Journal of Gastroenterology, McCalls,* and *Shape.* Dr. Robertson is an internist and gastroenterologist who trained at Princeton University, the University of Colorado, and Cornell University Medical School. He is the founder and medical director of the Southwest Bariatric Nutrition Center in Scottsdale, Arizona, and is a nationally recognized authority on nutrition and weight loss.

■ **Marcia Rorty, Ph.D.,** received her doctoral degree in Clinical Psychology from UCLA in 1993. She is currently Assistant Professor of Graduate Psychology at Azusa Pacific University in Azusa, California. She has conducted research and treatment in the area of eating disorders for 10 years, specializing in understanding and working with those individuals who have survived childhood trauma. She has published many theoretical and empirical articles in this area.

■ **Jan Rothman-Sickler, M.A.,** is a certified associate counselor with the group practice Psychological Pathways in Scottsdale, Arizona, specializing in the treatment of anorexia, bulimia, and compulsive overeating. She is the Family and Expressive Group therapist for Psychological Pathways' intensive outpatient program, Food for Thought. Her work with young people in the area of Expressive and Group Therapy is extensive. She has worked as a Drama Therapy consultant in school districts across the country. She acts as consultant to corporations and

schools, leading workshops to enhance creativity, problem solving, and teamwork among employees. She is a speaker and a workshop leader to professional and lay groups.

■ **Catherine Shisslak, Ph.D.,** is an associate professor in the department of family and community medicine and the Arizona Prevention Center at the University of Arizona College of Medicine. Her research on eating disorders has spanned both treatment and prevention-based investigations in children and adults. She has extensive clinical experience with eating disorders based on the development and direction of a multidisciplinary research, teaching, and clinical eating disorder inpatient and outpatient program at the University of Arizona Medical Center. Her most recent work focuses on identifying risk and protective factors associated with eating disorders through a longitudinal study of these factors in children and adolescents.

■ **Melissa D. Strachan, B.A.,** is a doctoral candidate at the Virginia Consortium Program in Clinical Psychology in Norfolk, Virginia. A body-image researcher and community consultant, she has conducted several investigations of the relationships between body image, eating disorders, and feminism. Her doctoral dissertation is a treatment outcome study of a recently published, cognitive-behavioral self-help program.

■ **Adrian H. Thurstin, Ph.D.,** is an associate professor in the department of psychiatry and behavioral neurobiology at the University of Alabama School of Medicine in Birmingham. He has contributed chapters regarding eating disorders to several clinical nutrition texts.

■ **Sheldon Wagman, D.O., F.A.C.N.,** is board-certified in psychiatry and is in private practice in Phoenix, Arizona. He is a psychiatric consultant with Psychological Pathways, Professional Psychological Associates, and Arizona Community Psychiatric Group. He is associate professor of psychiatry at the Arizona College Osteopathic Medicine. His specialties include eating disorders, psychiatric treatment of adolescents and adult disorders, and medication management of psychiatric disorders.

■ **Susan Wagner, Ph.D.,** maintains a private practice in White Plains, New York, and is a voluntary faculty member of the Eating Disorders unit of the Westchester division of New York Hospital-Cornell Medical Center. Her published works include the article "The Sense of Personal Ineffectiveness in Patients with Eating Disorders: One Construct or Several?"

■ **Lillie Weiss, Ph.D.,** is a clinical psychologist in private practice in Phoenix, Arizona, and is an adjunct associate professor in the department of psychology at Arizona State University in Tempe. Dr. Weiss has done extensive research and therapy with bulimic women.

▪ **Sharlene Wolchik, Ph.D.,** is a clinical psychologist and professor in the department of psychology at Arizona State University in Tempe. Dr. Wolchik has done extensive research and therapy with bulimic women.

▪ **Joel Yager, M.D.,** is professor and vice chair for education, department of psychiatry at the University of New Mexico School of Medicine Health Sciences Center. Previously, he was professor of psychiatry and associate chair for education at the UCLA Neuropsychiatric Institute and West Los Angeles Veterans Administration Medical Center for

20 years. He has edited or co-edited six books and published more than 200 articles, chapters, and reviews in the field of psychiatry. He is editor-in-chief of *Eating Disorders Review,* a professional newsletter, and serves on the editorial board of six professional journals. He has received numerous awards and honors, including the Joseph Goldberger Award in Clinical Nutrition from the American Medical Association.

▪ **Lela Zaphiropoulos, A.C.S.W.,** is a faculty member of the Women's Therapy Centre Institute in New York City, a training institute for the practice of feminist relational psychotherapy. She is coauthor of *Eating Problems: A Feminist Psychoanalytic Treatment Model* and *Preventing Childhood Eating Problems.* She is in private practice in New York City.

Glossary of Terms

achalasia: failure to relax; referring to visceral openings such as the pylorus and cardia.

amenorrhea: irregular or absence of menstrual periods.

anorexia nervosa: an eating disorder that is often life-endangering, characterized by a distorted body image, excessively low weight, and a relentless pursuit of thinness. There are two types: Restricting Type, involving low nutritional intake; and Binge-Purging Type with alternating episodes of binge eating or purging behavior, i.e., self-induced vomiting, laxative abuse, diuretic abuse, or enemas.

anxiety disorders: a group of disorders including panic attacks, agoraphobia (e.g., fear of being away from home or being in a crowd, etc.), specific phobias, social anxieties, obsessive-compulsive disorder, posttraumatic stress disorders, and generalized anxiety disorders involving excessive anxiety and worry.

at-risk groups: individuals belonging to a demographic group or participating in an activity (e.g., modeling, dance, gymnastics) that increases the risk for developing an eating disorder.

autonomic nervous system: the part of the nervous system that regulates automatic (i.e., involuntary) bodily functions.

basal metabolic rate: the rate at which the body uses calories at rest.

binge eating disorder (BED): recurrent episodes of binge eating in the absence of regular use of inappropriate compensatory behaviors characteristic of bulimia nervosa.

body mass index: the most commonly used measure to determine healthy weight, calculated by dividing an individual's weight in kilograms by height in meters squared.

borderline personality disorder: a specific type of personality disorder involving a pervasive pattern of instability in interpersonal relationships, self-identity problems, and difficulty regulating emotions. Real or imagined abandonment and impulsivity characterize this disorder.

bradycardia: slow heart rate, under 60 beats per minute, associated with starvation and low weight.

bulimia nervosa: recurrent episodes of binge eating characterized by an excessive intake of food in a discrete period of time with a lack of a sense of control during the episode. Binge eating is accompanied by inappropriate compensatory behavior to prevent weight gain such as self-induced vomiting or laxative abuse, etc. There are two types: Purging Type, with self-induced vomiting, laxative, diuretic, or enema abuse; and Non-purging Type, with other compensatory behaviors such as fasting or excessive exercise.

cardiac arrhythmias: irregular heart rhythms that can result in fatal conditions.

cognitive therapy: a method of treatment embracing a number of techniques that aim to change one's thinking in order to produce both behavioral and emotional changes. Some forms are known as "self-talk" therapy, reframing, and rational emotive therapy. Also known as Cognitive-Behavior Therapy when combined with techniques of behavioral change.

co-morbid: the presence of more than one illness in a defined period of time in a single individual.

compulsive overeating: overlapping with binge eating disorder, compulsive overeating involves "nervous eating" to soothe the emotions over a long period of time or binge eating in a discrete period. (*see also* binge eating disorder)

conversion disorder: an unconscious defense mechanism in which anxiety is hypothesized to be converted into somatic (body) symptoms.

critical weight: the minimum amount of body weight that an individual needs for healthy functioning.

delayed gastric emptying: a condition in which the time for digestion is increased and food is retained in the stomach resulting from chronic disordered eating.

diabetes mellitus: a dysfunction in insulin regulation of blood sugar involving Type I (insulin-dependent) and Type II (non-insulin-dependent).

differential diagnosis: the professional assessment to differentiate one psychological disorder from another.

diuretic: an agent that promotes water loss through excretion of urine.

drama therapy: the use of role-playing, improvisation, and other techniques of enactment to create emotional and behavioral change.

dynamic psychotherapy: a method of therapy deriving from psychoanalysis emphasizing cause and effect relationships in underlying motives and drives.

dysphoria: a depressed mood involving general dissatisfaction or demoralization.

edema: excessive watery fluid in the cells and tissues of the body.

electrolyte imbalance: an imbalance of one or more of several chemicals in the body that conduct electrical impulses controlling the muscles, including the heart, causing sometimes fatal conditions.

emetic: an agent that causes vomiting.

enteritis: inflammation of the intestines.

esophageal obstruction: an obstruction in the esophagus that occurs in conjunction with eating-disorder behaviors, often seen in bulimia nervosa.

expressive therapy: the use of art, drama, and movement to allow for projection of internal experiences—conscious and unconscious—outwardly to create new meanings and healthy adaptation.

family therapy: a school of therapy organized around the structure and function of the family system and on how interpersonal relationships determine behavior in both individuals and families.

group psychotherapy: psychotherapy involving a psychotherapist and group of individuals who offer support and feedback for behavioral change. The group as a whole often mirrors family relations and offers opportunities for understanding issues related to family of origin.

hepatic illness: a variety of medical conditions affecting liver function.

hypoglycemia: low blood sugar.

hypokalemia: a depletion of potassium ions associated with such purge behaviors as laxative abuse and vomiting, resulting in an electrolyte imbalance.

inflammatory bowel disease: a variety of conditions involving inflammation and dysfunction of the gastric intestine tract.

insight-oriented therapy: psychotherapy aimed at creating self-realization and awareness of unconscious impulses and motivations.

major depression: a disorder involving depressed mood and/or loss of interest or pleasure which may be a single episode or recurrent, and of mild, moderate, or severe proportions.

metabolic rate: *see* basal metabolic rate.

mood disorders: a group of disorders that involve deregulation of mood, usually depression, but also including bipolar disorder (manic-depressive) episodes.

narrative therapy: a system of psychotherapy that locates the "disorder" in the story an individual tells about one's self (i.e., belief system) and in its resulting unhealthy identity. The goal of treatment is to externalize the problem identity and to create a healthier self-view.

neurotransmitter: a number of chemical agents found in the brain that transmit electrical messages from one neuron to the other.

obesity: a condition in which a person weighs 20% more than his/her maximum desirable weight for his/her height.

obsessive compulsive disorder: an anxiety disorder that is expressed through excessive worry and obsessiveness and/or compulsive behavior such as counting, checking, cleanliness rituals, etc.

osteopenia: decreased calcification or loss of bone density.

osteoporosis: reduction in bone mass or atrophy of skeletal tissue. Associated with poor nutrition and loss of menses.

pancreatitis: inflammation of the pancreas.

personality disorders: enduring patterns of maladaptive behavior that may affect thinking, mood, and interpersonal functioning as well as impulse control. Often viewed as a problem or defect in character development.

primary pulmonary hypertension: a serious medical condition involving heart and lung complications recently associated with the use of certain diet pill products.

psychoactive: pharmacological agents that possess the ability to alter moods, anxiety, and behaviors.

psychotropic: *see* psychoactive.

refeeding syndrome/ refeeding edema: the physiological complications that often involve excessive water retention following replenishment of nutrition after starvation.

serotonin: a neurotransmitter involved in regulating emotions and linked with depression, bulimia nervosa, and premenstrual syndrome.

solution-oriented therapy: a system of psychotherapy that focuses on building competencies and solutions to psychological and interpersonal problems, rather than on the problems themselves or on psychopathology.

subclinical eating disorders: disordered eating behavior that does not meet diagnostic criteria for a "full-blown" eating disorder, yet is problematic for the individual and may be a precursor to a more serious eating disorder at a later date.

uremia: an excessive amount of urea in the blood, associated with renal failure.

PART 1
Understanding Eating Disorders: Symptoms and Causes

The Eating Disorders: An Introduction

by Barbara P. Kinoy, Ph.D., Adele M. Holman, D.S.W., and Ray Lemberg, Ph.D.

This chapter discusses the three eating disorders—anorexia nervosa, bulimia nervosa, and binge eating disorder (also referred to as compulsive overeating)—as well as "the obesities." For additional information, please see Adrien H. Thurstin's chapter, "Behavioral, Physical, and Psychological Symptoms of Eating Disorders," beginning on page 12.

ANOREXIA NERVOSA

Anorexia nervosa is an eating disorder characterized by a purposeful weight loss far beyond the normal range. Fear of being fat is almost always an overriding factor in this pursuit. A desire to perfect one's self through one's body, and by extension in every other way, is also a strong characteristic and can supersede the reality of body structure and function, resulting in a distorted body image. This pursuit can also displace or change other requirements of living, such as family and social relationships.

Listed below are behavioral, physical, and emotional symptoms and changes that are a part of the picture of anorexia nervosa. Symptoms of bulimia nervosa, or bulimia, will also be reviewed. Similar to anorexia nervosa, bulimia has often been linked with it, and the discussion of each will be overlapping. Finally, binge eating disorder will be discussed. Keep in mind, however, that people do not always fit exactly into the categories of anorexia, bulimia, or binge eating disorder, and thus the line between them may be a fine one.

Anorexia nervosa is officially classified into two categories: (1) the restricting type (characterized by low calorie intake and the absence of binge-eating or purging behavior) and (2) binge-eating/purging type (characterized by calorie restriction and binge and/or purge behaviors).

SYMPTOMS OF ANOREXIA NERVOSA

- Intense fear of becoming obese, which does not diminish as weight loss progresses.

- Disturbance in body image, for example, seeing one's self as fat even when one is bone thin or emaciated.

- Weight loss of at least 15 percent of expected body weight, adjusted for height, body build, and age.

- Refusal to maintain normal weight.

- A cessation of the menstrual cycle, which may occur before an appreciable weight loss.

- Hyperactivity (i.e., one is busy all the time, hardly ever coming to rest, especially in the initial stages).

- Fasting, vomiting, or laxative use, often following bingeing but sometimes after ordinary intake of food.

- Determined and/or repetitive rituals and thoughts called compulsive and obsessive behaviors; among them, a preoccupation with thoughts of food, weight, and exercise, to the extreme. Exercise goes far beyond the purpose of pleasure or fitness; it is used to "burn off" calories, to diminish whatever fat remains, and to affirm one's control over the nature of one's body.

- Often, the appearance of depression.

Proceeding from the above are the following changes, which are more marked and severe:

- A disturbance in cognitive ability (thinking).

- Deterioration or absence of family and social relationships or, conversely, poor family relationships contributing to the onset of the weight loss.

- Reduction, or absence of, social activity (i.e., social isolation).

- An overt increase in depression. Although some experts suggest this state is part of anorexia nervosa and/or an underlying cause, the disorder itself sometimes seems to act as a substitute for overt depression.

- The development of fine body hair (lanugo).

- The sensation of feeling cold (hypothermia).

- Lowered blood pressure.

- A slowed pulse rate.

- An imbalance in the body chemistry, called an electrolyte imbalance. For example, excessive purging or laxative use can reduce potassium content in the body to a dangerous degree. Medical attention is required to diagnose and treat this symptom.
- Occurrence of dental problems, most often in those who vomit, because the acid content of the vomitus erodes tooth enamel.
- The possible occurrence of death if the process remains unabated. Suicide is not an uncommon consequence of the despair and depression connected with this condition.

THE HISTORY OF ANOREXIA NERVOSA

The restrictive and bingeing aspects of diet control have been around for a long time. In early humans they served a purpose in times of sparse food and in times of plenty. Middle Ages civilization attached a religious connotation to starving one's self in the context of self-denial, sacrifice, and mortification of the flesh for holy and spiritual affirmation. By the late 1800s, anorexia nervosa was fairly well established as a medical condition with emotional factors. Although Sir William Gull in England described its physical attributes, it was Charles Lasegue in France, around the same time, who noted the marked emotional qualities accompanying the physical symptoms. He called it "anorexie hysterique"; Gull called it "anorexia nervosa." *Anorexia* actually means loss of appetite, which is a misnomer as appetite is denied, at least initially. Although a person with anorexic behavior may deny hunger, he or she will often feed others and become obsessive about everything related to food. The German term *Pubertatsmagersucht*, or "leanness passion of puberty," is perhaps most descriptive of a segment of the anorexic population.

CAUSES OF ANOREXIA NERVOSA

Anorexia nervosa mainly affects females, usually in the adolescent years, although the overt onset may occur as early as age 10 (and occasionally even earlier) or as late as the postmenopausal years. A trigger usually marks the acute onset, such as the refusal or inability to stop dieting; a critical remark about weight or appearance from a significant person, relative, or peer; a sexual threat; or a trauma such as the loss of a parent or sibling, a divorce, or illness.

The trigger, however, may not necessarily be the cause, only the last straw. Causation is very complex and may not always be known specifically or identified. This is an area where mind and body are closely interrelated. Medical experts, as described in other parts of this book, look for and have found certain physiological clues. Psychological experts have added their findings. It is important to understand that no one event causes anorexia nervosa. It is more likely that the exquisitely timed convergence of many external forces promotes the anorexic process and allows it to predominate.

Growing up is frightening for some girls as they watch their bodies become round, curvy, and capable of sexual activity and reproduction. One strives to perfect oneself for the monumental task ahead that is adulthood. A tendency to "hold back" the passage of time is noted as a resistance to maturing, as if to ensure that the early constellation of parent and child need not change.

In addition, there are indications that anorexia is unknowingly fostered in very close parental or family relationships that do not encourage the development of one's own thoughts or opinions. In some instances, certain issues are secret and simply not discussed.

Individuals with anorexia may have grown up with an inordinate need to please others before themselves, or may never have been sure of their own perceptions in relation to their parents'. Described as extra sensitive, they often have been the caretakers of other needy family members or of the family's emotional balance.

Families in which there have been alcoholic or addictive problems appear to be more at risk for eating disorders. Often the anorexia nervosa of a child replicates some form of impulse-control problem or depression in a parent or previous generation. The significance of these findings is uncertain. At most, they suggest a predisposition to eating disorders in certain families. High family expectations, or the perception of such expectations, may be instrumental in exerting pressure on the anorexic-to-be.

ANOREXIA NERVOSA AS A PRESENT-DAY DISORDER

Anorexia nervosa is found in postindustrial countries where the availability of food is generally assured. In these countries achievement and financial success are part of the cultural value system. The United States, for example, places tremendous emphasis on slim female bodies and using them as sexual, seductive charms to sell products as well as provide a romantic alliance of thinness/happiness/success. The bombardment of television programs, movies, and magazines conveying these cultural symbols has reinforced an ideal that only a few can achieve. Thus, the vulnerable find themselves striving for the perfection that is an impossible dream.

It is also thought that the status of females in Western society has contributed to the marked presence of anorexia nervosa. The new voices of assertion and independence in the last decade or two are additional challenges to be absorbed into the emerging female character. Often, sexuality, motherhood, achievement, assertion, independence, dependence, appearance, and weight all get mixed up in one confusing picture of "how to be." Anorexic thinking and behavior evolve as one way to retreat from this confusion and one way to handle the accompanying depression.

Men and boys who suffer from anorexia nervosa are much fewer in number. They exhibit similar vulnerabilities in their histories and similar struggles in today's world. Masculine identity is undergoing changes, too, as women change. The old concept of the macho male is not always the ideal or the reality. As young boys struggle to find their place in society, they often associate success, achievement, and maleness with fitness and slimness. This is a problem particularly among athletes. It is suspected that more males suffer from anorexia nervosa than come to health professionals' attention.

BULIMIA NERVOSA

Bulimia, or bulimia nervosa, as it is officially called, is an eating disorder that is closely linked to anorexia nervosa. The first descriptions of the binge-eating and purging symptoms of bulimia are from early Roman times. The French psychiatrist Pierre Janet wrote about a patient who binged and purged compulsively but never lost her appetite (Janet, 1903). An American authority on obesity, Dr. Albert Stunkard, was the first to identify bulimia in contemporary terms in 1959. The American Psychiatric Association (1994) first characterized bulimia nervosa as a distinct disorder in describing the following characteristics:

- Recurrent episodes of binge eating.
- A feeling of lack of control over eating behavior during the eating binges.
- The regular need to either self-induce vomiting, use laxatives or diuretics, diet severely or fast, or exercise vigorously to prevent weight gain.
- A minimum average of two binge eating episodes a week for at least three months.
- Persistent overconcern with body shape and weight.

Bulimia nervosa is divided into two categories or types: (1) use of vomiting, laxatives, diuretics, or enemas following a binge, and (2) nonpurging type—using other inappropriate compensatory behaviors to avoid weight gain, such as fasting or excessive exercise.

THE PSYCHOLOGY OF BULIMIA NERVOSA

Bulimia is an emotionally based disorder in which food is used as a means of satisfying inner needs. In contrast to anorexia, in which restriction of food is used as a means of gaining control, in bulimia, eating unusually large amounts of food, bingeing, and then purging is a response to distress. The word *bulimia* derives from the Greek, meaning "insatiable appetite." The troubled person feels a powerful urge to eat and is driven by the belief that only by giving in to a craving for food that is much more intense than normal feelings of hunger can satisfaction be achieved.

Bingeing usually involves the rapid consumption of high-calorie foods that are often sweet and of a texture that is easily swallowed. Binges may last several minutes or several hours and may be planned or unplanned. If the urge to eat comes on suddenly, available food may be devoured quickly. At other times, binges are planned, and the person decides in advance to binge at a specific time and place. For most people with this problem, an uncontrollable pattern of bingeing develops into a daily routine; as this becomes a habit, the body loses its ability to signal satisfaction, and consequently, eating is no longer in response to physiological hunger.

Rapid consumption of large amounts of food brings on considerable abdominal discomfort and a bloated feeling. Relief comes through purging, that is, ridding the body of the consumed food and fluids. Most often, this is accomplished by vomiting. Some individuals purge by using laxatives, diuretics, or a combination of means. Often tolerance to laxatives builds, leading to the use of extraordinarily large quantities, sometimes more than 100 doses a day. Usually purging reduces the physical discomfort, relieves stress, and reduces the fear of gaining weight. What the individual does not know is that most calories are absorbed, even with purging. What was begun as an "ideal" way to eat and lose weight frequently becomes the basis for a very persistent and disturbing self-reinforcing pattern of behavior.

Many individuals with bulimia engage in daily strenuous exercise routines as another means of controlling weight gain. The strong urge to exercise often contributes to a self-punishing regime. When half an hour is seen as good, an hour is seen as better, and more than that is better yet.

All of these behaviors are usually experienced as bizarre, unnatural, and shameful. Therefore, an element of secrecy evolves in carrying them out. Considerable effort is spent in obtaining food, consuming it, getting rid of it, and excessively exercising. Individuals often go to great lengths to conceal these activities from others to avoid shame and guilt, although these feelings become internalized anyway, adding to the vicious cycle.

A common form or stage of bulimia that combines restrictive aspects of anorexia with those of bulimia has sometimes been referred to as "bulimarexia." This form of bulimia is characterized by periods of starving to lose weight alternated with periods of bingeing and purging. Typically, the process begins with restrictions on food, then, either due to the individual feeling pressure to give it up from within or from an outside source, shifts to bingeing and purging. This stage is sometimes interspersed with periods of normal eating, but then the pattern of fasting or bingeing resumes. As a result, weight often fluctuates markedly.

A number of physiological effects of this self-inflicted behavior can prove serious, irreversible, and potentially fatal. These effects are discussed in greater detail in other chapters of this book but should be mentioned here as well. Medical problems include menstrual cessation and irregularities; digestive disturbances; brittle hair and nails; dry skin; dizziness; electrolyte imbalance; muscle cramps; fatigue; enlargement of the parotid (salivary) gland; dental problems, especially permanent erosion of the enamel; poor circulation; heart irregularities; and heart failure. When proper nutrition is restored, most of these problems are re-versible; however, permanent damage may be done. Therefore, early detection and treatment are extremely important.

WHO IS LIKELY TO DEVELOP BULIMIA NERVOSA?

Bulimia can be better understood by knowing who is likely to engage in this behavior and the underlying dynamic reasons that encourage people to develop it. Research has shown that most persons with bulimia are female, although a small percentage are male. Usually those with bulimia are within a normal weight range, although some weigh 10 to 15 pounds within normal weight range and struggle with weight fluctuation.

Although bulimia and anorexia nervosa are closely linked, significant differences exist between the two. In bulimia the individual is likely to have a more accurate perception of body image than in anorexia and is more likely to acknowledge abnormal eating patterns. Those with bulimia tend to be more impulsive and are more apt to refer themselves for treatment. They also are more likely to be in a relationship or to be married than persons suffering from anorexia nervosa.

The families of individuals with bulimia are drawn from various class and ethnic groups. A history of physical or sexual abuse exists in some of these families, along with a higher than usual incidence of substance abuse. Depression may be in one or both parents. It should be noted, however, that a significant percentage of families seem to be without dysfunction.

Generally, bulimia develops in the late adolescent or early adult years, but it may occur later in life. The early history of those with bulimia shows that they were always deeply concerned with weight and appearance, reacting to values of thinness expressed in movies and magazines, on television, and by friends and families. Frequently, people who develop bulimia have been overweight or have family members who have been overweight. Thus, weight and appearance become a focal point for feelings of self-consciousness and inadequacy.

These individuals have feelings of low self-worth and dissatisfaction with various aspects of life. Typically, they experience loneliness, fear, and lack of emotional fulfillment. Interest in sexual activity is often minimal. Significant depression over a period of time is common and sometimes so severe that suicide attempts are made.

Characteristically, those engaging in bulimic behavior tend to be dependent and compliant people who are especially concerned with acceptance and approval. They may adopt a confident and independent manner to mask their deep feelings of inadequacy. Also, they often show an eagerness to win approval by striving for perfection in the activities they undertake. Failure to achieve their goals creates disappointment and anxiety and often results in irresponsible and unreasonable actions. Escape is sought through the substitute satisfactions of eating large quantities of food and/or purging. Bingeing and purging become the means of taking control of one's world by providing temporary comfort and security. Paradoxically, attempts at over-control ultimately result in feelings of being out of control.

The pattern of seeking comfort and escape in binge eating can be compared with seeking relief from anxiety through the use of alcohol or drugs. Consequently, some theorists consider bulimia to be a "food addiction."

Psychologically, the gorging of food is understood to have a numbing effect on anger and anxiety. At the same time, the guilt that accompanies the eating and the self-disgust that accompanies the purging contribute to further distress. However, the physical and emotional relief from purging may be so great that it provides an emotional "high" and may become a desired end in itself. This, then, promotes a self-perpetuating habit akin to any destructive, obsessive-compulsive behavior.

BINGE EATING DISORDER

The third and most recently described eating disorder has been termed binge eating disorder. This pattern of disordered eating is characterized by episodes of binge eating *without* the use of compensatory behaviors, such as purging, that are characteristic of bulimia nervosa.

Many therapists and researchers refer to this disorder as compulsive overeating, a problem that unfortunately is exceedingly common. In fact, it has been reported that the average American adult binge eats at least twice a month, although this does not imply that all have an eating disorder.

Two common patterns characterize binge eating: compulsively snacking over long intervals (such as all day at work or all evening in front of the computer or television) and/or a consumption of large amounts of food at one time, significantly beyond the requirements to satisfy normal hunger.

Binge eating disorder often leads to problems with weight regulation and sometimes obesity. However, obesity itself is not considered an eating disorder as a large percentage of obese individuals are genetically programmed toward being overweight rather than practicing disordered eating patterns.

SUMMARY

Experience has shown that anorexia nervosa, bulimia nervosa, and binge eating disorder are complex disorders with physical and emotional complications, and it is essential to take them seriously. The eating-disordered individual must participate in one or more forms of therapy to recover. The various forms of treatment are medical, nutritional, and psychological. Psychological treatment includes individual, group, or family therapy or a combination of therapies. In addition to therapy, participation in a self-help group for people with eating disorders can be beneficial.

REFERENCES

American Psychiatric Association. (1994). *Diagnostic and statistical manual of mental disorders* (4th ed.). Washington, DC: American Psychiatric Association Press.

Janet, P. (1903). *Lee's obsessions et la psycasthenie.* Paris: Felix Alcan.

Stunkard, A. (1959). Eating patterns and obesity. *Psychiatric Quarterly 33*, 284–295.

What We Know About Eating Disorders: Facts and Statistics

by Carolyn J. Cavanaugh, Ph.D. and Ray Lemberg, Ph.D.

Obsessing over weight and attempting to alter the body have been pastimes for many women, both historically and today. During the 19th century women wore corsets to attain the ideal female body shape. Negative effects of wearing the corset were many: shortness of breath, restriction of movement, weakness, constipation and other digestive problems, fractured ribs, uterine prolapse, and displacement of the liver. Yet it was widely used, even during pregnancy (Boskind-White, 1991). The corset of the 19th century has given way to cosmetic surgery and disordered eating in the 20th century. It is estimated that Americans spend more than $33 billion annually on diets and diet-related products (The Eating Disorder Connection, 1997) and cosmetic surgery. Given this national obsession with body weight, it is not surprising that the prevalence of eating disorders has grown tremendously over the past few decades and has spread beyond upper-middle-class females to include males and members of ethnic minorities. This chapter provides information on the demographics of anorexia nervosa and bulimia, medical complications and mortality rates of these disorders, sociocultural precursors, and a summary of outcome studies.

PREVALENCE OF EATING DISORDERS

A recent survey of female high school and college students showed that 15.4 percent met the clinical criteria for an eating disorder; 4.2 percent of those respondents met the specific criteria for anorexia nervosa (Nagel & Jones, 1993). Current estimates of bulimia among female college students using strict diagnostic criteria range from 4 percent (Pyle, Neuman, Halvorson, & Mitchell, 1991) to 5.1 percent (Heatherton, Nichols, Mahamedi, & Keel, 1995). Although the proportion of females with eating disorders is far greater than the proportion of males, recent epidemiological studies estimate an increase in the prevalence of eating disorders among men to almost 10 per-

cent of all eating disorder cases (Andersen, 1995). Likewise, the proportion of minorities with eating disorders is rising. Hsu (1987) notes an increase in the prevalence of eating disorders among African American women, due, in part, to increased affluence among that population, and probable increased access to upper-middle-class, white values related to thinness. Lee (1995, 1996) reports an increase in the prevalence of eating disorders within the Asian population but suggests that prevalence rates may have been underestimated in the past because of differences in clinical presentation of eating disorders across cultures. For instance, fat phobia, which is commonly viewed as a hallmark of eating disorders in Western culture, is not an important component of eating disorders in Asian cultures (Lee, 1996). Wilfley, Schreiber, Pike, and Striegel-Moore (1996) raise the possibility that ethnicity itself may not be an important factor in the development of eating disorders, but that income and education level may be.

MEDICAL COMPLICATIONS

Many medical complications of eating disorders have been reported in the literature. Consequences of bulimia include erosion of tooth enamel, metabolic acid base imbalances, hypochloremia, hypokalemia, hyponatremia, hypomagnesia, hypocalcemia, hyperuricemia, esophageal ulcers, and edema (Hofland & Dardis, 1992). Specific side effects of laxative abuse include constipation; malabsorption of fat and fat-soluble vitamins A, D, E, and K; gastrointestinal bleeding; rectal prolapse; potassium and calcium depletion; and possible increased risk for colon cancer (Eating Disorders Review, May/June 1996).

Given the significant medical complications, it is ironic that primary purging methods of bulimia (see Figure 1) are not particularly effective in producing the desired weight loss. Studies on calorie retention after bingeing indicate that, re-

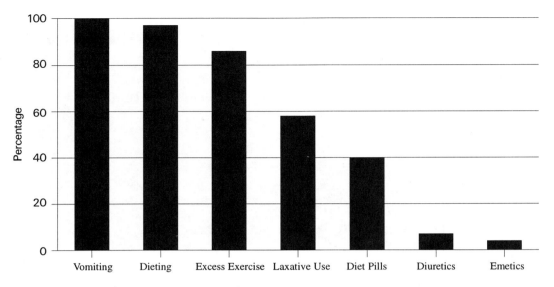

Figure 1. Methods of weight control among 50 women with bulimia.

gardless of binge size, approximately 1,100 to1,200 calories are retained and digested following self-induced vomiting (Kaye, Weltzin, Hsu, McConaha, & Bolton, 1993). Also, laxative use only decreases the number of calories retained by the body by approximately 12 percent (Bo-Linn, Santa Ana, Morawski, & Fordtran, 1983).

Anorexia carries its own medical consequences, including vitamin deficiencies that affect cognitive functioning, electrolyte imbalances, arrhythmias, bradycardia, hypotension, hypothermia and muscle weakness (Greenfield, Mickley, Quinlan & Roloff, 1995). More than 50 percent of anorexic patients have significant osteopenia, and at least some bone loss experienced during anorexia is irreversible even when nutritional status improves (Ward, Brown, & Treasure, 1997). A recent study noted that neurologic complications had been found in 47 out of 100 anorexic patients (Eating Disorders Review, May/June, 1997). It has also been found that patients with severe anorexia can suffer a loss of smell that does not necessarily return after weight gain (Fedoroff, Stoner, Andersen, Doty, & Rolls, 1995). Other medical complications and health risks are shown in Figure 2.

MORTALITY RATES

The many medical complications of eating disorders contribute to the significant mortality rate.

Mortality rates in 20-year studies have been approximately 18 percent (Goldbloom & Kennedy, 1995) and 20 percent at a 30-year follow-up (Hartman, 1995). The mortality rate for eating disorders is higher than for female psychiatric inpatients and females in the general population (Sullivan, 1995). Aggregate annual mortality rates associated with anorexia are more than 12 times higher than the annual death rate due to all causes for females 15 to 24 years old, and more than 200 times higher than the suicide rate of females in the general population (Eating Disorders Review, Nov/Dec 1995).

PRECURSORS TO EATING DISORDERS: THE FEMININE BEAUTY MYTH

Although eating disorders have many roots, the role of sociocultural pressures cannot be ignored. It is generally accepted that Western society is very appearance oriented (Boskind-White, 1991; Striegel-Moore, Silberstein, & Rodin, 1986). People learn at very early ages the importance of appearance, what is valued and what is stigmatized. For example, six-year-old children show an awareness of the stigma of obesity, attributing negative personal attributes (e.g., laziness, naughtiness, dishonesty, stupidity) to overweight children (Staffieri, 1967). Children as young as three years of age categorize other children based on weight, with female youngsters preferring normal-

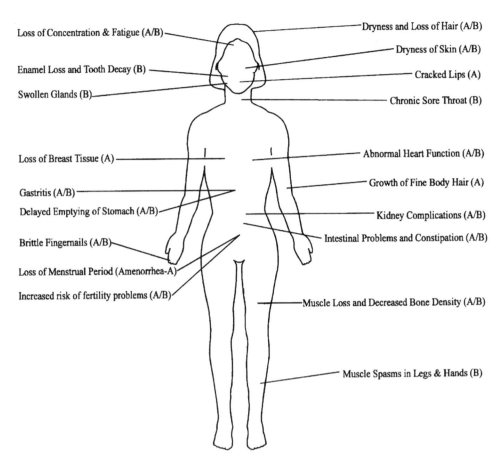

Loss of Concentration & Fatigue (A/B)

Enamel Loss and Tooth Decay (B)

Swollen Glands (B)

Loss of Breast Tissue (A)

Gastritis (A/B)

Delayed Emptying of Stomach (A/B)

Brittle Fingernails (A/B)

Loss of Menstrual Period (Amenorrhea-A)

Increased risk of fertility problems (A/B)

Dryness and Loss of Hair (A/B)

Dryness of Skin (A/B)

Cracked Lips (A)

Chronic Sore Throat (B)

Abnormal Heart Function (A/B)

Growth of Fine Body Hair (A)

Kidney Complications (A/B)

Intestinal Problems and Constipation (A/B)

Muscle Loss and Decreased Bone Density (A/B)

Muscle Spasms in Legs & Hands (B)

Figure 2. Selected health risks and medical complications associated with anorexia nervosa (A) and bulimia nervosa (B).

weight children to overweight ones (White, Mauro, & Spindler, 1985).

The current Western cultural conception of feminine beauty emphasizes thinness and attractiveness (Rodin, Silberstein, & Striegel-Moore, 1984). This ideal is reflected in the media's portrayal of the "model woman," which has grown thinner in recent years, well beyond what is physically attainable for most women. Garner, Garfinkel, Schwartz, and Thompson (1980) examined body measurements and weights of *Playboy* centerfolds and Miss America pageant contestants from the years 1959 to 1978, and discovered that while these "model" women had grown smaller over the time span, the average American woman's weight and body proportions had actually grown larger, creating an increasing discrepancy between the culturally endorsed ideal and reality. Likewise, Silverstein, Purdue, Peterson,

and Kelly (1986) surveyed major magazines and television programs from the 1930s to the 1980s and found that women in the 1970s and 1980s were portrayed as thinner and less curvaceous than in previous years. Boskind-White (1991) asserts that many of the female models whose figures are idealized are *literally* anorexic. The Barbie doll epitomizes this unrealistic ideal. According to a recent study conducted at Yale, if Barbie were life-size, she would be more than seven feet tall, and her measurements would be 40-22-36.

DIETING TO ATTAIN AN UNREALISTIC IDEAL

Schlosberg (1987) reports that 27 percent of American females are overweight, according to standard life insurance tables, but that more than 50 percent of American females are dieting. In addition, according to Schlosberg, many of the women who *are* overweight are *not* dieting. Thus, it would appear that at least half the women who are dieting are *not* overweight.

Furthermore, females are becoming more concerned about their weight at younger ages than previously (Boskind-White, 1991). A study of London schoolchildren found that most of the young women aged 12 to 17 thought they were overweight when they were actually normal weight or even underweight; most of them engaged in dieting behavior and experienced guilt when not dieting. Half as many boys of the same age group reported feeling overweight, and expressed less concern about weight and dieting (Wardle & Beales, 1986). Likewise, researchers (Salmons, Lewis, Rogers, Gatherer, & Booth, 1988) found that more than one-quarter of the 11- to 13-year-old females from a school in Birmingham, England reported "always" being terrified of gaining weight, while males of the corresponding age were unconcerned. In the United States, estimates of restrained eating in third-grade children range as high as 45 percent, and as high as 80 percent among fourth and fifth graders (Mellin, Irwin, & Scully, 1992). Gender differences in dieting frequency are also apparent, as a survey of obese children revealed that 49 percent of obese boys reported trying to lose weight in the previous year and 13 percent reported currently dieting, while 90 percent of obese girls reported a history of dieting and 72 percent reported currently trying to lose weight (Wadden, Steen, Foster & Andersen, 1996).

Given that concern about weight and dieting behavior is fairly common among children, it is not surprising that puberty, and the increase in body fat that accompanies it, is especially difficult for girls. Phelps and colleagues found that concern about body weight increased sharply when girls reached puberty, as did eating-disordered behaviors such as self-induced vomiting (Phelps, Andrea, Rizzo, Johnston, & Main, 1993). Likewise, Hayward and colleagues found that girls who experienced puberty early were twice as likely to develop eating disorders as those with average or late-onset puberty (Hayward, Killen, Wilson, Hammer, Litt, Kraemer, Haydel, Varady, & Taylor, 1997).

HOW MANY RECOVER?

Several outcome studies have been conducted to assess the recovery rate for anorexia and bulimia and to identify predictors of successful recovery. Keel and Mitchell (1997) found that approximately half of women diagnosed with bulimia were symptom-free 10 years later, while one-fifth continued to meet full criteria. The remaining group had experienced some relapse in bulimic symptoms (see Figure 3). Keel and Mitchell noted that the risk of relapse decreased four years after patients sought treatment. Herzog and colleagues (1993) reported that 56 percent of those with bulimia were in recovery one year after treatment, while only 10 percent of patients with anorexia were. They found that body weight was the critical factor in recovery: for every 10 percent that a patient was below her ideal body weight, her risk of relapse increased 18 percent. Several other factors have been found to heighten the probability of relapse in bulimia. These include: co-morbid substance abuse, suicide attempts, and increased bingeing and vomiting prior to treatment (Olmsted, Kaplan & Rockert, 1994); after treatment, factors found to increase likelihood of relapse are interpersonal distrust, poorer understanding and control of symptoms, a decision to start dieting, and inability to face and resolve difficulties when they initially arise (Olmsted et al., 1994). Positive predictors for bulimia include less severe bulimic behavior at the start of treatment, good friendships, and higher and more stable body weight at the end of treatment (Keel & Mitchell, 1997). Poorer outcome in anorexia has been linked to longer duration of the disorder and the presence of vomiting.

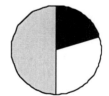

■ Met full criteria for bulimia
☐ Relapsed with some bulimic symptoms
☐ Fully recovered

Figure 3. Ten-year outcome of women with bulimia

Predictors of positive outcome include early treatment (Herzog et al., 1993).

SUMMARY AND CONCLUSIONS

The prevalence of eating disorders in the United States has increased significantly over the past few decades. Once thought to be found exclusively among upper-middle-class white females, anorexia and bulimia are spreading to males and members of minority groups. Although the outcome literature is somewhat optimistic about the success in treating bulimia, the treatment picture for anorexia is much more pessimistic. It appears that both disorders tend to be chronic and not particularly amenable to the short-term psychotherapy modalities encouraged by cost-cutting HMOs. It is particularly troubling that in the face of the increasing incidence of eating disorders, society continues to promote an unrealistic beauty ideal, and to encourage the use of diets, pills, surgeries, and other unhealthy practices to attain this ideal. The medical problems and increased mortality rates caused by these disorders are staggering and argue strongly for focusing attention on improving treatment and especially prevention efforts.

REFERENCES

Andersen, A. (1995). Eating disorders in males. In K. Brownell and C. Fairburn (Eds.), *Eating disorders and obesity: A comprehensive handbook*. New York: Guilford Press. pp. 177–182.

Bo-Linn, G., Santa Ana, C., Morawski, S., & Fordtran, J. (1983). Purging and calorie absorption in bulimic patients and normal females. *Annals of Internal Medicine* 99(1), 14–17.

Boskind-White, M. (1991, February). Gender and eating disorders. Paper presented at the Eating Disorder Conference, Tempe, AZ.

Fedoroff, I., Stoner, S., Andersen, A., Doty, R., & Rolls, B. (1995). Olfactory dysfunction in anorexia nervosa and bulimia nervosa. *International Journal of Eating Disorders*, 18(1), 71–77.

Garner, D., Garfinkel, P., Schwartz, D., & Thompson, M. (1980). Cultural expectations of thinness in women. *Psychological Reports*, 47, 483–491.

Goldbloom, D., & Kennedy, S. (1995). Medical complications of anorexia nervosa. In K. Brownell and C. Fairburn (Eds.), *Eating disorders and obesity: A comprehensive handbook*. New York: Guilford Press. pp. 266–270.

Greenfield, D., Mickley, D., Quinlan, D., & Roloff, P. (1995). Hypokalemia in outpatients with eating disorders. *American Journal of Psychiatry*, 152(1), 60–63.

Hartman, D. (1995). Anorexia nervosa—diagnosis, aetiology and treatment. *Postgraduate Medical Journal*, 71(842), 712–716.

Hayward, C., Killen, J., Wilson, D., Hammer, L., Litt, I., Kraemer, K., Haydel, F., Varady, A., & Taylor, C. (1997). Psychiatric risk factors associated with early puberty in adolescent girls. *Journal of the American Academy of Child and Adolescent Psychiatry*, 36(2), 255–262.

Heatherton, T., Nichols, P., Mahamedi, F., & Keel, P. (1995). Body weight, dieting and eating disorder symptoms among college students 1982 to 1992. *American Journal of Psychiatry*, 152(11), 1623–1629.

Herzog, D., Sacks, N., Keller, M., Lavori, P., VonRanson, K., & Gray, H. (1993). Patterns and predictors of recovery in anorexia and bulimia nervosa. *Journal of the American Academy of Child and Adolescent Psychiatry*, 32(4), 835–842.

Hofland, S., & Dardis, D. (1992). Bulimia nervosa: Associated physical problems. Journal of Psychosomatic Nursing and Mental Health Services, 30(2), 23–27.

Hsu, L. (1987). Are the eating disorders becoming more common in blacks? *International Journal of Eating Disorders*, 6(1), 113–124.

Joiner, T., Heatherton, J., & Keel, P. (1997). Ten-year stability and predictive validity of five bulimia-related indicators. *American Journal of Psychiatry*, 154, 1133–1138.

Kaye, W., Weltzin, T., Hsu, G., McConaha, C., & Bolton, B. (1993). Amount of calories retained after binge eating and vomiting. *American Journal of Psychiatry*, 150(6), 969–971.

Keel, P., & Mitchell, J. (1997). Outcome of bulimia nervosa. *American Journal of Psychiatry*, 154(3), 313–321.

Lee, S. (1995). Self starvation in context: Towards a culturally sensitive understanding of anorexia nervosa. *Social Science Medicine*, 41(1), 25–36.

Lee, S. (1996). Clinical lessons from the cross-cultural study of anorexia nervosa. *Eating Disorders Review*, 7(3), 1–3.

Mellin, L., Irwin, C., & Scully, S. (1992). Prevalence of disordered eating in girls: A survey of middle-class children. *Journal of the American Dietetic Association*, 92(7), 851–853.

Nagel, K. L., & Jones, K. H. (1993). Eating disorders: Prevention through education. *Journal of Home Economics*, 85(1), 53–56.

Olmsted, M., Kaplan, A., & Rockert, W. (1994). Rate and prediction of relapse in bulimia nervosa. *American Journal of Psychiatry*, 151(5), 738–743.

Phelps, L., Andrea, R., Rizzo, F., Johnston, L., & Main, C. (1993). Prevalence of self-induced vomiting and laxative/medication abuse among female adolescents: A longitudinal study. *International Journal of Eating Disorders*, 14(3), 375–378.

Pyle, R., Neuman, P., Halvorson, P., & Mitchell, J. (1991). An ongoing cross-sectional study of prevalence of eating disorders in freshman college students. *International Journal of Eating Disorders*, 10(6), 667–677.

Rodin, J., Silberstein, L., & Striegel-Moore, R. (1984). Women and weight: A normative discontent. *Nebraska Symposium on Motivation*, 32, 267–307.

Salmons, P., Lewis, V., Rogers, P., Gatherer, A., & Booth, D. (1988). Body shape dissatisfaction in schoolchildren. *British Journal of Psychiatry*, 153 (supp. 2), 27–31.

Schlosberg, J. (1987). The demographics of dieting. *American Demographics*, 9, 35–62.

Silverstein, B., Purdue, L., Peterson, B., & Kelly, E. (1986). The role of the mass media in promoting a thin standard of bodily attractiveness for women. *Sex Roles*, 14 (9/10), 519–532.

Staffieri, J. (1967). A study of social stereotypes of body image in children. *Journal of Personality and Social Psychology*, 7(1), 101–104.

Story, M., French, S., Resnick, M., & Blass, R. (1995). Ethnic/racial and socioeconomic differences in dieting behaviors and body image perceptions in adolescents. *International Journal of Eating Disorders*, 18(1), 173–179.

Striegel-Moore, R., Silberstein, L., & Rodin, J. (1986). Toward an understanding of risk factors for bulimia. *American Psychologist*, 41(3), 246–263.

Sullivan, D. (1995). Mortality in anorexia nervosa. *American Journal of Psychiatry*, 152(7), 1073–1074.

Wadden, T., Steen, S., Foster, G., & Andersen, R. (1996). Are obese adolescent boys ignoring an important health risk? *International Journal of Eating Disorders, 20*, 281–286.

Ward, A., Brown, N., & Treasure, J. (1997). Persistent osteopenia after recovery from anorexia nervosa. *International Journal of Eating Disorders, 22*(1), 71–75.

Wardle, J., & Beales, S. (1986). Restraint, body image and food attitudes in children from 12 to 18 years. *Appetite, 7*, 209–217.

White, D., Mauro, K., & Spindler, J. (1985). Development of body-type salience: Implications for early childhood educators. *International Review of Applied Psychology, 34*, 422–433.

Wilfley, D., Schreiber, G., Pike, K., & Striegel-Moore, R. (1996). Eating disturbance and body image: A comparison of a community sample of adult black and white women. *International Journal of Eating Disorders, 20*(4), 388–397.

Behavioral, Physical, and Psychological Symptoms of Eating Disorders

by Adrian H. Thurstin, Ph.D.

Although anorexia nervosa, bulimia nervosa, and binge eating disorder (compulsive overeating) share common features, each disorder is characterized by specific symptoms and signs. Although some of the symptoms of eating disorders are easily observable, others often go unnoticed. This chapter will discuss the behavioral, physical, and psychological features of anorexia, bulimia, and binge eating disorder. Each disorder will be examined separately to provide a complete picture of the disorder and to emphasize the similarities and differences among the disorders.

ANOREXIA NERVOSA

Behavioral Features

Anorexia nervosa, in its initial stages, may be difficult to distinguish from normal dieting. Like normal dieters, anorexics often avoid certain foods (e.g., fats, sweets, and breads) and reduce portions of other food groups. Unlike normal dieters, however, anorexics (usually young women) continue food restrictions after achieving a "normal" body weight. Whereas healthy dieters enjoy meals and eat what they are permitted (and sometimes more!), individuals with anorexia typically eat less than what is on the plate, perhaps no more than a few bites. Frequently, individuals with anorexia appear

to be eating when, in fact, they are simply moving food around on the plate, cutting food into tiny servings, or taking small bites while chewing slowly. While normal dieters appreciate their weight loss and the positive changes in their bodies, in contrast, individuals with anorexia describe themselves as overweight and fat, even after becoming severely emaciated. When confronted with their weight loss and eating problems, anorexic individuals often deny that they are restricting and that they have a problem with food. They may become quite defensive and even hostile.

Not only do individuals with anorexia display eating behaviors distinct from normal eating or typical dieting, but they also demonstrate unusual responses to eating or to eating situations. Instead of looking forward to being with others at meals, they often find excuses to eat alone. Initially, they may isolate themselves only at mealtimes; later, they begin to withdraw from social situations more completely. Commonly, individuals with anorexia demonstrate an exaggerated interest in recipes and cooking for others. Some individuals with anorexia go to great lengths to prepare gourmet meals that they serve to others, but not to themselves. Some individuals with anorexia also deny feelings of hunger or cravings for food. Often, after eating a small meal, or hardly anything at all, individuals with anorexia become anxious and complain of feeling "stuffed." In part, the feeling of fullness following little food intake is associated with physiological adjustments to caloric restriction.

In addition to the eating behaviors that characterize anorexia nervosa, specific exercise behaviors are also common. Just as with eating, initial exercise patterns may appear appropriate. Over time, however, the amount and degree of exercise may become excessive. For a person with anorexia, three to four hours of exercise per day is not uncommon. For example, a young woman with anorexia may participate in an aerobics class, walk or run for an hour, and complete a series of calisthenics. In anorexia, the level of daily activity is often directly related to caloric intake. For instance, if on a certain day the individual has consumed a low (no)-fat, sparse diet, then an hour of aerobics may be sufficient. Alternatively, the person who believes he or she has overeaten that day may substantially increase the amount of exercise to compensate for the extra calories. Occasionally, individuals with anorexia exercise more subtly, such as walking stairs, running in place while watching television, tensing or tightening muscles while in class or studying, or stretching.

In general, individuals with anorexia nervosa act in ways to minimize caloric consumption and maximize energy output. In this context, the restrictive dieting, unusual eating behaviors, and excessive exercise are easily understood. Because the body's instinct is to preserve itself, the individual with anorexia often engages in even greater caloric restriction and exercise activity as the disorder progresses. Furthermore, individuals with anorexia may use other compensatory behaviors, such as vomiting and taking laxatives or diuretics, to control their weight.

Physical Features

The physiological changes associated with anorexia nervosa are similar to those that follow a prolonged period of malnutrition and starvation. Some of the effects of nutritional restriction appear early in the course of the illness, while others are not apparent until the disorder has significantly progressed. The most readily recognized change in anorexia is the very rapid weight loss. It is not unusual for a young person with anorexia to lose 20 pounds in a month and as much as 20 to 25 percent of total body weight over several months. With the serious decline in body weight and nutritional status, women with previously regular menstrual cycles often cease menstruating.

Anorexia also contributes to problems in regulation of bodily functions. Related to severe weight loss, individuals with anorexia often demonstrate difficulty in maintaining appropriate fluid balance. Symptoms of fluid depletion include muscle cramping, fatigue, and "dizziness" due to low blood pressure on standing. These symptoms are exacerbated by the use of laxatives or diuretics. Individuals with anorexia also have difficulty regulating body temperature. Because the body cannot warm itself without fuel or needed layers of fat, individuals with anorexia are often overly sensitive to cold. In fact, individuals with anorexia may need to wear a sweater to be comfortable when others are in shorts and T-shirts. As the condition progresses, some people grow fine hair, called lanugo, over much of the body to maintain warmth.

Given the emphasis that individuals with anorexia place on physical appearance, it is ironic that many of the effects of anorexia tend to diminish physical attractiveness. The protein deficiency that accompanies caloric restriction often results in lackluster hair, skin, and nails. Both hair and nails become brittle, resulting in damage and breakage. The hair may also appear thin, as new hair is not grown to replace lost hair. Dry, scaly skin develops from the lack of nourishment. Another problem in anorexia is the declining condition of teeth and gums. Cavities and gum disease frequently occur secondary to the lack of calcium and nutrient intake, or as a consequence of vomiting in some individuals.

Although the physical features discussed to this point constitute serious health problems, they are generally not life-threatening. However, the long-term consequences of anorexia do affect the quality and quantity of life. Prolonged starvation impairs nearly all major bodily functions as the body begins burning muscle and organs for fuel. Anorexia can result in damage to vital organs, including the heart, liver, kidneys, stomach and bowels, muscles and bones, reproductive system, and brain. Potential long-term health problems related to organ and tissue damage include kidney failure, heart failure, osteoporosis (loss of bone density), infertility, intellectual decline, and chronic bowel impairment in laxative abusers.

Psychological Characteristics

Psychological symptoms of anorexia consist of those characteristics that are related to the development of the disorder and those that are secondary to the disorder. Several characteristics, including high achievement orientation, perfectionism, and acquiescence, are common in women who develop anorexia. Individuals with anorexia often desire to be "the best" in everything, including school, recreational activities, and personal appearance. Pressure to achieve the ideal body may lead to preoccupation with even the most minor physical "flaws." In addition to being perfectionists, individuals with anorexia tend to be "people pleasers." Parents often describe them as "model" children, willing to do what is asked without complaining. Individuals with anorexia attempt to please others in any way possible to avoid conflict and anger, fearing that others will dislike them if they fail to meet their expectations.

In addition to the psychological symptoms that typically precede anorexia (as anorexia progresses), the individual may develop depression, increased feelings of worthlessness, and lowered self-esteem. Many individuals with anorexia feel unloved, unaccepted, and deficient. These feelings become magnified as the disorder progresses, and as the individual becomes more isolated, withdrawn, and obsessed with losing weight. Concentration difficulties related to malnutrition, preoccupation with food and exercise, and depression are also common and often interfere with schoolwork or job performance.

BULIMIA NERVOSA

Behavioral Features

The eating behaviors associated with bulimia nervosa differ from anorexia nervosa and from healthy dieting. Bulimia is characterized by two primary symptoms: binge eating and purging through vomiting, excessive exercise, laxative use, and/or diuretic use. The binge-eating episodes that are the hallmark of the disorder are rarely observed. Individuals with bulimia usually demonstrate restrained, controlled eating behavior in public. In fact, the restraint displayed by young women with bulimia is so extreme that others may wonder how they can keep from losing weight. During public meals, individuals with bulimia may avoid fats, sweets, and junk foods, while consuming vegetables, fruits, and small amounts of lean meat. The public exhibition of self-control masks the bulimic's private, chaotic, and uncontrolled eating patterns, as well as his or her fears of food.

Similar to anorexia, social isolation is a common behavioral feature of bulimia. Often individuals with bulimia become more socially withdrawn as binge eating and purging consume more of their time and energy. A once outgoing, sociable young woman may begin declining invitations to parties, dinners, or other activities involving food. Individuals with bulimia who live with family or friends may isolate themselves by withdrawing to their rooms rather than watching television, playing games, or conversing. Frequent excuses include studying, fatigue, or housework. Typically, it is during such isolation that a binge occurs. A parent, sibling, or friend may later discover empty food containers hidden under a bed, stuffed in a closet, or tossed in a trash can.

Another common behavior in bulimia is a quick exit after eating. Individuals with bulimia often excuse themselves to the bathroom immediately after a meal to vomit even modest amounts of food. If prevented from purging, bulimics may experience extreme anxiety, which can evolve into distress and panic.

Physical Features

The numerous physiological problems associated with bulimia vary, based on the frequency and intensity of binge eating and the methods of purging used by the individual. Physical problems associated with binge eating include stomach pain, bloating, flatulence, constipation, and diarrhea. With more extreme binges, the stomach may rupture and result in death.

Purging is also associated with specific physical symptoms. The alternation between binge eating and purging may result in observable weight fluctuations. More significant weight cycling may occur with laxative and/or diuretic abuse, which alters the individual's fluid balance. Because the vast majority of women who develop bulimia are at normal weight or slightly above normal weight, nutritional irregularities and amenorrhea (absence of menstrual periods) often occur as a result of weight cycling and nutritional deficiencies related to the disorder. Purging may also contribute to an electrolyte imbalance, which is primarily related to depletion of potassium. Potassium is necessary for proper functioning of muscle tissue; a deficiency results in muscle fatigue and cramping, heart rhythm irregularities, kidney damage, and, in severe cases, paralysis. Replacement of potassium is essential to correct fluid imbalances and to restore regular organ functioning. However, such replacement must be monitored by a physician, because too much or too little potassium may lead to heart or kidney failure.

Some physical symptoms of bulimia are specific to the method of purging used by the individual (e.g., self-induced vomiting, laxative use, diuretic use). Purging through self-induced vomiting has some potentially serious physical consequences, including sore throats, mouth and gum ulcers, dry and cracked lips, tooth decay, generalized swelling, salivary gland irregularities, and constipation. Although seemingly innocuous, these side effects often signify more serious damage. For instance, a chronic sore throat with occasional blood in the vomit may be a sign of esophageal tearing or ulcers. Constipation in women with bulimia may indicate serious colon damage. Frequent vomiting may "paralyze" the digestive tract, so that food cannot move through the body efficiently. As a result, individuals with bulimia often complain of "feeling full" for a longer period of time than most people, and may have bloating without the relief of a bowel movement.

Purging through laxative use also has specific physical consequences, including abdominal cramping, nausea, vomiting, bloating, constipation, and bowel dysfunction. With severe laxative abuse, the colon may sustain serious damage in the form of inflammation (colitis), atrophy and ulcers (cathartic colon), and/or discoloration (melanosis coli). Although rare, the damage may be permanent and may necessitate a colonectomy.

Purging through diuretic use can result in dehydration and kidney impairment. Diuretic use is especially dangerous because of its effects on electrolyte regulation. Severe and chronic diuretic abuse increases the potential for hypertension, kidney failure, and heart failure.

Psychological Characteristics

The predominant psychological characteristics of individuals with bulimia include obsession with thinness, a diminished perception of self-worth, and an impaired sense of self-confidence. Compared with individuals with normal eating habits, bulimic individuals demonstrate a greater interest in dieting and are more likely to associate thin-

ness with success, attractiveness, and happiness. Related to their overvaluation of thinness, many individuals with bulimia believe that when they become thin, they will finally be good enough and attractive enough to feel worthwhile. Individuals with bulimia tend to see themselves as less attractive, less capable, and less interesting than others.

Some research indicates that the low self-esteem associated with bulimia is related to a strong achievement motivation and perfectionism. Because bulimics believe that they are not as competent as others, they may attempt to compensate by doing things perfectly. By being perfect, they believe they can escape any possible criticism. Unfortunately, individuals with bulimia are neither able to recognize their own successes nor accept the recognition of their successes by others. For most individuals with bulimia, the security of doing well lasts only until the next task is undertaken or until the next request is made. Although coworkers may describe individuals with bulimia as compulsive, demanding, and rigid, most bulimics have trouble setting limits on what is asked of them. They are terribly afraid that they will disappoint someone and, subsequently, be disliked. Not surprisingly, individuals with bulimia often suffer from anxiety and depression. Because they are so concerned about their performance and others' acceptance of them, individuals with bulimia tend to be tense, high-strung, and worried. They are particularly sensitive to any indication that someone is dissatisfied, because they assume that it is their responsibility to make sure everyone is happy. Consequently, the individual with bulimia is continuously vigilant for sources of potential conflict or frustration in others. He or she fears anger and its expression. If others are angry or upset, the individual with bulimia frequently accepts the "blame" and tries to correct the problem. As it is impossible to anticipate all of the needs of others, bulimics encounter constant frustration in their efforts to control the environment. Guilt and depression are often the direct result of this personal "failure." Specific frustrations leading to guilt and depression in women with bulimia include failure to control their weight, inability to stop binge eating, difficulty maintaining healthy relationships, and failure to "do a good job" (according to their own standards). As bulimia progresses and frustrations become more intense, the individual may become increasingly hostile and irritable toward others. Once compliant, passive, and accommodating, he or she may become aggressive and hostile. The emergence of resentment and anger represents only the tip of the iceberg of the rage harbored within, resulting from feeling unloved, unappreciated, and abused by others.

BINGE EATING DISORDER (COMPULSIVE OVEREATING)

Behavioral Features

Binge eating disorder (compulsive overeating) shares several characteristics with bulimia. Like bulimics, binge eaters experience loss of control over food, frequently resulting in binge-eating episodes. Both bulimics and binge eaters tend to overvalue thinness and the importance of thinness in achieving success, happiness, and popularity. Similar to bulimics, binge eaters often demonstrate observable weight fluctuations directly related to the alternation between restriction and binge eating.

Although binge eating and bulimia share some symptoms, significant differences exist. Individuals with compulsive overeating habits do not purge. Furthermore, the nature of binges differs between bulimia and binge eating. For individuals with bulimia, a binge generally consists of food that is of limited nutritional value, such as sweets or junk food. For compulsive overeaters, binge eating may also involve foods that are otherwise healthy. The compulsive overeater may sit with others and consume an appropriate amount during a meal but may lose control later while clearing the table of leftovers. He or she may eat what other people leave on their plates, finish what remains in the serving dishes, or continue to eat while putting food away. Another pattern of the binge eater involves continuous snacking, especially during evening hours, when food takes on the role of a "soothing companion." Many binge eaters eat very little during the day in the presence of others, but then binge at night when they are alone.

Individuals with compulsive overeating habits demonstrate some behavioral characteristics similar to those of anorexia and bulimia. For instance, compulsive overeaters often have trouble denying the requests of others, dropping their own plans to meet the needs of others. Rarely will a compulsive overeater suggest that a request is inconvenient or an imposition. At work, compulsive overeaters often assume extra responsibility and are always ready to be of assistance, no matter how heavy the workload. The simplest description of the binge eater's attitude is "people pleasing." If it makes someone else happy, he or she will do it.

Physical Features

Compulsive overeaters often have weight problems or difficulty maintaining a stable weight. In fact, some research suggests that as many as 50 percent of obese individuals presenting for treatment meet criteria for compulsive overeating. Teenagers and younger adults who are just developing compulsive overeating habits may not have reached the stage of serious obesity, but they tend to be significantly overweight. The physical effects of binge eating are initially not as observable as those of anorexia and bulimia, and are generally indistinguishable from those of obesity. Long-term consequences of compulsive overeating are related to obesity, including diabetes, hypertension, dyslipidemia, gallbladder disease, respiratory disease, cancer, and arthritis. Thus, individuals with compulsive eating habits must not only contend with the direct effects of their disorder but with the consequences of obesity, which may result in more medical problems and shorter life spans than individuals at healthy weights.

Psychological Characteristics

The psychological features of binge eating disorder are similar to those of anorexia and bulimia. They include dysphoria (feeling unwell or unhappy), anxiety, low self-esteem, the need for approval and acceptance by others, difficulty expressing anger and frustration, and feelings of disgust and guilt in relation to their binges. Outwardly, individuals with compulsive overeating habits may appear happy and content. However, when they are alone, they report feeling sad, lonely, and frustrated. Individuals with binge eating disorder are insecure in their identities and in their acceptance by others. Compulsive overeaters attempt to ensure acceptance by others by being "people pleasers" or by completing tasks perfectly. They are chronically tense, as they are afraid that their behavior will not be satisfactory to others.

Finally, individuals with binge eating disorder tend to have a low tolerance for frustration. This is especially evident in their expectations for, and reactions to, weight loss or gain. Often individuals with binge eating disorder set unrealistic weight loss goals and interpret weight gain as a personal failure—control. Binge eaters are generally unable to express anger or frustration. Like bulimics, compulsive overeaters often have difficulty placing limits on the demands of others. Although they may become frustrated and angry when they overextend themselves or cave in to those who take advantage of them, they tend to conceal their feelings for fear that expressing them will result in rejection. After concealing negative feelings, compulsive overeaters may turn to food for comfort.

CONCLUSION

Anorexia nervosa, bulimia nervosa, and compulsive overeating share some similar behavioral, physiological, and psychological characteristics.

Becoming familiar with the features that typify the disorders may be helpful to friends, relatives, and health care professionals in the identification and differentiation of the disorders.

SUGGESTED READING

Boskind-White, M., & White, W. C. (1987). *Bulimarexia.* New York: Norton.

Brisman-Siegel, M., & Winshel, M. (1997). *Surviving an eating disorder: Strategies for families and friends.* New York: HarperCollins.

Cooper, P. J. (1992). *Bulimia nervosa and binge eating.* New York: New York University Press.

Fairburn, C. (1995). *Overcoming bulimia.* New York: Guilford Press.

Pipher, M. (1995). *Hunger pains.* New York: Ballantine.

Sandbeck, T. J. (1993). *The deadly diet.* Oakland, CA: New Harbinger.

Sucker, I. M. (1987). *Dying to be thin.* New York: Warner.

Causes, Symptoms, and Effects of Eating Disorders: Child Development As It Relates to Anorexia Nervosa and Bulimia Nervosa

by Irene Chatoor, M.D.

There is growing evidence in the Western world that the prevalence of eating disorders among young girls is on the rise. To understand why this is happening in our culture requires answering this question: Why are increasing numbers of young girls susceptible to eating disorders while others who diet are able to undertake the developmental tasks of adolescence?

People with anorexia nervosa and bulimia nervosa have these characteristics in common: gross disturbances in eating behavior, intense fear of obesity and disturbance of body image, and a feeling of being fat even when slim or emaciated. However, these two disorders differ in the eating pattern displayed. Whereas anorexics restrict their food intake by counting calories and forcing themselves into eating less and less, bulimics tend to alternate among dieting, fasting, and binge eating. They display a roller-coaster type of eating pattern with great variations in the timing and amount of food eaten. The hallmark of bulimia is recurrent episodes of binge eating characterized by the rapid consumption of a large amount of usually high-calorie, easily ingested food, such as ice cream, cookies, cakes, and breads. Whereas the binge eating appears to serve as a distraction and to provide comfort and pleasure, at the end of the episode the individual usually experiences physical and emotional distress and severe guilt and panic over the amount of food eaten. This panic frequently leads to purging in the form of vomiting or taking laxatives or diuretics; it may also lead to a new cycle of starvation followed by another binge episode. Both eating disorders can upset hormonal regulation. Anorexia nervosa, as it progresses toward malnutrition, leads to amenorrhea (the absence or suppression of menstruation). The menstrual pattern in bulimia nervosa tends to be irregular.

CAUSES AND ORIGINS OF ANOREXIA AND BULIMIA

Both eating disorders begin most commonly during adolescence, a time when a young person needs to meet major developmental tasks and master the developmental issues of separating from the family and becoming an individual. A young girl needs to adapt to puberty when her body proportions change from those of a child to those of a young woman. She needs to make the transition between loosening the ties with her parents and increasing her dependency on her peers. To find her place in her peer group she needs to deal with personal and cultural values regarding body image, sexuality, and achievement—key areas where young girls with eating disorders appear to struggle.

Although the exact etiology, or causes, and mechanisms of anorexia nervosa and bulimia nervosa are not known, most experts agree with Garfinkel and Garner (1982) that these eating disorders are the product of the interplay of a number of forces. *Predisposing factors* appear to combine with *precipitating events* in the individual's life to lead to an eating disorder. One way to understand the developmental crisis of adolescence as it shows up in these eating disorders is to look at the individual, family, and cultural factors that enhance or interfere with the preparation of the child for the developmental tasks of adolescence.

SIGNALS IN INFANCY

Hilde Bruch, a pioneer in the field of eating disorders, hypothesized that anorexia nervosa and juvenile onset of obesity are related to a disturbed

awareness of inner processes among these individuals. They do not recognize when they are hungry or satiated, nor do they differentiate the need for food from other uncomfortable sensations and feelings (Bruch, 1973). These individuals need external signals to know when and how much to eat because their own inner awareness has not been programmed correctly. Reconstructing the developmental histories of her patients, Bruch concluded that there was a lack of appropriate and confirming responses by the parents to the child's signals that reflected his or her needs and other forms of self-expression. Bruch hypothesized that appropriate responses to cues from the infant, whether biological, intellectual, social, or emotional, are necessary for the child to organize the significant building blocks for the development of self-awareness and self-effectiveness. If a parent's reaction is frequently inappropriate, be it neglectful, overly solicitous, inhibiting, or indiscriminately permissive, the child will experience confusion (Bruch, 1973).

Bruch's hypothesis was confirmed through a prospective study by Leon, Fulkerson, Perry, and Early-Zald (1995). They followed 852 girls and 815 boys from grades 7 through 10. Poor interoceptive awareness (difficulty in identifying internal feeling states) was the one factor in girls that had the most predictive strength for disordered eating over the three-year period. Lyon et al. (1997) also confirmed that feelings of ineffectiveness and poor interoceptive awareness are risk factors for anorexia nervosa.

In my own work with infants and toddlers with feeding disorders and failure to thrive I also found evidence confirming Bruch's hypothesis. James Egan and I have observed an eating disorder in infants and toddlers that closely resembles anorexia nervosa in the adolescent. Initially we called it a separation disorder. Because of the similarities with anorexia nervosa we named it infantile anorexia nervosa (Chatoor, Egan, Getson, Menvielle & O'Donnell, 1988), but recently we renamed it infantile anorexia to emphasize the lack of appetite and the early onset of the disorder (Chatoor, Hirsch & Persinger, 1997). The onset of infantile anorexia is usually between 9 months and 3 years, with a peak onset between 9 months and 18 months of age when infants usually begin using a spoon and self-feeding. The disorder occurs with the infant's thrust for autonomy during the first period of separation and individuation. As the infant develops motor skills, parent (usually the mother) and infant need to negotiate who is going to put the spoon in the infant's mouth. The parent's appropriate responses to the infant's signals of hunger and fullness versus the infant's cues for autonomy and self-control in the feeding situation create an essential interplay in successfully negotiating this period of transition to self-feeding. The mother needs to determine whether the infant wants to nurse because of hunger or for comfort, and whether he or she refuses to open the mouth because of anger, desire for attention, or satiety. If the mother is unable to interpret the infant's cues correctly, because of her own anxiety or conflicts over issues of control, and thus overrides the infant's signals by trying to coax, cajole, or force it into eating her way, the infant will confuse internal signals of hunger and satiety with intense emotions aroused by the interactions with the mother. As a result, meals become a battle-ground between parent and child, where the infant's food intake is controlled by emotions instead of physiological sensations of hunger and fullness. The infant does not develop *somatopsychological differentiation* or interoceptive awareness, which in this case is the ability to differentiate between feelings, such as anger, frustration, love, and affection on the one hand, and sensations of the body, such as hunger and fullness, on the other.

DIFFERENTIATING BETWEEN MIND AND BODY SIGNALS

Difficulty with somatopsychological differentiation appears to be a primary basis of all eating disorders. In the eating-disordered individual, eating is controlled by emotions and external cues instead of internal physiological signals. Interestingly, data from our recent research reveal a striking tendency of anorexic, restricting individuals to be unable to eat when they experience negative emotions, such as anger, frustration, or anxiety, whereas bulimic individuals report that they seek food and eat in response to the same feelings. In addition, both eating-disordered groups reported significant confusion over feelings of hunger and fullness.

TEMPERAMENT OF CHILDREN WHO BECOME ANOREXIC

The question remains as to what might have gone wrong in the development of mind-body differentiation in individuals with eating disorders. In recent years, a number of studies have pointed to temperament or personality characteristics that might predispose individuals to develop eating disorders. First, several studies of identical and fraternal twins, where one or either of the twins was diagnosed as having anorexia nervosa or bulimia nervosa, consistently demonstrated a significantly higher concordance rate in the expression of the same eating disorder in identical twins compared with fraternal twins. This finding led to the assumption of high heritability of these eating disorders and to a search for what these heritable factors predisposing certain individuals to develop an eating disorder might be. A number of studies of temperament and personality characteristics have further explored this question.

Casper (1990) reported that recovered anorexic women showed a temperamental disposition toward greater restraint in emotional expression and initiative and rated higher on risk avoidance when compared with their sisters and a control group without eating disorders. Other authors have found obsessive-compulsive traits (Rastram, 1992), harm avoidance, and reward dependence (Kleifeld, Sunday, Hurt, & Halmi, 1994) to be associated with anorexia nervosa, whereas higher scores on novelty seeking have been reported in individuals with bulimia nervosa (Bulik, Sullivan, Welzin, & Kaye, 1995).

In my own work, I have observed a striking difference in temperament between infantile and adolescent anorexics. Whereas the infants tend to be strong-willed, persistent, and demanding in the expression of their wants (which leads to conflicts in the early phase of separation and individuation), adolescent anorexic girls are usually described to have been compliant and obedient infants and children. The parents usually do not remember strong oppositional behaviors or temper tantrums during the early phase of separation and individuation. This difference in temperament appears to determine infantile versus adolescent onset of anorexia nervosa.

However, both groups of children are difficult to read when it comes to the expression of their emotional cues versus physiological signals of hunger and fullness. The infantile anorexics display only low hunger cues and very intense emotionality, which usually overrides their interactions with their parents. In contrast, parents' reports about adolescent anorexics indicate that during infancy and childhood, they did not challenge their parents by expressing their own wishes and wants in opposition to the parents' demands. They usually ate what was put on their plate and performed in school according to what was expected from them. Just as they have failed to express their feelings and wants in a determined way, they also have failed to receive distinct confirmation or rejection of what they wanted or did not want. They have remained unaware of their inner feelings and strivings and consequently have failed to develop a sense of self.

In my work with adolescent anorexic girls I have been impressed by their simultaneous sensitivity to verbal and nonverbal cues of others and their unawareness of their own feelings. It appears that these youngsters have perfected the art of focusing on others and reading their cues while remaining unaware of their own needs and emotions. Their intense interpersonal sensitivity and assumed passivity to avoid conflict (harm) fostered a submissive style that allowed them to grow up as extensions of their mothers and to fulfill their parents' wishes and expectations without developing a sense of self.

THE ROLE OF DEPRESSION AND ANXIETY

Another factor that can contribute to the disturbance in mind-body differentiation and lead to confusion between the feelings of anger, sadness, loneliness, and fear of rejection and hunger and satiety is an anxiety or depressive disorder. Several studies have reported the presence of mood disturbances among patients with anorexia nervosa or bulimia nervosa. Herzog's (1984) research revealed that 55 percent of anorexic patients and 23 percent of bulimic patients met criteria for major depressive disorders. Piran et al. (1985) reported on the high incidence of panic disorder in patients with bulimia nervosa. Many studies have reviewed the frequency of psychiatric illness among relatives of patients with anorexia nervosa or bulimia nervosa.

Whether depression or the eating disorder comes first, however, can vary from patient to patient. Evidence exists that malnutrition leads to

mood disturbances and that binge eating is frequently followed by intense negative emotion. On the other hand, depressive and anxious moods affect the awareness of hunger and fullness and can interfere with eating. Whatever comes first, the eating or the mood disorder, one affects the other with a compounding effect.

FAMILY INFLUENCE ON EATING DISORDERS

If temperament and mood disorders are considered risk factors for these eating disorders, certain family and cultural factors have been implicated as well. Parents of children with any type of psychiatric disorder frequently feel responsible for, or guilty about, the child's problems. However, family studies of patients with anorexia nervosa indicate that some of these families reveal no specific psychopathology and demonstrate no more interactional problems than other families with healthy adolescents. Family distress may be an effect of the adolescent's eating disorder rather than its cause. However, certain family characteristics seem to join with cultural factors to contribute to the adolescent's conflicts. Families in which there is rigid adherence to rules and conservative values, avoidance of open conflict, and lack of conflict resolution seem to produce more patients with anorexia nervosa (Minuchin, Rosman, & Baker, 1978). On the other hand, families with severe parental conflict and inconsistency of rules and values also threaten the adolescent process of identity formation (Kog & Vandereycken, 1989). Observations by Humphrey (1989) of family interactions among anorexic, bulimic, and normal families showed that parents of anorexics communicated a double message of nurturant affection combined with neglect of their daughters' needs to express themselves and their feelings. Anorexic daughters, in turn, were ambivalent about disclosing their feelings versus submitting to their parents. In contrast, bulimics and their parents were hostilely enmeshed, and, for them, this appeared to undermine the daughter's separation and self-assertion.

Interestingly, many families of eating-disordered patients appear preoccupied with food and gourmet cooking, weight, and dieting, thus drawing attention to food as representing more than nutrition. A study by Miller, McCluskey-Fawcett, and Irving (1993), which explored the relationship of early mealtime experiences to later bulimia nervosa, revealed significant group differences among bulimics, nonbulimics, and repeat dieters, with the bulimic group reporting the most negative experiences. Women with bulimia reported high levels of stress and conflict during meals, the use of food as a tool for punishment or reward, and emphasis on dieting and weight by their parents. In the recent study of adolescent anorexics, bulimics, and a control group of high school students, we also found that the eating-disordered adolescents reported significantly more parental control over eating, more parental affection expressed through food, and more parental preoccupation with dieting and weight. In our study we also found that bulimics reported the highest degree of disturbed parental eating patterns and child-rearing practices in regard to food.

CULTURAL CHANGES AND EATING DISORDERS

Finally, the cultural changes over the last 20 years, the sexual revolution, the entrance of more women into the workforce, the emphasis on thinness as the ideal for women, and the general indulgence in food have led to a potpourri of values and ideals with which most young persons would have difficulty. Young girls confront food at home, at parties, at the movies, wherever they go. At the same time, they are expected to embody the ideal of thinness modeled in the fashion magazines. They have been brought up to believe in religious and interpersonal values that often clash with a world of violence, fast food, and fast sex. Many have grown up in a home where the mother fulfilled everybody's needs while foregoing her own ambitions. As adolescents they confront choices of careers as professionals or as housewives, the conservative roles their own mothers may have filled. They tend to think that, to be perfect, they must master both roles at the same time.

One can see how adolescents with temperamental vulnerabilities or tendencies for depressive and anxiety disorders, when exposed to conflicting family and cultural values, become frightened of growing up. When subjected to what might seem a minor trauma, such as the loss of a best friend, a change of school, or rejection by a peer group, they often find control of their eating and weight a welcome escape and turn it into their solution to the overwhelming task of growing up and finding their place in a world that appears so frightening. Their eating and their body size are two things they strive to control when the rest of their life seems so much out of control.

REFERENCES

Bruch, H. (1973). *Eating disorder: Obesity, anorexia nervosa, and the person within.* New York: Basic Books.

Bulik, C. M., Sullivan, P. F., Weltzin, T. E., & Kaye, W. H. (1995). Temperament in eating disorders. *International Journal of Eating Disorders, 17*(3), 251–261.

Casper R. G. (1990). Personality features of women with good outcome from restricting anorexia nervosa. *Psychosomatic Medicine, 52*, 156–170.

Chatoor, I., Egan, J., Getson, P., Menvielle, E., & O'Donnell, R. (1988). Mother-infant interactions in infantile anorexia nervosa. *Journal of the American Academy of Child and Adolescent Psychiatry, 2*, 535–540.

Chatoor, I., Hirsch, R., & Persinger, M. (1997). Facilitating internal regulation of eating: A treatment model for infantile anorexia. *Infants and Young Children, 9*(4), 12–22.

Garfinkel, P. E., & Garner, D. M. (1982). *Anorexia nervosa: A multidimensional perspective.* New York: Brunner/Mazel.

Herzog, D. (1984). Are anorexic and bulimic patients depressed? *American Journal of Psychiatry, 141*, 1594–1596.

Humphrey, L. L. (1989). Observed family interactions among subtypes of eating disorders using structural analysis of social behavior. *Journal of Clinical and Consulting Psychology, 57*(2), 206–214.

Kleifield, E. I., Sunday, S., Hurt, S., & Halmi, K. A. (1994). The Tridimensional Personality Questionnaire: An exploration of personality traits in eating disorders. *Journal of Psychiatric Research, 28*(5), 413–423.

Kog, E., & Vandereycken, W. (1989). Family interaction in eating disorder patients and normal controls. *International Journal of Eating Disorders, 8*, 11–23.

Leon, G. R., Fulkerson, J. A., Perry, C. L., & Early-Zald, M. B. (1995). Prospective analysis of personality and behavioral vulnerabilities and gender influences in the later development of disordered eating. *Journal of Abnormal Psychology, 104*(1), 140–149.

Lyon, M., Chatoor, I., Atkins, D., Silber, T., Mosimann, J., & Gray, J. (1997). Testing the hypothesis of the multidimensional model of anorexia nervosa in adolescents. *Adolescence, 32*(125), 101–111.

Miller, D. A. F., McCluskey-Fawcett, K., & Irving, L. M. (1993). Correlates of bulimia nervosa: Early family mealtime experiences. *Adolescence, 28*(111), 621–635.

Minuchin, S., Rosman, D., & Baker, L. (1978). *Psychosomatic families: Anorexia nervosa in context.* Cambridge, MA: Harvard University Press.

Piran, N., Kennedy, S., Garfinkel, P. E., & Owens, M. (1985). Affective disturbance in eating disorders. *Journal of Nervous and Mental Disorders, 173*, 395–400.

Rastram, M. (1992). Anorexia nervosa in 51 Swedish adolescents: Premorbid problems and comorbidity. *Journal of the American Academy of Child and Adolescent Psychiatry, 31*(5), 819–829.

Childhood Abuse and Other Trauma in the Histories of Eating-Disorder Patients

by Marcia Rorty, Ph.D., and Joel Yager, M.D.

Persons who have been abused or otherwise traumatized in childhood are at significant risk of developing psychological disorders in adulthood, including but not limited to eating disturbance. Child abuse may include sexual, physical, emotional, or psychological abuse. Emotional and physical neglect, parental major mental illness or alcoholism, significant separations from caregivers, and witnessing of spousal abuse are among the many other forms of childhood trauma that may have lasting, debilitating effects (Herman, 1992). Among this range of adverse experiences, child sexual abuse (CSA) has been the main type of trauma studied thus far in relation to the eating disorders. Still, some researchers have expanded the types of experiences considered to include physical and psychological abuse of the patient (Rorty, Yager, & Rossotto, 1994), controlling or indifferent parental treatment, chaotic family environments, and family violence involving members other than the patient herself (Schmidt, Tiller, and Treasure, 1993). Almost all research in this area to date has examined female eating-disordered patients. However, there is no reason to believe that males would not be similarly affected.

Eating-disordered individuals traumatized in childhood and their care providers face many challenges, such as increased likelihood of co-morbid conditions including dissociation, depression, anxiety, posttraumatic stress disorder, alcohol and substance use disorders, and personality disorders (Vanderlinden & Vandereycken, 1997). These disorders may precede, occur concurrently with, or follow the eating disorder. Patients also almost uniformly experience profound interpersonal distrust emerging from early abandonment and betrayals of trust. Consequently, treatment and recovery may be very complex for these patients.

PREVALENCE OF TRAUMA HISTORIES AMONG EATING DISORDER PATIENTS

Research on traumatic histories among eating disorder patients is in its relative infancy, beginning with any frequency in the mid- to late-1980s, when case reports and reports on clinical series appeared (Root & Fallon, 1988). Clinicians noted the critical connections made by their patients (Goldfarb, 1987), whereas some researchers doubted the veracity of these connections on empirical grounds (Pope & Hudson, 1992).

Although the methods used have varied greatly, studies have demonstrated a child sexual abuse (CSA) rate of approximately 20 to 50 percent in eating-disordered women (Vanderlinden & Vandereycken, 1997), approximately the rate found among other groups of nonpsychotic psychiatric outpatients. Conversely, studies of trauma victims show elevated levels of eating disturbance (Vanderlinden & Vandereycken, 1997). Rates of CSA histories among inpatient psychiatric samples converge roughly on two-thirds or more, although the range may vary considerably by study and disorder (e.g., rates for dissociative identity disorder typically exceed 90 percent). Individuals reporting a greater number of types of abuse or severity of abuse tend to demonstrate higher levels of dysfunction (Rorty, Yager, & Rossotto, 1994). Research has demonstrated fairly conclusively that CSA is a risk factor for bulimic disorders, though it is apparently not specific to the eating disorders as opposed to other psychiatric disorders (Fairburn, Welch, Doll, et al., 1997). The role of CSA in restricting anorexia nervosa, at least in a statistical sense, is less clear (Vanderlinden & Vandereycken, 1997). Nonetheless, self-starvation may be a very important posttraumatic response in individual cases, where the symbolic meaning of the trauma in the patient's eating disorder is often profound.

LONG-TERM EFFECTS OF CHILDHOOD ABUSE AND OTHER TRAUMA

Trauma researchers Herman, van der Kolk, and their colleagues have observed a cluster of symptoms consistently found in victims of interpersonal trauma, particularly trauma beginning at an early age and continuing over time (Herman, 1992a,b; Vander Kolk & Fisler, 1994). Among several names, this cluster of symptoms has been described as "complex posttraumatic stress disorder" (Herman, 1992b), reflecting its association with and elaboration upon the major signs of PTSD, which include intrusive recollections of the trauma, a numbing of responsiveness, and chronic autonomic hyperarousal. First, according to these experts, there are alterations in the regulation of affect and impulses. Patients may feel chronic dysphoria and be preoccupied with death or thoughts of suicide. Their anger expression may be inhibited, explosive, or alternate between the two. They often feel chronically "out of control" of their emotions, which may be highly variable and intense. Second, trauma victims frequently experience alterations in attention or consciousness, such as amnesia, dissociative experiences, and reliving experiences. Third, they often have a high number of explained and unexplained somatic pains and problems.

Fourth, according to Herman and her colleagues, trauma survivors may carry distorted perceptions of themselves and others. Survivors of abuse and trauma often feel as though they are damaged, shameful, evil, or somehow fundamentally different from the rest of the human race. They may have great difficulty trusting others, simultaneously yearning for deep human connection yet fearing the potential of relationships for exploitation, abandonment, and betrayal. They may demonstrate poor interpersonal judgment, placing their trust in the hands of undeserving individuals and rejecting or sabotaging relationships with those who would relate to them in a healthy manner. Many women describe entering into psychologically or physically destructive relationships because it is all they know experientially or they believe they do not deserve better. Because it is foreign to their relational history, to take part in a healthy relationship would be to enter into territory that is unknown and therefore potentially terrifying. Finally, victims of trauma experience alterations in systems of meaning. For instance, many suffer from chronic feelings of emptiness, meaninglessness, and lack of a sense of life purpose (Herman, 1992a).

Psychobiological Effects. It is critical to note that overwhelming life experiences may have lasting biological effects that will significantly affect the traumatized eating disorder patient (McFall, Murburg, Roszell, et al., 1989). These effects include excessive arousal, including generalized hyperarousal (e.g., exaggerated startle response in relation to innocuous stimuli), as well as specific fight, flight, or freeze responses in relation to reminders of the trauma. A number of studies have documented higher levels of stress hormone by products in victims of trauma, even long after the trauma has ended (Yehuda, Kahana, Binder-Byrnes, et al., 1995). Survivors may be much more easily "thrown" by stressful situations in general, and in particular by those that bear resemblance to the original trauma. Often these reminders are long forgotten in conscious memory and not obvious to observers. However, as van der Kolk aptly states, "the body keeps score" (van der Kolk, 1994). Thus, overwhelming physical and psychological reactions may occur as if out of the blue, with no apparent trigger, leading the traumatized patient to feel as though she is "crazy" and increasing her sense of basic difference from others.

RELEVANCE TO EATING DISORDERS

Eating disorders may represent a powerful response to and means of coping with the psychological and biological effects of trauma outlined above. When viewed as a means of coping, as well as a possible symbolic representation of the trauma, eating disturbances become more comprehensible to the patient and clinician alike.

Dieting

First, the process of dieting often represents the desire to transcend human need (for, in the trauma survivor's experience, to need is dangerous) or "purify" the damaged self. In cases of sexual abuse, some individuals starve themselves in a deliberate effort to repulse the perpetrator and any future perpetrator. Additionally, starving can bring on dissociative-like states, permitting a level of removal from the here-and-now. Finally, refusing food can give one the illusion of power when one has repeatedly faced powerlessness, as occurs in cases of abuse, including the power to say "no" to others' wishes, expectations, or demands. Many women with anorexia nervosa comment that the consumption or lack of consumption of food is the one area in life in which they feel a sense of efficacy and personal power. Removal of this symptom, as a result, is unlikely to succeed in the long run unless personal efficacy and agency are developed in other areas of life.

Western culture's preoccupation with slenderness in women adds yet another dimension to these issues. The desire for a slender physique among women is highly culturally sanctioned, representing "control," having it all "together," happiness, success, and internal equanimity. For the trauma patient lacking a fundamental sense of meaning and life purpose, this pursuit of thinness may take on added importance, representing a quest for meaning and the hope of equanimity amidst internal confusion, chaos, and inter- and intrapersonal pain (Rorty & Yager, 1996).

Binge Eating

When most patients eventually lose dietary restraint in binge eating, their voracious appetites speak not only of their biological need for food (a normal physiological response to caloric deprivation), but also of the wish to fill forever their deep internal emptiness and existential aloneness. Food initially promises comfort and nurturance not supplied by the self or others. Many patients, in fact, binge on "comfort foods" such as pastries and other sweets. Binge eating to the point of painful fullness may also represent punishment for "wrongdoings" or basic badness, notions originally instilled by the perpetrator(s) but internalized over time by the patient herself. Abuse of other substances like alcohol and drugs, self-mutilation, and engaging in other damaging behaviors such as risk-taking activities often serve a similar function and are frequently present (Vanderlinden & Vandereycken, 1997).

Some women describe how binge eating provides an escape by providing a means through which they dissociate, going into trance-like periods, during which they feel removed from painful affective states like anger and dysphoria. However, having binged, the woman often feels intense self-recrimination, because in her mind her basic unworthiness has been confirmed in her lack of "control" and "excessive" neediness. The lack of

self-forgiveness for normal human responses (e.g., eating in response to intense hunger) is often striking. Many patients further chastise themselves for having a disorder that can only exist amidst ample food supplies; thus, according to this reasoning, the psychological needs of which their powerful physical appetite speaks are not valid or worthy of compassion or attention.

For women who compulsively overeat or binge without purging, developing an armor of excess weight can serve a similar function to emaciation, in that the patient may feel her weight will repel potential perpetrators and/or make her more powerful and formidable. In a society that holds individuals responsible for their body weight and portrays overweight individuals as slothful, lazy, and lacking in "willpower," excess weight can also symbolize to the patient and the world that she is unworthy of love and respect as she "wears" the bodily shame and self-contempt she gained as a result of abuse.

Purging

For women who purge, purging not only serves to rid oneself of unwanted calories, but also provides the autonomic "jolt" that is a reinforcing sensation to many trauma survivors (Herman, 1992a), piercing through a dead ennui, akin for some patients to self-cutting or other forms of self-mutilation. On a psychological level, many patients describe a sense of being purified or cleansed by purging.

TREATMENT ISSUES

Given the enormous psychological and biological complexities involved in working with patients with eating disorders, and the almost universal presence of associated co-morbid conditions, treatment planning requires full appreciation of and attention to each person's total needs. The eating disorder may not even be the most prominent syndrome demanding attention.

A multimodal approach involving professionals from several disciplines is often indicated. Therapeutic modalities helpful in the treatment of the traumatized patient include individual psychotherapy, groups for eating-disordered women victimized as children, couples therapy, family therapy, pharmacologic interventions, and adjunctive self-help groups for addictions (e.g., Alcoholics Anonymous) or for other problems, such as compulsive sexual behavior.

Individual psychotherapy. The first goal of individual psychotherapy is to provide a safe, empathic, and appropriately boundaried therapeutic relationship in which a deeply painful past may be safely explored. A second goal is to help the patient understand the connection between her disturbed eating behavior and prior experiences of victimization and helplessness. Education about the psychobiology of trauma may help the patient understand her "overreactions" and the way in which some of her responses are virtually preprogrammed in her body. A third goal is to help her regain (or gain for the first time) her sense of mastery and life purpose. The severity of her symptoms may actually increase as she approaches the traumatic material in greater depth (Root & Fallon, 1989). Thus, it is crucial that therapist and patient prepare for such an eventuality by making plans to ensure her safety. Hospitalization may be indicated in severe cases. A therapeutic contract that allows both client and therapist to feel safe is often critical.

Because the abuse occurred in the context of a human relationship, usually an intimate one, an intensive relational focus in psychotherapy can bring tremendous healing, though many struggles will naturally occur in the process for both parties. Therapeutic "neutrality" has little or no place in this therapy. Instead, neutrality may only serve to recapitulate a caregiver's failure to protect and intervene, despite observing the child's suffering. It also reinforces the patient's sense that her perception of reality is distorted and that the abuse "really wasn't that bad." (In the patient's mind, if her feelings and memories were accurate, the therapist would surely react.) As psychotherapy proceeds, the external soothing and containing functions provided by the therapist are gradually internalized and can be increasingly called upon in the therapist's absence.

Couples Therapy

For patients with relatively supportive spouses or partners, couples therapy may be an important intervention. The partner of the traumatized eating disorder patient can be educated about the long-term effects of childhood trauma as well as about the eating disorder. Traumatic recapitulations occurring in the love relationship may be explored. It can be helpful for the couple to learn to parti-

tion the piece of their conflicts occurring in the here-and-now from the piece that is primarily a posttraumatic response. As the couple develops methods of dealing effectively with difficult issues, not only will the relationship become more fulfilling for both parties, but also the healing power of human connection can be experienced by the patient. The therapist is wise to congratulate the patient for taking such an interpersonal risk, given her history of interpersonal harm.

In cases of destructive relationships, such as battering or emotionally abusive relationships, therapy should obviously proceed differently. In the process of couples work, the patient may begin to see that relational problems are not all her fault. Recapitulations may become more obvious to her, particularly if she is being re-victimized. She may feel empowered to leave a destructive relationship or to demand certain changes to make the relationship healthier. The clinician must attend to signs of potential danger in an abusive relationship, because the risk to the patient often increases with increased assertiveness and self-esteem on her part.

Family Therapy

Family therapy with the patient's family of origin may be helpful in certain cases. For example, if the abuse occurred within the family, it may help restore the relationship between the patient and the nonoffending parent. In cases of extrafamilial abuse, family therapy may be used to educate the family about the long-term effects of trauma and to address issues that hamper family members from providing much-needed support. However, this modality must be used with caution. If not handled carefully, the therapy may recapitulate the trauma of familial denial and disbelief. Together, therapist and patient must weigh the risks and benefits of such interventions. It is probably unwise to proceed until the patient feels she has sufficient internal capacity and social support to cope with a possible negative outcome.

Group Therapy

Group therapy for survivors of childhood abuse can be especially effective for decreasing the desperate feelings of isolation and aloneness typical of both eating-disordered and traumatized individuals. Group work allows members to interact

with others who have "been there" and to be helpful to others as well as to be helped.

Psychologists Wooley and Kearney-Cooke
recommend using experiential techniques to cut
through intellectualization and denial (Wooley &
Kearney-Cooke, 1986). Some techniques include
body-image work, guided imagery, role-playing,
sculpting or painting abuse images, and describing abusive experiences in the present tense. Many
experts believe that group patients should always
be engaged concurrently in individual psychotherapy.

Pharmacotherapy

Pharmacologic therapy can play a critical role in
stabilizing the patient's physical symptoms and
propensity toward intense psychobiologic
dysregulation. Psychotropic medications may decrease the patient's suffering, allow a degree of
stabilization of a chaotic internal and external life,
and therefore permit her to engage more intensively and productively in psychotherapy. Psychiatrists often prefer to use the selective serotonin
reuptake inhibitors (SSRIs) because of their demonstrated efficacy with post-traumatic stress symptoms, binge eating, and depression (Fluoretine
Bulimia Nervosa, Collaborative Study Group,
1992; van der Kolk, Dreyfuss, Michaels, et al.,
1994), all of which are common among these patients. Trauma survivors may have brief psychotic
or quasi-psychotic episodes in times of extreme
stress. In some cases, low levels of antipsychotic
medications may be helpful on an as-needed basis to halt the process of biological "hijacking"
that occurs. Whatever the pharmacologic intervention, it is crucial that the traumatized patient be an
informed collaborator, rather than a passive recipient of treatment. It is critical that she experience
changes, even those produced by medications, as
emanating from her (e.g., she elected to undergo a
particular course of pharmacotherapy in a well-
informed manner), rather than locating positive
changes in an external agent, be it the therapist or
a medication.

Self-Help Groups

Some patients find the additional support of self-
help groups, such as "12-step" groups like Alcoholics Anonymous, tremendously beneficial, while
other patients find them quite alienating. When

recommending this form of adjunctive help, the
clinician is wise to counsel patients to be informed
consumers, taking care to find groups that are reputable and feel "safe" to the patient.

CONCLUSION

Deficits in the ability to regulate emotional states
are among the most devastating effects of childhood trauma (van der Kolk & Fisler, 1994). For
some individuals with eating disorders, the eating
disturbance represents a desperate, though highly
damaging, effort to soothe painful effects, escape
from remembrances and reminders of abuse, and
take the place of comfort that would normally be
provided by close personal relationships. Binge
eating, purging, and starving become apt metaphors for the boundless hunger, the wish to fulfill
needs together with the wish to rid oneself forever of need, the desire to "purify" the damaged
psychic and physical self, and the hope of restor-
ing meaning. For many women (and probably
men), a traumatic personal history, the resulting
posttraumatic biology, and a culture that promises
that thinness will bring "control," equanimity, and
life meaning, converge to make disturbed eating a
comprehensible outcome of abuse. Treatment is
almost always challenging, yet ultimately highly
rewarding, for patients and mental-health providers alike.

REFERENCES

Fairburn, C. G., Welch, S. L., Doll, H. A., et al. (1997). Risk factors
for bulimia nervosa. *Arch Gen Psychiatry 54*, 509–517.

Fluoxetine Bulimia Nervosa Collaborative Study Group (1992).
Fluoxetine in the treatment of bulimia nervosa: A multicenter,
placebo-controlled, double-blind trial. *Arch Gen Psychiatry
49*, 1379–147.

Goldfarb, L. A. (1987). Sexual abuse antecedent to anorexia nervosa,
bulimia, and compulsive overeating: Three case reports. *Int J
Eat Disorders 6*, 675–680.

Herman, J. L. (1992a). *Trauma and recovery*. New York Basic Books.

Herman, J. L. (1992b). Complex PTSD: A syndrome in survivors of
prolonged and repeated trauma. *J Trauma Stress 5*, 377–391.

McFall, M. E., Murburg, M., Roszell, D. K., et al. (1989). Psycho-
physiologic and neuroendocrine findings in posttraumatic stress
disorder: A review of theory and research. *J Anxiety Disorders 3*, 243–257.

Pope, H. G., & Hudson, J. I. (1992). Is childhood sexual abuse a risk
factor for bulimia nervosa? *Am J Psychiatry 149*, 455–463.

Root, M. P. P., & Fallon, P. (1988). The incidence of victimization
experiences in a bulimic sample. *J Interpers Violence 3*, 161–
173.

Root, M. P. P., & Fallon, P. (1989). Treating the victimized bulimic.
Journal of Interpersonal Violence 4, 90–100.

Rorty, M., & Yager, J. (1996). Histories of childhood trauma and complex post-traumatic sequelae in women with eating disorders. *Psychiatric Clin North America 19*, 773–791.

Rorty, M., Yager, J., & Rossotto, E. (1994). Childhood sexual, physical, and psychological abuse in bulimia nervosa. *Am J Psychiatry 151*, 1122–1126.

Schmidt, U., Tiller, J., & Treasure, J. (1993). Setting the scene for eating disorders: Childhood care, classification and the course of illness. *Psychol Med 23*, 663–672.

van der Kolk, B. A. (1994). The body keeps score: Memory and the evolving psychobiology of PTSD. *Harvard Review of Psychiatry 1*, 253–265.

van der Kolk, B. A., Dreyfuss, D., Michaels, M., et al. (1994). Fluoxetine in posttraumatic stress disorder. *J Clin Psychiatry 55*, 517–522.

van der Kolk, B. A., & Fisler, R. E. (1994). Childhood abuse and neglect and loss of self-regulation. *Bull Menninger Clin 58*, 145–168.

Vanderlinden, J., & Vandereycken, W. (1997). Trauma, dissociation, and impulse dyscontrol in eating disorders. Bristol, PA.

Wooley, S. C., & Kearney-Cooke, A. Intensive treatment of bulimia and body-image disturbance. In K. D. Brownell and J. P. Foreyt (eds). Handbook of eating disorders, New York, Basic Books, 1986, pp. 476–502.

Yehuda, R., Kahana, B., Binder-Brynes, K., et al. (1995). Low urinary cortisol excretion in Holocaust survivors with posttraumatic stress disorder. *American Journal of Psychiatry 152*, 982–986.

Body Images, Eating Disorders, and Beyond

by Thomas F. Cash, Ph.D. and Melissa D. Strachan, B.A.

"It's what's inside that counts." Although most of us wish to believe this cliché, our societal reality is that, for better or worse, appearance matters (Cash & Pruzinsky, 1990; Jackson, 1992). The media bombard us with extreme, often unattainable images of the "body beautiful." One need only watch television, glance at the covers and contents of most women's magazines, or catch a glimpse of the omnipresent ads for dieting, fitness, and cosmetic surgery to get the message: *"It's what's outside that counts."*

Perhaps even more striking than these media messages is the extent to which people absorb them and pursue bodily perfection. These images fuel American women's aspirations for a slender yet busty, well-toned physique and a lofty level of physical attractiveness. Understandably, many women feel cheated by the body of their birthright. Their inner image of their looks is lacking. They have a "negative body image," which refers, most simply, to dissatisfaction with one's physical appearance. Individuals with a negative body image often dislike one or more of their physical features, have thoughts or worries about their looks that lead to despondency, frustration, or self-consciousness, or to diminished self-esteem. Not surprisingly, these difficulties place people at greater risk of developing depression, interpersonal discomfort, sexual difficulties, and eating disorders.

Much of the contemporary popular and professional discussion of body image focuses on its linkage with eating disorders, such as anorexia nervosa and bulimia nervosa. However, this chapter will explore body image in a manner that includes and transcends its association with eating disorders. We will examine this multifaceted concept, its psychological correlates, scientific assessment, and professional treatment. The chapter will first summarize research on body image, its dysfunctions, and their development. Then, we will delineate a structured therapeutic program that combines cognitive and behavioral interventions to bring about positive body-image change.

HISTORY AND COMPONENTS OF THE BODY-IMAGE CONSTRUCT

The study of body image has its roots in the turn of the century when physicians were trying to understand the causes of neurological patients' strange bodily sensations. From 1914 to 1940, the writings of Paul Schilder shifted the focus from neurological phenomena to the attitudes and feelings patients had about their bodies (Fisher, 1990). Concurrently, psychoanalytic thinkers were examining the body-related experiences of their patients and expanding Freud's psychosexual theory of development to include an emphasis on patients' perceptions of the body as the "boundary" between themselves and their external world (Fisher, 1986).

In recent decades, a clinical and scientific interest in body image has flourished, in part because of the need to understand the increasing prevalence of eating disorders. Body image is now viewed as a multidimensional construct consisting of two key components: perception and attitude (Cash & Pruzinsky, 1990; Thompson, 1996). The perceptual facet of body image typically concerns the extent to which an individual is able to judge his or her body size accurately. Researchers have developed a variety of instruments to measure individuals' degree of body-size distortion, whether based on perceptions of the whole body or discrete areas of the body (Cash & Deagle, 1997; Thompson, 1996). Attitudinal body image, on the other hand, is typically assessed by self-report questionnaires to measure people's beliefs and feelings about their looks. Thompson (1990) states that the Multidimensional Body-Self Relations Questionnaire (MBSRQ) may be one of the best of the attitudinal body-image measures. The 69-item MBSRQ contains 10 subscales to assess specific attitudes toward one's appearance, fitness, and health (Brown, Cash, & Mikulka, 1990; Cash, 1994a). Other widely used, well-validated measures of body satisfaction are the Body Cathexis Scale (Secord & Jourard, 1953) and the Body Esteem Scale (Franzoi & Shields, 1984).

Attitudinal body image itself consists of at least two relatively distinct components (Cash, 1994b)—evaluation/affect and investment. Body-image evaluation refers to one's level of satisfaction or dissatisfaction and one's evaluative thoughts or beliefs about one's looks. The degree of body satisfaction depends on the degree of congruence (or discrepancy) between one's view of one's actual body or body parts and one's physical ideals (Cash & Szymanski, 1995; Szymanski & Cash, 1995). Relatedly, body-image affect refers to the emotional experiences that result from this physical self-evaluation. When a person evaluates his or her appearance unfavorably, dysphoric body-image emotions may result. Body-image investment is the extent to which one's attention, thoughts, and actions focus on one's own looks, including how much one relies on physical appearance to define one's sense of self. A negative body image occurs as a joint function of a negative evaluation and excessive investment.

THE PREVALENCE AND DEMOGRAPHICS OF BODY-IMAGE DISCONTENT

Survey research indicates that negative body-image experiences are not only commonplace in America, but their prevalence is increasing. From a national *Psychology Today* magazine survey of 30,000 people, Cash and his colleagues (1986) sampled 2,000 individuals representing the United States population for age and gender. The survey revealed that 38% of women and 34% of men were dissatisfied with their overall appearance. While most respondents were content with their face and their height, body weight and shape were clear sources of discontent. Data further indicate that the prevalence rates of body dissatisfaction are on the rise, especially among women. In a 1993 national survey, 48% of American women reported experiencing dissatisfaction with overall appearance, in addition to a fear of being or becoming overweight (Cash & Henry, 1995). Garner's 1997 *Psychology Today* survey determined that 56% of female respondents and 43% of the men evaluated their overall appearance negatively. Eighty-nine percent of the women wanted to lose weight, and 15% reported that they would sacrifice five years of their life to do so. Attesting to growing body-image problems among American women, a recent meta-analysis of 222 body-image studies from the past 50 years reveals continual increases in women's body dissatisfaction (Feingold & Mazzella, 1998).

These and other surveys confirm significant gender differences in body satisfaction. Prevalence rates are significantly higher among women in our society, especially young women (Drewnowski & Yee, 1987; Pliner, Chaiken, & Flett, 1990). Muth and Cash (1997) examined body-image investment, evaluation, and affect among college women and men. Gender comparisons indicated that women were more invested in their looks, experienced more negative affect, and had greater self-ideal discrepancies. Hence, while many men struggle with a negative body image, dissatisfaction with and distress about one's looks is more common among women, who are more invested in their appearance vis-à-vis self-definition.

In addition to age and gender differences, race is relevant to body satisfaction. In general, African American women hold more favorable body images than do Caucasian or Hispanic women. For example, Black college women's self-evaluations were more positive both with respect to global appearance and to weight-related satisfaction (Rucker & Cash, 1992). Perhaps because a larger female body size is idealized within African American culture, they experience less of a self-ideal discrepancy, even at heavier body weights. Relative to Caucasian women, they also have a higher threshold for perceiving a body as "fat." Moreover, they exhibit lower rates of eating pathology. Cash and Henry's (1995) survey data extend these findings to a national sample, also indicating that Black women are more satisfied with their looks and are less preoccupied with gaining weight than their White and Hispanic counterparts.

THE EMERGENCE OF A NEGATIVE BODY IMAGE

How does one's body image, positive or negative, develop? According to a cognitive social learning perspective, it unfolds as a complex function of various historical and present influences (Cash, 1995b, 1996, 1997; Cash & Grant, 1996). Historical factors largely pertain to one's early socialization about the meaning of physical appearance and one's experiences of one's body during childhood and adolescence. These events foster the acquisition of basic body-image attitudes which, in turn, serve to predispose how the individual views and reacts to current life events.

Media Messages

American culture's emphasis on beauty and thinness as standards for women permeates all levels of media communication (Fallon, 1990; Wooley, 1994). Technological advancement has enabled widespread dissemination of these cultural expectations, increasing the drive for the "ideal female shape" in girls and women. This quest to achieve the societal standard is so common that it has been referred to as a "normative" process (Fontaine, 1991; Rodin, Silberstein, & Striegel-Moore, 1985).

Complicating women's desire to resemble the media images of the female shape is the fact that

the standards for women are changing over time (Heinberg, 1996; Mazur, 1986). Garner, Garfinkel, Schwartz, and Thompson (1980) suggest that beginning in the early 1970s, a shift occurred from a voluptuous ideal to a more lean, angular body type. The researchers examined the evolution of norms of weight and shape among Playboy models and contestants of the Miss America beauty pageant, finding that the average weight of both groups of women had significantly decreased over two decades. Both models and pageant contestants weighed significantly less than the average American woman, and pageant winners were thinner than their competitors. Further research revealed that Miss America contestants from 1979 to 1988 weighed between 13% and 19% less than the "normal" weight for women their height (Wiseman, Gray, Mosimann, & Ahren, 1992). Moreover, the researchers observed that over the 30-year period from 1959 to 1989, the prevalence of women's magazine articles focusing on weight-loss dieting and exercise have grown. Advertising on television medium has similarly increased its emphasis on weight-loss products and services (Wiseman, Gunning, & Gray, 1993).

What bearing do such media images and messages have on women's body-image experiences? Research has demonstrated that exposure to these images and body dissatisfaction are related. The more a woman internalizes cultural standards of beauty, the higher the likelihood that she will feel dissatisfied with her own appearance (Stice, Schupak-Neuberg, Shaw, & Stein 1994; Stormer & Thompson, 1996). In fact, media messages of the beauty ideal are particularly damaging to women who are highly invested in their looks or who view their bodies negatively. For example, women with bulimic symptoms who were exposed to slides of thin models reported significantly lower levels of self-esteem and weight satisfaction than those who viewed slides of normal or overweight women (Irving, 1990). Even in women with subclinical levels of body-image disturbance, the media's portrayal of the "thin is beautiful" standard has been shown to have a negative impact on body acceptance (Heinberg & Thompson, 1995). This impact occurs in two ways: First, girls are encouraged to adopt these salient and extreme standards as their own. Second, exposure to such messages serves to remind the appearance-invested, dissatisfied person of her body's inadequacies vis-à-vis the standard.

Familial Expectations and Experiences

Expectations, opinions, and verbal and nonverbal messages within the family also contribute to the formation of body image (Rieves & Cash, 1996; Striegel-Moore, Silberstein, & Rodin, 1986). Parental role modeling communicates the degree to which physical appearance is valued within the family, establishing a standard against which a child compares himself or herself. Highly appearance-invested mothers who value dieting behavior, strive for weight loss, or engender family competition based on physical attractiveness may promote the development of a negative body image in their daughters (Striegel-Moore et al., 1986). Rozin and Fallon (1988) have noted a correspondence between the degree of body dissatisfaction and weight/dieting concerns of mothers and their college-aged daughters. Rieves and Cash (1996) also found that daughters' perceptions of their mothers' levels of body satisfaction, weight preoccupation, and investment in appearance correlated with their own.

Not surprisingly, the attractiveness of siblings may play a role in body-image development. Having a more attractive sibling may lead to a less favorable self-evaluation of appearance, just as having a less attractive sibling may produce the opposite effect (Rieves & Cash, 1996). Siblings apparently provide a social-comparison standard for the evaluative appraisal of one's own looks. Siblings, especially brothers, are also frequent perpetrators of appearance-related teasing or criticism (Cash, 1995a; Rieves & Cash, 1996). Thus, family members represent important teachers of the lessons learned about the meaning and acceptability of one's physical characteristics.

Appearance Teasing

Being teased about one's physical appearance is a common childhood and adolescent experience. For many individuals, such interpersonal ridicule by peers predisposes body dissatisfaction. Researchers have found correlations between previous appearance teasing and the existence of a negative body-image in adulthood (Cash, 1995a; Cash et al., 1986; Fabian & Thompson, 1989; Grilo, Wilfley, Brownell, & Rodin, 1994; Rieves & Cash, 1996). Furthermore, such experiences have been proposed to play a causal role in body-image development (Thompson & Heinberg, 1993), as a significant and consistent predictor of eating disturbance and body dissatisfaction.

Bodily Changes during Puberty

Pubertal maturation during adolescence, a period marked by rapid physical change, can significantly affect body-image development. For girls, puberty takes place at 9 or 10 years of age and brings with it adipose weight gain in the hips, abdomen, and breasts (Papalia & Olds, 1992). Boys enter puberty somewhat later, at around age 12, and experience a broadening of the shoulders, changes in voice, and overall body growth. Puberty, while a universal experience, affects the body images of boys and girls differently. For boys, gaining weight, strength, and muscle is a positive change because it brings them closer in line with society's standard of "masculinity" for men, and as a result, boys evaluate their looks more positively (Striegel-Moore et al., 1986). However, the weight gain that girls experience during adolescence, or what some refer to as the "fat spurt," is seen as a movement away from society's thinness ideal, resulting in increased dieting efforts and dissatisfaction with weight (Attie & Brooks-Gunn, 1989).

Obesity

In the context of our society's emphasis on thinness as a standard of beauty, it is not surprising that obese children, teenagers, and adults often struggle with a poor body image (Cash & Roy, in press; Friedman & Brownell, 1995). Moreover, Cash and Hicks (1990) concluded that the inaccurate self-perception of being overweight is associated with body dissatisfaction to practically the same degree as actually being overweight. The effects of obesity on body image are more deleterious for females than males (Cash & Hicks, 1990; Cash & Roy, in press; Tiggemann & Rothblum, 1988). The body images of obese individuals are also significantly affected by whether or not eating pathology is present. Obese binge-eaters have a more negative body image than obese nonbingers (Cash, 1991).

The age of onset of obesity may exert differential effects on adult body image. Stunkard and Burt (1967) proposed that juvenile-onset obesity engenders a more negative body image than adult-onset obesity. Cash, Counts, and Huffine (1990) extended these findings by comparing formerly overweight women with currently overweight and normal-weight participants. A powerful vestigial influence of overweight was observed. The formerly overweight group continued to perceive themselves as fat and were dissatisfied with their appearance and anxious about their weight nearly as much as the currently overweight group and more than the never-overweight group. Termed "phantom fat," the experience of having been heavy may persist as a body-image vulnerability even after weight loss.

Gender Attitudes

Are there personality factors that may predispose individuals to a problematic body-image? Recent research has explored the relationship between body-image satisfaction and attitudes toward gender roles, including feminist identity. Investigators have theorized that possessing more traditional gender-role attitudes and values might foster greater appearance investment and body dissatisfaction. However, this link between body image and gender-role attitudes has proved to exist only on the level of ideology about male-female social relations (Cash, Ancis, & Strachan, 1997). Regardless of their extent of feminist identity, women who endorsed traditional gender attitudes in their social relationships with men exhibited greater investment in their appearance, had more fully internalized cultural standards of beauty, and held more maladaptive assumptions about their looks. An emphasis on feminine role enactment in male-female interactions is also correlated with eating disturbance (Cash, Strachan, & Roy, 1997). Women who believe that it is their "feminine duty to be what men want" not only put their body image in jeopardy, they also are more apt to view other women ambivalently, as their "beauty competitors" (Cash, Roy, & Strachan, 1997).

CURRENT CAUSAL PROCESSES

Thus far, we have examined the historical, developmental contexts that predispose the acquisition of negative body-image attitudes. Now we must briefly consider how such attitudes operate within the context of everyday life. According to a cognitive-behavioral perspective, specific situational cues or events activate cognitive processing of information about and self-appraisals of one's appearance, especially among individuals who are highly invested in (or schematic for) physical appearance. Such precipitating events may entail, for example, body exposure, mirror exposure, social scrutiny, social comparisons, wearing certain clothing, weighing, exercising, mood states, and so forth. The resultant internal dialogues involve emotion-laden automatic thoughts, inferences, interpretations, and conclusions about one's looks. Often, due to problematic body-image attitudes and assumptions, these inner dialogues are habitual, faulty, and dysphoric. Subsequently, to manage or cope with these distressing body-image thoughts and emotions, individuals engage in defensive, self-regulating actions. Such adjustive actions include avoidant and body-concealment behaviors, appearance-correcting rituals, social reassurance seeking, and compensatory strategies. These maneuvers serve to maintain body-image problems via negative reinforcement, as they enable the individual temporarily to escape, reduce, or regulate body-image discomfort.

BODY-IMAGE PSYCHOPATHOLOGY

Body-image dysphoria may be conceptualized as falling on a continuum, ranging from mild discontent to clinical pathology. For many people, the negative feelings they have about their looks are only a mild annoyance, yet for others their distress greatly compromises their quality of life. When a negative body image reaches a critical level of severity, it may contribute to several disorders included in the *DSM-IV* (American Psychiatric Association, 1994). Specifically, body-image disturbance is a diagnostic criterion for body dysmorphic disorder and certain eating disorders.

Body Dysmorphic Disorder

Body dysmorphic disorder (BDD) is known as the disorder of "imagined ugliness" by virtue of the fact that its essential feature is a preoccupation with a perceived defect or minor flaw in one's appearance (Phillips, 1996). For individuals experiencing BDD, their appearance-related distress is excessive and can cause constant torment. Their obsessive worry and compulsive appearance-checking significantly interferes with daily functioning, particularly with participation in social interactions.

BDD involves both perceptual and attitudinal body-image dysfunctions. Individuals who show no blemish perceive one to exist, and those who do exhibit a minor physical defect experience it as considerably more noticeable and "uglier" than the objective observer. Attitudinally, persons with BDD rigidly adhere to distorted thoughts and maladaptive assumptions related to their perceived defect (Rosen, 1995). Although these persons typically can recognize the exaggerated nature of their complaints, their feelings of unattractiveness are so pronounced that they feel perpetually embarrassed and repulsive to others. The body-image symptoms of BDD border on delusional; however, the distortions are usually not bizarre and tend to be related only to situations requiring an attentional focus on appearance. Behavioral manifestations of BDD may involve avoidance of social situations, grooming to conceal the perceived defect, recurrent appearance-checking rituals, and efforts to improve their looks, including the pursuit of plastic surgery.

Eating Disorders

When an individual's dissatisfaction with appearance, particularly body weight and shape, causes considerable distress, he or she will take steps to eliminate or ameliorate the feelings of anxiety. For some, this means drastically altering eating habits so as to control weight. Most researchers and clinicians regard a negative body-image to be the cardinal feature of eating disorders, such as anorexia and bulimia nervosa (Bruch, 1962). A multitude of studies have documented both attitudinal and perceptual body-image disturbances among eating disordered patients (for reviews, see Cash & Brown, 1987; Cash & Deagle, 1997; Rosen, 1990). This research further suggests that the extent of body-image disturbance may determine the severity of eating disordered symptoms and body-image dysfunctions predisposing, precipitating, and maintaining causes of eating disorders.

Nevertheless, scientists have debated the specific nature of body-image difficulties in eating disorders. Some researchers contend that perceptual distortion (i.e., size overestimation) is not synonymous with body-image disturbance (Hsu, 1982; Hsu & Sobkiewicz, 1991). Others contend that perceptual distortion is less central to the eating disorders, and that body-image attitudes play a more essential role (Cash & Brown, 1987).

In an effort to resolve this controversy, Cash and Deagle (1997) conducted a meta-analysis of 66 investigations (from 1974 to 1993) of percep-

tual and attitudinal body image among patients with anorexia nervosa or bulimia nervosa. Relative to "normal" controls, eating-disordered women exhibited greater body dissatisfaction and perceptual body-size distortion. Affect sizes for perceptual distortion were moderate, ranging from .61 to .64 among women with eating disorders compared to control groups. Body dissatisfaction measures yielded consistently larger affect sizes, ranging from 1.10 to 1.13. Thus, women with clinical eating disorders experience attitudinal body dissatisfaction to a much greater degree than they perceptually overestimate their body size. Furthermore, although anorexics' and bulimics' perceptual distortions were comparable, bulimics clearly held more negative body-image attitudes than anorexics. The meta-analysis also indicated that such size overestimation appears unlikely to reflect a more generalized tendency to overestimate the size of nonbody objects.

Cash and Deagle (1997) argued for more sophisticated studies of body image and eating disorders—studies that examine the investment (or schematicity) dimension of body-image attitudes and studies that capture the cognitively mediated and emotional processing of body-related information in meaningful life situations. Such research is especially important in view of the fact that in the absence of body-image changes following eating disorder treatment, these patients remain at substantial risk for relapse (see Cash & Deagle, 1997; Rosen, 1990, 1997).

CO-MORBID DISORDERS AND DIFFICULTIES OF BODY-IMAGE DISCONTENT

Most people with a negative body-image do not have BDD, nor do they have a clinical eating disorder. Neither does a negative body image exist in isolation from other psychosocial problems. Whether as cause or consequence, a negative body-image is related to poor self-esteem, social anxiety, depression, and sexual difficulties.

Self-Esteem

Body-image attitudes and self-esteem are interdependent, such that "a distortion of one will affect the other" (Freedman, 1990, p. 274). Indeed, body-image is a key component of self-concept. Many researchers have noted a strong and positive correlation between body image and self-esteem. Children, adolescents, or adults who feel negatively about their appearance typically report lower self-esteem, including social self-esteem (e.g., Ben-Tovim, Walker, Murray, & Chin, 1990; Cash & Labarge, 1996; Mable, Balance, & Galgan, 1986; McCaulay, Mintz, & Glenn, 1988; Mendelson & White, 1982; Rosen & Ross, 1967). Put simply, if one dislikes one's body, it's difficult to like the person who lives there.

Lavallee and Cash (1997) examined changes in self-esteem among body-dissatisfied women who completed bibliotherapeutic self-help programs. One group completed a body-image program, while the other used a program focused on self-esteem. Interestingly, both conditions produced significant gains in social self-esteem, reporting greater feelings of confidence during social interactions, and both enhanced body image. Thus, effectively treating body-image disturbance will improve self-esteem. Conversely, self-esteem enhancement can cause body-image to become more positive as well.

Depression

Depression has also been linked to feelings of dissatisfaction with one's appearance. Marsella, Shizuru, Brennan, and Kameoka (1981) demonstrated that, regardless of age and gender, depressed individuals had increased levels of body dissatisfaction. A later study by Noles, Cash, and Winstead (1985) found that depressed college students experienced less body satisfaction and judged their attractiveness less favorably than did those who were not depressed. Among psychiatric inpatients, a poor self-evaluation of appearance is related to anxiety, depression, and interpersonal difficulties (Archer & Cash, 1985).

Interpersonal Anxiety

Individuals who feel that their looks are personally unacceptable are apt to feel that their looks are also socially unacceptable and that others view them more negatively. A negative body image would be expected to engender more discomfort in interpersonal relations, as was noted above (Archer & Cash, 1985). Cash and Szymanski (1995) examined this hypothesis by assessing the extent to which college women evaluated their physical characteristics as discrepant from their physical ideals and their degree of investment in these ideals. Women with greater self-ideal discrepancies and women who were more psychologically invested in their looks reported significantly higher levels of social-evaluative anxiety.

Sexual Dissatisfaction and Dysfunction

Research on body-image dysphoria and sexual dysfunction suggests that the two are related, and that a negative body image can contribute to physiological dysfunction, a restricted range of sexual experiences, and avoidance of sexual contact (Faith & Schare, 1993; Schiavi, Karstaedt, Schreiner-Engel, & Mandeli, 1992). For example, Hangen and Cash (1991) found that, for both sexes, a more negative body image was associated with a narrower variety of sexual experiences and decreased sexual satisfaction. For women, body-image discontent was related to lower rates of orgasm and more sexual difficulties in general. The researchers found that these relationships were especially evident with their new measure of body image that assessed the extent to which participants experienced anxiety about and sought to conceal their body's appearance during sexual activities. Thus, a self-conscious, anxious focus on one's body may interfere with sexual pleasure and responsivity.

Cognitive-Behavioral Body-Image Therapy

Because a negative body image is a widespread problem with consequences that can impair the psychosocial quality of life, professionals have developed a variety of treatments for this problem. Among these therapies, cognitive-behavioral treatment (CBT) has emerged as an effective, empirically sound intervention. CBT has proven efficacy within the modality of individual therapy (Butters & Cash, 1987; Dworkin & Kerr, 1987), group treatment (Fisher & Thompson, 1994; Grant & Cash, 1995; Rosen et al., 1989, 1990) and a self-help modality (Cash & Lavallee, 1997; Cash & Grant, 1995; Lavallee & Cash, 1997). The remainder of this chapter will provide an overview of Cash's eight-step CBT program for a negative body image. Based on empirical research, the program has gone through four generations of development. The first was an unpublished treatment manual used in the seminal investigation by Butters and Cash (1985). The second version was

Cash's (1991) published audiotape program available to mental health practitioners, *Body-Image Therapy: A Program for Self-Directed Change*, which includes four one-hour cassettes, client manual, and clinician's manual. In the third version of the program, Cash (1995) expanded its contents into an eight-step self-help book for the public, entitled *What Do You See When You Look in the Mirror?: Helping Yourself to a Positive Body-Image*. Most recently, the program has been refined based on empirical data and client feedback and is published as *The Body Image Workbook: An Eight-Step Program for Learning to Like Your Looks* (Cash 1997). It is presented in a user-friendly format that contains over 40 "Self-Discovery Helpsheets" and "Helpsheets for Change." The components of this current version of Cash's body-image CBT are summarized as follows (for more detail, see Cash, 1996, 1997; Cash & Grant, 1996):

- The *Workbook*'s introduction provides a description of body-image problems and gives an overview of the program, including evidence of its effectiveness. Difficulties that require professional assistance (e.g., BDD, eating disorders, clinical depression) are identified.

- **Step 1** takes the participant through a series of scientific self-assessments which are self-scored and normatively compared to ascertain one's body-image strengths and weaknesses. The participant then sets specific goals for body-image change, based on the interpretations offered for elements of the body-image assessment profile.

- **Step 2** is principally a psychoeducational component of the program. Detailed information is provided on the nature of body image and the past and present causes of a negative body image. This step continues the self-discovery process with mirror exposure activities and an autobiographical summary of participants' own body-image development. Using a "Body-image Diary," participants learn to systematically monitor the sequence of their current body-image experiences—attending to and recording the triggers of distress and the effects of these activating events on their thought processes ("Private Body Talk"), their emotions, and behavioral reactions. This diary is completed throughout the program.

- **Step 3** teaches participants "Body and Mind Relaxation," combining muscle relaxation, dia-phragmatic breathing, mental imagery, and positive self-talk to develop skills for controlling body-image dysphoria. These skills are incorporated into systematic body-image desensitization to increase comfort with distress-provoking body areas.

- **Step 4** identifies 10 dysfunctional "appearance assumptions." These are unquestioned beliefs or schemas about appearance that affect an individual's daily body-image experiences. Examples of these assumptions are: "Physically attractive people have it all." "If I could look just as I wish, my life would be much happier." "If people knew how I really look, they would like me less." "I should do whatever I can to always look my best." "The only way I could ever like my looks would be to change them." Participants learn to become aware of the operation of these core assumptions in daily life and to question and refute these beliefs.

- **Step 5** assists participants in identifying eight cognitive distortions in their Private Body Talk and provides strategies for monitoring and modifying them. Such distortions include comparing one's appearance to more attractive persons, thinking of one's looks in dichotomous extremes (e.g., fat or thin, ugly or good-looking), and arbitrarily blaming one's appearance for past or future adversities. Participants now expand the body-image diary to incorporate cognitive restructuring exercises to correct distortions and record the effects.

- **Step 6** details specific behavioral strategies to alter avoidant behaviors, which might include avoiding the beach or pool due to appearance dissatisfaction, wearing only body-concealing clothing, or being unable to be seen in public without facial cosmetics. Participants also identify and alter "appearance-preoccupied rituals," such as repeated mirror checking or excessive grooming regimens.

- **Step 7** applies a metaphor of human relationship satisfaction to promote one's proactive, positive relationship with one's body. Participants carry out specific activities of "body-image affirmation" and body-image enhancement. For example, in developing a healthy, pleasurable relationship with his or her body, the participant engages in self-prescribed, reinforcing activities that pertain to bodily fitness and health, sensate pleasure, and grooming for enjoyment.

- **Step 8** concludes the program by having individuals retake the body-image assessments to receive feedback about positive changes and to set goals for further change. Within a framework of relapse prevention, participants learn to identify and prepare for situations that place their body image at risk, especially troublesome interpersonal events.

As previously cited, numerous studies attest to the effectiveness of body-image CBT conducted as individual therapy, group therapy, and self-administered treatment. The observed outcomes not only reflect body-image improvements but also indicate a generalization of positive effects to self-esteem, social functioning, sexual experiences, depressive symptoms, and eating pathology. Although most of these treatment studies were carried out with extremely body-dissatisfied college women, additional research points to the efficacy of body-image CBT with obese persons (Rosen, Orosan, & Reiter, 1995) and individuals with BDD (Rosen, Reiter, & Orosan, 1995). Although the utility of this treatment with eating-disordered individuals certainly holds promise, the fruition of its potential requires systematic scientific verification.

CONCLUSIONS

As a multidimensional psychological concept, body-image has considerable importance in the understanding of human behavior. This chapter has attempted to elucidate this concept beyond its familiar association with the eating disorders. All too often, the quality of our embodied lives is diminished by the views we hold of our own physical appearance. How this unfortunate fact comes to be and continues to be is certainly worthy of sustained scientific inquiry. Equally valuable is the professional pursuit of answers concerning how body-image disorders and difficulties can be prevented and overcome.

REFERENCES

American Psychiatric Association. (1994). *Diagnostic and statistical manual of mental disorders* (4th ed.). Washington, DC.

Archer, R.P., & Cash, T.F. (1985). Physical attractiveness and maladjustment among psychiatric inpatients. *Journal of Social and Clinical Psychology, 3,* 170–180.

Attie, I., & Brooks-Gunn, J. (1989). Development of eating problems in adolescent girls: A longitudinal study. *Developmental Psychology, 25,* 7–79.

Ben-Tovim, D., Walker, M.K., Murray, H., & Chin, G. (1990). Body size estimates: Body-image or body attitude measures? *International Journal of Eating Disorders, 9,* 57–67.

Brown, T.A., Cash, T.F., & Mikulka, P.J. (1990). Attitudinal body-image assessment: Factor analysis of the body-self relations questionnaire. *Journal of Personality Assessment, 55,* 135–144.

Bruch, H. (1962). Perceptual and conceptual disturbances in anorexia nervosa. *Psychosomatic Medicine, 24,* 187–194.

Butters, J.W., & Cash, T.F. (1987). Cognitive-behavioral treatment of women's body-image dissatisfaction. *Journal of Consulting and Clinical Psychology, 55,* 889–897.

Cash, T.F. (1991a). *Body-image therapy: A program for self-directed change.* New York: Guilford.

Cash, T.F. (1991b). Binge-eating and body images among the obese: A further evaluation. *Journal of Social Behavior and Personality, 6,* 367–376.

Cash, T.F. (1994a). *The users' manual for the Multidimensional Body-Self Relations Questionnaire.* Available from the author, Old Dominion University, Norfolk, VA.

Cash, T.F. (1994b). Body-image attitudes: Evaluation, investment, and affect. *Perceptual and Motor Skills, 78,* 1168–1170.

Cash, T.F. (1995a). Developmental teasing about physical appearance: Retrospective descriptions and relationships with body image. *Social Behavior and Personality, 23,* 123–130.

Cash, T.F. (1995b). *What do you see when you look in the mirror?: Helping yourself to a positive body image.* New York: Bantam.

Cash, T.F. (1996). The treatment of body-image disturbances. In J.K. Thompson (Ed.), *Body-image, eating disorders, and obesity* (pp.83–107). Washington, DC: American Psychological Association.

Cash, T.F. (1997). *The body-image workbook: An 8-step program for learning to like your looks.* Oakland, CA: New Harbinger Publications.

Cash, T.F., Ancis, J.R., & Strachan, M.D. (1997). Gender attitudes, feminist identity, and body images among college women. *Sex Roles, 36,* 433–447.

Cash, T.F., & Brown, T.A. (1987). Body image in anorexia nervosa and bulimia nervosa: A review of the literature. *Behavior Modification, 11,* 487–521.

Cash, T.F., Counts, B., & Huffine, C.E. (1990). Current and vestigial effects of overweight among women: Fear of fat, attitudinal body image, and eating behaviors. *Journal of Psychopathology and Behavioral Assessment, 12,* 157–167.

Cash, T.F., & Deagle, E.A. (1997). The nature and extent of body-image disturbances in anorexia nervosa and bulimia nervosa: A meta-analysis. *International Journal of Eating Disorders, 21,* 2–19.

Cash, T.F., & Grant, J.R. (1996). Cognitive-behavioral treatment of body-image disturbances. In V.B. Van Hasselt & M. Hersen (Eds.), *Sourcebook of psychological treatment manuals for adult disorders* (pp. 567–614). New York: Plenum.

Cash, T.F., & Henry, P.E. (1995). Women's body images: The results of a national survey in the U.S.A. *Sex Roles, 33,* 19–28.

Cash, T.F., & Hicks, K.L. (1990). Being fat versus thinking fat: Relationships with body-image, eating behaviors, and well-being. *Cognitive Therapy and Research, 14,* 327–341.

Cash, T.F., & Labarge, A.S. (1996). Development of the Appearance Schemas Inventory: A new cognitive body-image assessment. *Cognitive Therapy and Research, 20,* 37–50.

Cash, T.F., & Lavallee, D.M. (1997). Cognitive-behavioral body-image therapy: Extended evidence of the efficacy of a self-directed program. *Journal of Rational-Emotive and Cognitive-Behavior Therapy, 15,* 281–294.

Cash, T.F., & Pruzinsky, T.P. (Eds.). (1990). *Body images: Development, deviance, and change.* New York: The Guilford Press.

Cash, T.F., & Roy, R.E. (in press). Pounds of flesh: Weight, gender, and body images. In J. Sobal & D. Maurer (Eds.), *Interpreting weight: The social management of fatness and thinness.* Hawthorne, NY: Aldine de Gruyter.

Cash, T.F., Roy, R.E., & Strachan, M.D. (1997, May). *How physical appearance affects relations among women: Implications for women's body images.* Poster presented at the convention of the American Psychological Society, Washington, D.C.

Cash, T.F., Strachan, M.D., & Roy, R.E. (1997). *Women's attitudes about male-female relations: Relevance to body-image and eating disturbances.* Poster session presented at the annual meeting of the American Psychological Society, Washington, D.C.

Cash, T.F., & Szymanski, M.L. (1995). The development and validation of the Body-Image Ideals Questionnaire. *Journal of Personality Assessment, 64,* 466–477.

Cash, T.F., Winstead, B.A., & Janda, L.H. (1986). The great American shape-up. *Psychology Today, 20,* 30–37.

Drewnowski, A., & Yee, D.K. (1987). Men and body image: Are males satisfied with their body weight? *Psychosomatic Medicine, 49,* 626–634.

Dworkin, S.H., & Kerr, B.A. (1987). Comparison of interventions for women experiencing body-image problems. *Journal of Counseling Psychology, 34,* 136–140.

Faith, M.S., & Schare, M.L. (1993). The role of body image in sexually avoidant behavior. *Archives of Sexual Behavior, 22,* 345–356.

Fallon, A.E. (1990). Culture in the mirror: Sociocultural determinant of body-image. In T.F. Cash & T. Pruzinsky (Eds.), *Body images: Development, deviance, and change* (pp. 80–105). New York: Guilford.

Feingold, A., & Mazzella, R. (1998). Gender differences in body image are increasing. *Psychological Science, 9,* 190–195.

Fisher, E., & Thompson, J.K. (1994). A comparative evaluation of cognitive-behavioral therapy (CBT) versus exercise therapy (ET) for the treatment of body-image disturbance. *Behavior Modification, 18,* 171–185.

Fisher, S. (1986). *Development and structure of the body image* (Vols. 1 & 2). Hillsdale, NJ: Erlbaum.

Fisher, S. (1990). The evolution of psychological concepts about the body. In T.F. Cash & T. Pruzinsky (Eds.), *Body images: Development, deviance, and change* (pp. 3–20). New York: Guilford.

Fontaine, K.L. (1991). The conspiracy of culture: Women's issues in body size. *Nursing Clinics of North America, 26,* 669–676.

Franzoi, S.L., & Shields, S.A. (1984). The body-esteem scale: Multidimensional structure and sex differences in a college population. *Journal of Personality Assessment, 48,* 173–178.

Freedman, R. (1990). Cognitive-behavioral perspectives on body-image change. In T.F. Cash and T. Pruzinsky (Eds.), *Body images: Development, deviance, and change* (pp. 272-295). New York: Guilford.

Friedman, M.A., & Brownell, K.D. (1995). Psychological correlates of obesity: Moving to the next research generation. *Psychological Bulletin, 117,* 3-20.

Garner, D.M. (1997). The 1997 body-image survey results. *Psychology Today,* 30-44, 75-80, 84.

Garner, D.M., Garfinkel, P.E., Schwartz, D., & Thompson, M. (1980). Cultural expectations of thinness in women. *Psychological Reports, 47,* 483-491.

Grant, J.R., & Cash, T.F. (1995). Cognitive-behavioral body-image therapy: Comparative efficacy of group and modest contact treatments. *Behavior Therapy, 26,* 69-84.

Grilo, C.M., Wilfley, D.E., Brownell, K.D., & Rodin, J. (1994). Teasing, body image, and self-esteem in a clinical sample of obese women. *Addictive Behaviors, 19,* 443-450.

Hangen, J.D., & Cash, T.F. (1991, November). *Body-image attitudes and sexual functioning in a college population.* Paper presented at the meeting of the Association for Advancement of Behavior Therapy, New York.

Heinberg, L.J. (1996). Theories of body-image disturbance: Perceptual, developmental, and sociocultural factors. In J.K. Thompson (Ed.), *Body-image, eating disorders, and obesity* (pp. 27-47). Washington, D.C.: American Psychological Association.

Heinberg, L.J., & Thompson, J.K. (1995). Body image and televised images of thinness and attractiveness: A controlled laboratory investigation. *Journal of Social and Clinical Psychology, 14,* 325-338.

Hsu, L.K.G. (1982). Is there a disturbance in body image in anorexia nervosa? *Journal of Nervous and Mental Disease, 5,* 305-307.

Hsu, L.K.G., & Sobkiewicz, T.A. (1991). Body-image disturbance: Time to abandon the concept for eating disorders? *International Journal of Eating Disorders, 10,* 15-30.

Irving, L.M. (1990). Mirror images: Effects of the standard of beauty on the self- and body-esteem of women exhibiting varying levels of bulimic symptoms. *Journal of Social and Clinical Psychology, 9,* 230-242.

Jackson, L.A. (1992). *Physical appearance and gender: Sociobiological and sociocultural perspectives.* Albany: SUNY Press.

Lavallee, D.M., & Cash, T.F. (1997, November). *The comparative efficacy of two cognitive-behavioral self-help programs for a negative body image.* Poster presented at the convention of the Association for Advancement of Behavior Therapy, Miami Beach.

Mable, H.M., Balance, W.D.G., & Gaigan, R.J. (1986). Body-image distortion and dissatisfaction in university students. *Perceptual and Motor Skills, 63,* 907-911.

Marsella, A.J., Shizuru, L., Brennan, J., & Kameoka, V. (1981). Depression and body-image satisfaction. *Journal of Cross-Cultural Psychology, 12,* 360-371.

Mazur, A. (1986). U.S. trends in feminine beauty and overadaptation. *The Journal of Sex Research, 22,* 281-303.

McCaulay, M., Mintz, L., & Glenn, A.A. (1988). Body image, self-esteem, and depression-proneness: Closing the gender gap. *Sex Roles, 18,* 381-391.

McKay, M., & Fanning, P. (1992). *Self-esteem: A proven program of cognitive techniques for assessing, improving, and maintaining your self-esteem.* Oakland, CA: New Harbinger.

Mendelson, B.K., & White, D.R. (1982). Relation between body-esteem and self-esteem of obese and normal children. *Perceptual and Motor Skills, 54,* 899-905.

Muth, J.L., & Cash, T.F. (1997). Body-image attitudes: What difference does gender make? *Journal of Applied Social Psychology, 27,* 1438-1452.

Noles, S.W., Cash, T.F., & Winstead, B.A. (1985). Body-image, physical attractiveness, and depression. *Journal of Consulting and Clinical Psychology, 53,* 88-94.

Papalia, D.E., & Olds, S.W. (1992). *Human Development* (5th ed.). McGraw-Hill, Inc.: New York.

Phillips, K.A. (1996). *The broken mirror: Understanding and treating body dysmorphic disorder.* New York: Oxford University Press.

Pliner, P., Chaiken, S., & Flett, G.L. (1990). Gender differences in concern with body weight and physical appearance over the life span. *Personality and Social Psychology Bulletin, 16,* 263-273.

Rieves, L., & Cash, T.F. (1996). Social developmental factors and women's body-image attitudes. *Journal of Social Behavior and Personality, 11,* 63-78.

Rodin, J., Silberstein, L., & Striegel-Moore, R. (1984). Women and weight: A normative discontent. *Nebraska Symposium on Motivation, 32,* 267-307.

Rosen, G.M., & Ross, A.O. (1967). Relationship of body image to self-concept. *Journal of Consulting and Clinical Psychology, 32,* 100.

Rosen, J.C. (1990). Body-image disturbance in eating disorders. In T.F. Cash & T. Pruzinsky (Eds.), *Body images: Development, deviance, and change* (pp. 190–216). New York: Guilford.

Rosen, J.C. (1995). The nature of body dysmorphic disorder and treatment with cognitive behavior therapy. *Cognitive and Behavioral Practice, 2,* 143–166.

Rosen, J.C. (1997). Cognitive-behavioral body-image therapy. In D.M. Garner & P.E. Garfinkel (Eds.), *Handbook of Treatment for Eating Disorders, 2nd Edition* (pp. 188–201). New York: Guilford.

Rosen, J.C., Cado, S., Silberg, N.T., Srebnik, D., & Wendt, S. (1990). Cognitive behavior therapy with and without size perception training for women with body image disturbance. *Behavior Therapy, 21,* 481–498.

Rosen, J.C., Orosan, P., & Reiter, J. (1995). Cognitive behavior therapy for negative body image in obese women. *Behavior Therapy, 26,* 25–42.

Rosen, J.C., Reiter, J., & Orosan, P. (1995). Cognitive-behavioral body-image therapy for body dysmorphic disorder. *Journal of Consulting and Clinical Psychology, 63,* 263–269.

Rosen, J.C., Saltzberg, E., & Srebnik, D. (1989). Cognitive behavior therapy for negative body image. *Behavior Therapy, 20,* 393–404.

Rozin, P., & Fallon, A. (1988). Body image, attitudes to weight, and misperceptions of figure preferences of the opposite sex: A comparison of men and women in two generations. *Journal of Abnormal Psychology, 97,* 342–345.

Rucker, C.E., & Cash, T.F. (1992). Body images, body-size perceptions, and eating behaviors among African-American and White college women. *International Journal of Eating Disorders, 12,* 291–299.

Schiavi, R., Karstaedt, A., Schreiner-Engel, P., & Mandeli, J. (1992). Psychometric characteristics of individuals with sexual dysfunction and their partners. *Journal of Sex and Marital Therapy, 18,* 219–230.

Secord, P.F., & Jourard, S.M. (1953). The appraisal of body-cathexis: Body-cathexis and the self. *Journal of Consulting Psychology, 17,* 343–347.

Stice, E., Schupak-Neuberg, E., Shaw, H., & Stein, R. (1994). Relation of media exposure to eating disorder symptomatology: An examination of mediating mechanisms. *Journal of Abnormal Psychology, 103,* 836–840.

Stormer, S.M., & Thompson, J.K. (1996). Explanations of body-image disturbance: A test of maturational status, negative verbal commentary, social comparison, and sociocultural hypotheses. *International Journal of Eating Disorders, 19,* 193–202.

Striegel-Moore, R.H., Silberstein, L.R., & Rodin, J. (1986). Toward an understanding of risk factors for bulimia. *American Psychologist, 41,* 246–263.

Stunkard, A., & Burt, V. (1967). Obesity and the body image: II. Age at onset of disturbances in the body-image. *American Journal of Psychiatry, 123,* 1443–1447.

Szymanski, M.L., & Cash, T.F. (1995). Body-image disturbance and self-discrepancy theory; Expansion of the body-image ideals questionnaire. *Journal of Social and Clinical Psychology, 14,* 134-146.

Thompson, J.K. (1990). *Body-image disturbance: Assessment and treatment.* Emsford, New York: Pergamon.

Thompson, J.K. (1996). Assessing body-image disturbance: Measures, methodology, and implementation. In J.K. Thompson (Ed.), *Body image, eating disorders, and obesity* (pp. 49–82). Washington, DC: American Psychological Association.

Thompson, J.K., & Heinberg, L.J. (1993). Preliminary test of two hypotheses of body-image disturbance. *International Journal of Eating Disorders, 14,* 59–63.

Tiggemann, M., & Rothblum, E.D. (1988). Gender differences in social consequences of perceived overweight in the United States and Australia. *Sex Roles, 18,* 75–86.

Wiseman, C.V., Gunning, F.M., & Gray, J.J. (1993). Increasing pressure to be thin: 19 years of diet products in television commercials. *Eating Disorders: The Journal of Treatment and Prevention, 1,* 52–61.

Wiseman, C.V., Gray, J.J., Mosimann, J.E., & Ahren, A.H. (1992). Cultural expectations of thinness in women: An update. *International Journal of Eating Disorders, 11,* 85–89.

Wooley, O.W. (1994). . . . and man created "woman": representations of women's bodies in Western culture. In P. Fallon, M.A. Katzman, & S.C. Wooley (Eds.), *Feminist perspectives on eating disorders* (pp. 17–52). New York: Guilford Press.

Father Hunger and Eating Disorders
by Margo Maine, Ph.D.

Girls and their dads: What an incredibly important relationship. Yet, in the field of eating disorders, it is a little-discussed topic, be the conversations personal and casual or professional and clinical. If you listen closely, however, to the stories of women who struggle with their body image, weight, self-esteem, and eating, you hear a great deal about fathers. You especially hear about Father Hunger, that deep desire of eating-disordered women to feel close to and connected with their dads, and to feel respected and loved by them. For many women with eating disorders, Father Hunger is a powerful experience that they need to understand as they recover.

Theorists and mental-health specialists have neglected the father's influence on children because of our expectations and beliefs about the role men should have in families. In essence, Western culture has normalized Father Hunger. We expect little from men, especially as parents of daughters. Thus, we have ignored a very important part of human experience and have unconsciously accepted Father Hunger and all the disastrous results. Those fortunate few whose Father Hunger has been satisfied are more likely to grow up feeling confident, secure, and "good enough." More often, Father Hunger is not satisfied, and the yearning grows into self-doubt, pain, anxiety, depression, and low self-worth. For boys, this usually leads to acting out behaviors and emotional detachment. For girls, this usually leads to self-punitive feelings, including feeling unworthy of food or wanting to please others by losing weight or having a "perfect" body. Their desire to please men, their need for attachment and relationships, and their negative feelings about themselves can easily lead to eating disorders.

THE CONTEXT OF FATHER HUNGER

The socially accepted role for men in families in Western countries like the United States has discouraged active parenting or involvement in children's lives until recently. Since the industrial revolution in the 1700s, men have been valued for their productivity, success, and earning power outside the home. Being a "good-enough" father meant providing for the family economically and maintaining an image of respect in the community. Their value to the family was connected to their absence from home. Simultaneously, mothers became solely responsible for the emotional life, health, and care of the children and family. That is why we so often blame mothers when children have problems, and ignore the father's influence.

Before the industrial revolution, men and women shared family responsibilities. For example, in the hunting and gathering societies, fathers were away "on the hunt" only when the food supply demanded it. The rest of the time, they were at home, participating in the daily work of the family and community. Also, the older men who could no longer hunt were available to the children; in general, men were present and involved. Later, in agrarian societies, men and women worked together on the farm. Similarly, in the preindustrial

era of the cottage industries (small, home-based factories), children saw their fathers throughout the day, and parenting was not just left up to women. In these eras, fathers were a vital part of the parenting process.

The industrial revolution brought tremendous economic and social advances, but also changed the family structure significantly. Specifically, dads were no longer part of the daily life of children and families, a change that has persisted until the end of the twentieth century. Now fathers are somewhat more involved, with the increase in dual working couples, single-parent households, and joint custody arrangements. But dads are still learning what their families need from them. Too often, with their daughters, they haven't a clue. And, too often, the results are devastating, with girls feeling unloved, "not good enough," and hungry for male approval.

FATHER HUNGER AND EATING DISORDERS

Often girls feel distant from their fathers at the exact point in their development when they most need a connection with the man who represents the outside world and the male experience. Fathers and daughters have an easier time feeling close and connected when the daughter is young and plays the role of "daddy's little girl," doing anything and everything for him. But, as girls mature into preadolescence and adolescence, become more involved with their peers and their own activities, and develop their own sense of self, the tie to dad becomes more fragile.

At this point, men are often uncomfortable around their daughters. Seeing their little girls as emerging young women is a major transition for fathers. Many men distance themselves in response to seeing their daughters mature sexually. They no longer know how to show affection and love, and they long to have their little girls back. They also may feel jealous of their daughters' interest in peers, boys, and other age-appropriate activities. Feeling displaced, dads often give up, rather than try to find new ways to maintain relationships. Or, they may not be able to tolerate their daughters' emerging ideas and potentially contrary opinions and beliefs. Again, too often, the response of fathers is to distance themselves, a response interpreted by the daughter as disapproval.

In some father-daughter relationships, it is the father's developmental issues rather than the daughter's that disrupt the relationship. Men may experience identity issues at mid-life, doubting their attractiveness, sexuality, or self-worth. They may become more focused on their individual happiness and withdraw from the family. Or they may become dissatisfied with their appearance as they age and invest their time and energy in losing weight, controlling their bodies, or exercising excessively. In many families I have treated, fathers developed concern about potential cardiac disease or other health problems, becoming overly rigid in their eating or exercise habits. If fathers are struggling with these issues at the same time that their daughters are experiencing self-doubt and increased sensitivity to their weight and appearance, the daughters are likely to develop significant problems with food, body image, and self-esteem.

At mid-life, men also may begin to experience illnesses and problems that interfere with relationships. Many fathers of my patients had been ill or depressed during their daughters' adolescence. In response, the girls became depressed themselves or tried to cheer dad up by taking care of him, being the best and the brightest in school and sports, and maintaining complete control over their bodies and weight. An eating disorder is a painful way to please dad, but it may be the answer to questions like "Am I good enough?" or "Does Daddy really love me?"

The father-daughter relationship may also be disrupted by parents' marital issues, family conflicts, separation, or divorce. In some families, the eating-disorder symptoms serve to keep the parents together or to distract them from other conflicts. Anorexia and bulimia are powerful behaviors that frighten most parents, so they may begin to focus solely on the problems. Unfortunately, the individual may feel she has to be sick to keep parents or family together. Or, she may feel her illness is the only way to get her father's attention, to create some closeness between them, and to fill the void that Father Hunger creates.

FATHER HUNGER AND GENDER

Research and clinical work in mental health, as well as in eating disorders, has focused on the impact of mothers on their children. When research examines the role of the father, it is usually in terms of paternal absence and its effects on boys. Only rarely have researchers examined the influence, positive or negative, that fathers have on daughters. Mental health has overemphasized the connections with the same-sex parent. In this framework, boys need their dads and girls need their moms to develop into healthy adolescent and adult men and women. Identity formation and comfort with issues related to gender and sexuality have been seen as a function of a girl's relationship with her mom, not her dad.

In fact, girls learn much about femininity and women's roles from their fathers. Interacting with the opposite sex facilitates understanding of what is unique or important about one's own gender. How their father treats women, especially their mothers, colors their feelings about what men expect women to be.

Because fathers are generally less involved in the family and more involved with the world of work, their opinions and beliefs have a special authority in children's lives. Furthermore, men have more economic and political power, so girls will try to please them and win their approval. Fathers also play a special role in their daughters' lives by helping them to move from childhood into the adult world. Learning how to negotiate issues, communicate, and disagree with men is important for girls. Feeling safe and accepted by one's father makes it much easier to enter into more mature relationships with boyfriends, teachers, coaches, and bosses. If a girl feels valued and respected by her dad, she will be less anxious in her other relationships with men and will be less likely to struggle with self-esteem, body image, and eating disorders.

When boys develop eating disorders, the underlying dynamics, self-esteem issues, and Father Hunger are similar. Both genders share a desire for connection with their dads and other father figures. Whether male or female, a positive relationship with their father produces confidence, security, and a positive sense of self. These qualities prevent eating disorders.

Girls are at greater risk to develop problems with food for several reasons. First, they have a closer relationship to food, as women tend to be responsible for the cooking and nutrition of their families. Second, women experience more pressure from the media and society to look a certain way. The dieting, cosmetic, and fashion industries all target women, trying to foment dissatisfaction with their looks and encourage them to buy products to make themselves more acceptable. Third, women are admonished throughout development to please others ahead of themselves. If this means seeking others' approval by maintaining the ideal body, weight, and appearance, it is nearly impossible to feel "good enough." Eating disorders are a logical outcome.

SOLUTIONS TO FATHER HUNGER

If you suffer from an eating disorder, it is useful to explore any unresolved issues with your father. This can be painful: You probably have done many things to avoid the emptiness of your Father Hunger. But addressing these issues may help you to move on in your recovery and feel better about yourself. Begin to explore these questions in therapy, a support group, or directly with your family.

- How do you feel about your relationship with your father?
- Do you feel "good enough" for your dad?
- How have you been trying to win his approval?
- Can you talk to your father or other key men in your life about feelings? If not, what stops you?
- How well do you know your father? Do you wish to know him better?
- What would you like to change in your relationship with him?
- What has your dad conveyed to you about your weight, appearance, and eating?
- Does your father have trouble with his own body, food intake, or exercise?
- How much has Father Hunger been a part of your life and your eating disorder?

You can work on these questions in a variety of ways. Talking to other family members if your father is not available will help you to understand your father. Writing in a journal as you consider these issues will also be helpful. Or, consider writing a letter to your father about his impact on you. You may choose not to send it, if the time does not feel right or you do not feel ready to process these issues together.

More frequently than not, men do not understand the impact they have on their children, especially their daughters. Because their role in the family has generally been more peripheral, they often feel unimportant. It may surprise both you and your father to realize how he has affected you.

It may be worth the risk to acknowledge your Father Hunger and try to heal this relationship.

A MESSAGE TO FATHERS

It is hoped that many men, not just their daughters, are reading this book. Here are some questions for fathers to address.

- What kind of relationship did I want with my children? How close have I come to that goal?
- Have I given my children unconditional love and approval?
- Have I been critical of their appearance?
- What do I value in women? Are appearance and weight more important than other attributes?
- Do I often make comments about women's bodies?
- Can I tolerate my daughter's differences with me, or do I want her views and attitudes to mirror mine?
- Do I respect women? Have I sent messages that girls are less important than boys or don't need to know the same things?
- How do I show interest in my daughter as a person?

For men as well, the best way to deal with these problems is in therapy. If you are not in family therapy, consider it, or consider individual treatment or a support group for parents. Get in touch with your own feelings about Father Hunger and how these may have affected your parenting. Most important, show your daughter that you know you must also change—that change is not just up to her. But you also must honor her boundaries—she may not want you to be involved in her treatment or she may need to keep you at a distance as she wrestles with other feelings. Respect her wishes and you will be more likely to develop a healthy father-daughter relationship in the future.

BIBLIOGRAPHY

Levine, M. (1994). Beauty myth and the beast: What men can do and be to help prevent eating disorders. *Eating Disorders: The Journal of Treatment and Prevention* 2(2), 101–113.

Maine, M. (1991). *Father Hunger: Fathers, daughters & food.* Carlsbad, CA: Gurze Books.

Osherson, S. (1992). *Wrestling with Love: How men struggle with intimacy.* New York: Fawcett-Columbine.

Differential Diagnoses, Co-Morbidities, and Complications of Eating Disorders

by Linda P. Bock, M.D.

Anorexia nervosa and bulimia nervosa can be confused with other illnesses, occur with other illnesses, and be complicated by certain illnesses. In medical terminology, the appropriate descriptors for these respective occurrences are differential diagnoses, co-morbidities, and complications of eating disorders.

DIFFERENTIAL DIAGNOSES

Illnesses that can present with one or several of the symptoms of anorexia nervosa include brain tumor, hyperthyroidism, depression, anxiety disorder, diabetes mellitus, Crohn's disease, celiac disease, ulcerative colitis, malabsorption disorders, body dysmorphic disorder, bipolar disorder, obsessive-compulsive disorder, poisoning, amphetamine abuse, tuberculosis, AIDS, cancer, medication side effect, and starvation state.

Other illnesses sometimes mistaken initially for bulimia nervosa include hepatic illnesses (mononucleosis, hepatitis), chronic alcohol use, pancreatitis, pregnancy, hyperemesis gravidairum, esophageal obstruction, achalasia, peptic ulcer disease, brain tumor, increased intracranial pressure, poisoning, uremia, enteric infections, viral or bacterial infections, tuberculosis, neoplasm (cancer-lymphoma), chronic appendicitis, conversion disorders, schizophrenia, poisoning, medication toxicities, and diabetes mellitus.

A thorough medical history, including a family history, and a physical examination can eliminate most of these diagnostic considerations. Laboratory tests can also be helpful. The important point here is that eating disorders can be diagnosed incorrectly and a significant illness overlooked. Because these psychiatric illnesses of anorexia nervosa and bulimia nervosa have such an impact on the body, it is necessary to evaluate medically all people who have suspected or confirmed eating disorders (Powers, 1997).

CO-MORBIDITIES

Co-morbid literally means "sick together" and can be defined as the presence of more than one illness in a defined period of time in a single individual. For this discussion, it is helpful to separate the co-morbidities of anorexia and bulimia into two groups: physical and psychiatric (Wittchen, 1996).

Physical Illnesses Occurring with Anorexia Nervosa or Bulimia Nervosa

Certain medical illnesses tend to occur often with the eating disorders and make treatment of both the medical and the psychiatric illnesses more difficult than the treatment of either illness alone (Seller, 1996). These medical conditions include

- diabetes mellitus,
- cystic fibrosis,
- inflammatory bowel disease, and
- thyroid disease.

Eating-disordered diabetic patients can withhold insulin to cause wasting of sugar into the urine and eventual weight loss and even vomiting. Eating-disordered cystic fibrosis patients can omit their pancreatic enzyme medications and thereby lose their ability to absorb food, thus losing weight. Unchecked inflammatory bowel diseases, such as Crohn's disease and ulcerative colitis, cause severe weight loss. If a person with both an eating disorder and an inflammatory bowel disease fails to take the medications to control the inflammation, malabsorption and weight loss will occur. Thyroid illnesses that cause an overactive or an underactive thyroid can enhance an eating disorder in unusual ways. An eating-disordered person with an overactive thyroid who stops taking the medication designed to "cool down" the thyroid will lose weight because the untreated overactive thyroid will keep the metabolic "heat" up. A patient with slow thyroid hormone production who is given a supplemental thyroid hormone to treat the thyroid illness can force an unsafe and dangerous weight loss by overdosing on the thyroid hormone.

Psychiatric Illnesses Occurring with Anorexia Nervosa or Bulimia Nervosa

If a person has one psychiatric illness, it is common to have a second psychiatric illness (Kaplan, 1995, pp. 1367–1371). Thus, about half of the people with anxiety disorders will eventually develop depression. About 40 percent of those with anorexia nervosa will also have obsessive-compulsive disorder, or OCD, which is characterized by various unwanted, intrusive, and repetitive thoughts or behaviors that are senseless or unhelpful. Common compulsions in OCD are excessive hand washing, counting, checking, and cleaning. Almost all starving people, including patients with anorexia nervosa, are depressed. Many times the depressive symptoms lift when the starving people eat. About half of anorexic patients are clinically depressed even after eating is reestablished. Of those with depression, many have a special form of depression, called bipolar depression or bipolar disorder. The old term for bipolar disorder was manic depression, a term that is no longer used. Anxiety disorders are frequent both in people with anorexia nervosa and in their family members.

Among bulimics, major depression and bipolar disorder are very common. Almost half of all bulimics are substance abusers, typically of alcohol, marijuana, or cocaine. Impulse disorders with symptoms such as kleptomania, sexual promiscuity, or gambling addiction often occur with bulimia. Some patients with bulimia also have Attention Deficit Hyperactivity Disorder, or ADHD, aggravating inattention to appetite and satiety cues. Sometimes a person with an anxiety disorder will vomit after eating, partly as a result of the anxiety disorder and partly as a result of the bulimia. Some patients with bulimia also have OCD with involvement of elaborate rituals about food as well as rituals about other parts of their lives.

Both anorexia nervosa and bulimia nervosa are seen commonly among traumatized persons. Sexual abuse and physical abuse may be as high as 50 percent to 80 percent in female inpatients with eating disorders. It is important, however, to note that this incidence of abuse is similar to the incidence of abuse among all psychiatric inpatients; the incidence of sexual abuse in the general population is 25 percent to 40 percent of women and 10 percent to 15 percent of men.

Co-morbidities do not imply any causal relationship. Thus, depression does not cause alcoholism, even though they may frequently occur together. It is important to know about co-morbid conditions so that treatment can focus appropriately on all areas of concern to achieve full recovery.

COMPLICATIONS

Numerous complications, or illnesses, can arise from the underlying eating disorder. For instance, one common complication of anorexia nervosa is bulimia. About 50 percent of anorexics eventually become bulimic.

Physical Illnesses That Can Complicate Anorexia Nervosa

The irreversible complication of anorexia nervosa is osteoporosis (loss of bone mass) and, of bulimia nervosa, the irreversible complication of loss of tooth enamel. All other medical complications usually disappear when the eating disorder ends unless death intervenes before recovery. Common causes of death include electrolyte abnormalities, refeeding syndrome, cardiac arrhythmias, inanition (wasting away from generalized organ failure), and suicide (Goldbloom & Kennedy, 1997). Refeeding syndrome occurs when inadequate electrolyte and mineral supplements are given to starving people when they are given food. Without appropriate supplements, starving people will die, literally with food in their hands, because of lethal drops in potassium, sodium, calcium, phosphorous or magnesium.

Reversible complications of anorexia nervosa include low thyroid function, hair loss, lanugo, hypoglycemia (low glycogen stores in the liver), general and cardiac muscle weakness and wasting, delayed gastric emptying time, gastric dilatation, pancreatitis, jaundice, constipation, laxative abuse, diarrhea, partial diabetes insipidus (low vasopressin production), dehydration, poor kidney function, atonic bladder, electrolyte disturbances (hypokalemia), mitral valve prolapse, cardiac arrhythmias (bradycardia, EKG abnormalities, hypotension), blueness of fingertips (acrocyanosis), pneumothorax, infertility, loss of menses (hypogonadotrophic hypogonadism), elevated cholesterol, various laboratory abnormalities, anemia, low white blood cell and platelet counts, mineral deficiencies (iron, zinc, magnesium), vitamin deficiencies (folate, B12, C, D, E), and decreased brain volume (increased ventricular size).

Reversible complications of bulimia nervosa include easy bruisability, enlarged salivary glands, delayed gastric emptying time, gastric dilatation, hypoglycemia, abnormal liver function, inflammation of the pancreas, constipation, laxative abuse, ipecac poisoning, cardiomyopathy, mitral valve prolapse, pneumomediastinum, aspiration pneumonia, periodontal disease, esophagitis, Mallory-Weiss tears (cuts in the esophageal-gastric junction with consequent bleeding), gastrointestinal ulcers, infertility, irregular menses (low estradiaol and progesterone levels), low thyroid function, kidney stones, renal damage, dehydration, and electrolyte abnormalities (hypochloremia, hypokalemia, alkalosis, hyponatremia, hypophasphatemia, hypocalcemia).

SUMMARY

Anorexia nervosa and bulimia nervosa are psychiatric illnesses with significant and frequent interplay with many other associated medical illnesses. These associated conditions make successful treatment of the eating disorders all the more difficult and complex. The involvement of knowledgeable and experienced medical clinicians on the treatment team is essential to the welfare of patients with eating disorders.

REFERENCES

Goldbloom, David S., & Kennedy, Sidney H. Medical complications of anorexia nervosa. In *Handbook of treatment of eating disorders, second edition* (pp. 266–270). New York: Guilford Press.

Kaplan, Harold I. (1995). *Comprehensive textbook of psychiatry/VI sixth edition.* Philadelphia: Williams & Wilkins.

Mitchell, James. Medical complications of bulimia nervosa. In *Handbook of treatment of eating disorders, second edition* (pp. 271–275). New York: Guilford Press.

Powers, Pauline. (1997). Management of patients with co-morbid medical conditions. In *Handbook of treatment of eating disorders, second edition* (pp. 421–436). New York: Guilford Press.

Seller, Robert. (1996). *Differential diagnosis of common complaints, third edition.* Philadelphia: W.B. Saunders.

Wittchen, Hans-Ulrich. (1996, June, Suppl). What is co-morbidity—Fact or artifact? *British Journal of Psychiatry 168,* 7–8.

Secrets and Denial: The Costs of Not Getting Help

by Linda P. Bock, M.D.

Chris was becoming dangerously thin. She avoided going out with her friends, especially if the event involved food. At school Jane worried about Chris's not eating lunch. Jane confronted Chris: "You're not eating!" Chris replied calmly, "I'm fine. There's nothing wrong."

Jennifer always seemed to eat a lot. One day she ate a double cheeseburger, large fries, a shake, and a large soda, then quickly went to the bathroom; later she and her friends went to an ice cream parlor where she had two banana splits and again went to the bathroom. Then, at home she ate a whole bag of cookies. When Jennifer came out of the bathroom, her friend Carol said, "Why do you go to the bathroom every time you eat?" Jennifer was scared but confessed, "I throw up." She told her story and ended by saying, "You're my friend and I trust you. Don't tell anyone, it's our secret."

THE COSTS OF SECRETS AND DENIAL

The secrets of bulimia and the denial of anorexia take many forms, but both defend the sufferer from the truth that he or she is actually ill.

Giving up the denial or trusting the secret to open view makes the person feel vulnerable and anxious. If recovery is to occur, secrecy and denial must stop.

A true friend or a loving sister, mother, father, or brother will confront their sick loved one: "I'm sorry, Chris, you are not fine. You are alone all the time, you never have fun, and you seem so tense and worried. I miss you."

Or: "Jennifer, I can't keep this a secret. Throwing up your food is dangerous. Can I go with you to talk to your parents, or do you want me to tell them myself?"

WHAT LOVED ONES CAN DO

Communicating with someone who has anorexia nervosa or bulimia nervosa and who is in denial is not easy. Jerry Kreisman, M.D., who wrote a book entitled *I Hate You, Don't Leave Me* (Kreisman & Straus, 1989) describes a communication technique that applies to people who, by their illness, say, "I'm hungry; don't feed me." In this technique, the concerned loved one has three tasks: show support and concern, express empathy or understanding, and tell a truth.

Kreisman believes one must complete all three tasks to achieve full communication. If you omit the support statement, you will seem uncaring. Or if the empathic statement is left out, the usual response is, "You don't understand." If you don't tell your truth statement, you are of no help and the denial persists.

To someone whose anorexia has made her dull, tired, and weak, a complete communication may be, "Susan, you seem so tired and exhausted, and you know I care about you. I know you must be afraid to realize it, and I am a little afraid too, but I need to insist that you are not well. You must get some help. We can work together on finding some help."

In this paragraph is a statement of love and support: "I care about you." Several statements recognize the anorexic's point of view: "You seem so tired . . . afraid." The truth is saved for last and consists of a statement that calls for action.

Although very ill people with anorexia nervosa may refuse the truth and rage or bluster, you have said your truth in the most acceptable way. The positive effect may not come until much later. Wait. Pray, if you choose. Be ready to act at the moment when the denial finally weakens.

For someone who suffers with bulimia nervosa, the out-of-control eating and purging is readily felt as abnormal. The secrecy is the way bulimics hide and defend themselves.

"Sharon, you know that I love you. I can't be a detective or policeman about your eating. My mother's heart tells me that these ways of yours—all the food, all the trips to the bathroom, your reddened eyes—you can't feel safe or normal. I'm certain you could feel very embarrassed perhaps, but my love will never be embarrassed by you. The truth is, all this is dangerous. Please let us take you for some help."

If such a speech falls on a ready heart, the journey to recovery can begin. You may have to repeat your intervention several times and wait for results. Remember that the illness did not begin overnight and that recovery will take time. Be prepared with the names and phone numbers of resources. Be ready to rearrange your schedule to accompany the person to the first appointment. Plan how to overcome the financial obstacles. Pray. And as soon as you can, act.

To some, anorexia nervosa and bulimia nervosa can seem like devastating failures in living. The only failure in these illnesses is *not* to learn from them. Henry Ford said, "Failure is simply an opportunity to begin again, more intelligently." Those who face their illness and learn how to defeat it are in fact stronger than those who have never faced a challenge in their life. These illnesses are present because some things need to be changed. Maintaining denial and secrecy makes change impossible.

The secrets and denial must be set aside so that reality can be clearly visible. Only with such clarity of vision can real recovery begin.

REFERENCE

Kreisman, J. J., & Straus, H. (1989). *I hate you, don't leave me: Understanding the borderline personality.* Los Angeles: Price Stern Sloan.

BIBLIOGRAPHY

Bennett, William, et al. (1982). *The dieter's dilemma: Eating less and weighing more.* New York: Basic Books.

Garner, David, et al. (1997). *Handbook of treatment for eating disorders.* New York: Guilford Press.

PART 2
Physiological and Medical Issues

Medical Dangers of Anorexia Nervosa and Bulimia Nervosa

by Diane W. Mickley, M.D.

Eating disorders involve a complex interplay of physical and emotional factors. The medical complications of anorexia and bulimia can be life-threatening even when they give no outward warning symptoms. Thus, attention to health realities must accompany (or even precede) therapy to resolve an eating disorder.

ANOREXIA NERVOSA: UNDERSTANDING THE EFFECTS OF STARVATION

Most patients with anorexia nervosa do not see themselves as starved because they do often eat very healthy foods such as salads. But just as a car with the best tires and oil can't run without gas, so no amount of healthy foods can make up for inadequate calories. Without enough calories, the body slows its metabolism, compromises vital functions such as circulation, and uses up its muscle to provide the fuel that isn't coming from food.

A well-known study done by the U.S. military simulated prisoner-of-war camps by subjecting healthy men to starvation. The men in Ancel Keyes's "Minnesota Experiment" (cited in *The Biology of Human Starvation*, 1950) soon exhibited many anorexic behaviors: They obsessed about food constantly, ate their meals slowly and with strange rituals, felt depressed and tired, and, once allowed to resume normal eating, binged for months afterwards. Some anorexic symptoms serve as a biologic defense against starvation—preoccupation with food, fatigue, and sometimes depression—and may disappear with weight gain.

Patients with anorexia often find that constant thinking about food and weight becomes plaguing. They may experience depression, fatigue, and sleep difficulty as well as feel cold, bloated, or constipated, or they may grow fine hair on the body (called lanugo). Many anorexics, however, insist that they feel fine, or minimize their discomforts and continue to work hard, get good grades at school, perform athletically, or exercise compul-sively. This makes it hard for patients, family, and friends—and sometimes even doctors—to realize the danger of their situation.

Not only do anorexic patients perform in a vigorous fashion, which may hide the severity of their illness, but the effects of starvation may not show on simple exam; the electrocardiogram may not reveal the kind of heart weakening that occurs, and blood tests often are normal or only seem mildly amiss. Because of this, anorexics often insist that they are healthy or are mistaken to be healthy when they are not.

When Is Low Weight Unhealthy?

Being underweight takes a major toll on the body. But what is underweight? Anorexics often believe that the fact that other women or models are underweight proves that very low body weight is acceptable. To estimate ideal weight, a young woman of average bone size should weigh 100 pounds plus approximately four pounds for every inch over five feet in height (108 pounds for a female 5' 2", 116 pounds for a female 5' 4", 124 pounds for a female 5' 6", and so on). For a female with a very slight bone size, this formula adjusts to add three pounds for every inch (106 pounds for a female 5' 2", 112 pounds for a female 5' 4", etc.). For a female with a very large frame, the formula adjusts to five pounds for every inch over five feet (110 pounds for a female 5' 2", 120 pounds for a female 5' 4", etc.).

The term *critical weight* defines a minimum required weight for the body to function healthily. Critical weight is about 90 percent of ideal weight. An average-sized, 5' 5" female would have an ideal weight of 120 pounds and a critical weight of 108 pounds (120-12 [10 percent of 120] = 108). Even at critical weight, a person may not have menstrual periods or may be unable to participate in competitive sports. Certainly, a person below critical weight will experience major physical compromises, regardless of how well he or she feels.

Two other factors are important in evaluating weight. First, youngsters still in puberty may not lose weight; they may just get taller. These preteens will fail to gain weight and ultimately stop growing. Second, individuals who are overweight to begin with may lose dangerous amounts of weight and show some of the physical damages of anorexia but may not seem as dramatically underweight because of the extra pounds with which they began.

Physical Tolls of Anorexia

One of the most obvious consequences of anorexia for women is the cessation of menstrual periods. For up to a third of anorexics, periods stop before weight loss begins. We used to consider the absence of periods a harmless reminder that an anorexic had work to do to recover. Now, however, we know that the subsequent absence of estrogen causes bone thinning after as little as six months' time. This may lead to osteoporosis and a lifelong risk of fractures. Hormone replacement is sometimes part of the medical treatment for anorexics with prolonged absence of periods. However, recent evidence suggests that estrogen replacement does not prevent osteopenia in the absence of weight restoration.

Anorexia's effects on the heart are especially worrisome. Heart muscle diminishes with malnutrition, just as arm and leg muscles do. The heart is smaller and weaker. Blood pressure falls, and the heart cuts back on circulation to the periphery to protect vital central organs. This is seen in the bluish-purplish appearance (called acrocyanosis) of the toes and then the fingers (especially in cold weather) of anorexic patients. Another serious consequence of cardiac impairment is the inability of the heart to increase oxygen delivery to the tissues in response to exercise. Because of this, continued exercise in underweight patients is especially dangerous. Acquired mitral valve prolapse and even fatal arrhythmias also can occur in low weight patients.

The metabolism slows progressively as weight is lost. Patients with underactive thyroids often complain of feeling cold, tired, constipated, and depressed, and anorexic patients often have low values on screening tests of thyroid functions. In fact, however, this reflects compensatory phenomena, not intrinsic thyroid malfunction, and improves without treatment once caloric intake increases.

The stomach is also affected by anorexia. Many patients feel full easily or bloated, and indeed there is delayed stomach emptying so that food may remain in the stomach many hours beyond normal. Liquids are better digested than solids, and frequent small portions are more comfortable than large meals. Postprandial fullness corrects with better nutrition, but medication (usually cisapride) is sometimes useful temporarily if symptoms are severe.

All sorts of other abnormalities can occur in anorexia. CT scans often show a loss of brain mass at very low weights. Cholesterol may increase, liver tests may indicate abnormal function, and blood counts may be low (both for red cells and white cells). Nerve palsies can occur, causing "foot drops."

The important thing is not to remember specific symptoms but the simple fact that being underweight is physically dangerous, often in ways that are not apparent. Most physical problems resolve completely with recovery. But regaining weight is critical for both safety and recovery. It may be possible for anorexics to gain weight by working with a physician and a dietitian on an outpatient basis, but sometimes hospitalization is necessary. Exercise should usually be stopped temporarily. Going to therapy to understand the causes of weight loss is of great importance. But restoration of weight cannot be put off in the meantime—it is the cornerstone of recovery.

UNDERSTANDING BULIMIA NERVOSA

Anorexia nervosa and bulimia nervosa sometimes overlap. About half of patients with anorexia develop bulimic symptoms during their illnesses, but the great majority of patients with bulimia are of normal weight; in fact, some have been overweight. Bulimics binge—sometimes on large volumes of food—but sometimes just a normal meal or a forbidden kind of food is experienced as a binge. Fearing weight gain, bulimics then purge, sometimes through strict fasting or excessive exercise, but most often by vomiting. Laxatives, diet pills, or water pills may also be used in futile efforts to lose weight.

Though some patients with bulimia feel well, many do not. Most patients feel uncomfortable emotionally: ashamed, secretive, isolated, depressed, out of control. Like anorexics, most bulimics are preoccupied with food and weight in a constant, bothersome way that soon intrudes on other spheres of their lives. Patients with bulimia may also experience a wide range of physical symptoms, including weight swings, insomnia, weakness, abnormal menstrual periods, heartburn, bloating, swollen cheeks, and dental decay.

Physical Tolls of Bulimia

Bulimia can have pervasive physical consequences. Patients who fast between binges slow their metabolisms and set up a cycle in which their undereating drives the body to binge again. Thus, treatment often involves learning to regulate eating to avoid excess dieting.

Bulimia may cause women to have irregular or no menstrual periods. However, this usually does not impair fertility. Because of the myth that birth control pills may cause weight gain, many patients with eating disorders avoid them, and often become pregnant. In fact, the very low doses of hormones in most modern oral contraceptives can be taken without fear of weight gain. Some studies show worrisome consequences of eating disorders during pregnancy, and patients with such disorders clearly require special care.

Most bulimic patients purge by vomiting, which causes many physical dangers. The teeth develop cavities, and the lingual surfaces erode. The loss of electrolytes during vomiting may reduce potassium levels, which may produce muscle weakness or, without symptoms, lead to fatal cardiac arrhythmias or respiratory paralysis. Detection requires periodic blood tests to monitor the need for potassium replacement. The likelihood of low potassium is compounded by low weight or abuse of diuretics or laxatives.

In patients with bulimia, the parotid glands often swell, producing a "chipmunk cheek" appearance. The submandibular glands under the chin may enlarge as well. Such swelling often affects both sides of the face, but it is painless and usually lessens once patients stop vomiting.

The esophagus often becomes inflamed from being bathed in stomach acid during vomiting. This can cause heartburn, which may be helped by medication. Tears (or even rupture) of the esophagus, which cause vomiting of blood, as well as pain, are another feared complication. The stomach tends to empty poorly in bulimics, causing a feeling of bloating after eating.

Most patients who abuse laxatives choose those with phenolphthalein, a drug that tends to work for the bowel, causing it to be unable to function on its own after a while. The very high doses used by some patients can even cause pancreatitis or encephalitis in rare cases. Ironically, though laxatives are believed to reduce weight, studies show that laxatives do not remove calories. They only cause water loss, as calories are already digested by the time food gets to the part of the colon affected by laxatives. Both laxatives and diuretics do cause loss of potassium. In addition, the dehydration they produce causes rebound fluid retention each time they are stopped. This leads to uncomfortable weight swings in many bulimic patients. Recent research raises the possibility that phenolphthalein may be carcinogenic, so a number of laxative preparations are being revised to omit it.

Most deadly among the forms of purging is the abuse of ipecac, a syrup used to treat poison victims. Many patients who try it once find it so unpleasant they avoid further use. However, the emetine in this medicine accumulates in the body, so repeated use, even on a two- or three-times-a-week basis, can cause high levels in the body. This in turn can produce a myopathy, with arm and leg weakness, or affect the heart and cause sudden death.

Up to 20 percent of patients with bulimia have problems with alcohol or drug abuse. Sometimes the patient has dealt with this by the time he or she comes for eating-disorder treatment. Obviously, however, patients who have active alcohol excess in their systems have a whole additional set of medical risks, especially to their liver and blood count. In-hospital treatment can be especially useful for such patients.

SUMMARY

Both anorexia and bulimia have specific physical dangers, and both require careful medical monitoring. Some patients will feel quite ill, others deceptively well. All should have a physical examination, including blood tests and an electrocardiogram when indicated. Other special studies are sometimes useful as well. Although these exam results may appear to be normal, we know that this in no way shows the patient to be free of danger. Medical treatment is geared to averting these risks, lessening symptoms, and promoting recovery.

REFERENCE

Keyes, A. (1950). *The biology of human starvation.* Minneapolis: University of Minnesota Press.

The Hazards of Chronic Undernutrition
by Linda P. Bock, M.D.

The extreme forms of undernutrition seen in anorexia nervosa and bulimia nervosa patients commonly begin with simple dieting. Dieting, or caloric restriction, leads to nutritional deprivation and eventually to serious problems. The fine line between the normative social behaviors of dieting and the abnormal behaviors of illness is marked by the autonomous nature of a diet that "develops a life of its own," sometimes referred to as a "runaway diet." When the dieter has "lost control," the dieting has become pathologic or abnormal.

Along this pathway to full-blown anorexia nervosa and bulimia nervosa are signs and symptoms—some psychological and others physical. The classic scientific observation of human starvation in 1944 by Ancel Keyes illustrates the interplay of body and mind during starvation. In this "Minnesota Experiment," 32 normal-weight men—all conscientious objecting soldiers—volunteered to lose 25 percent of their body weight. The weight-loss phase of the experiment demonstrated both psychological and physical responses to starvation.

PSYCHOLOGICAL RESPONSES TO STARVATION

The men in the "Minnesota Experiment" were content with their bodies and only chose to participate in this study to help prepare for the rescue of starving Europeans as World War II was ending. As the men began to experience chronic undernutrition, they became preoccupied with food. They saved food coupons and recipes, activities highly unusual for Army recruits. Their dreams and much of their spontaneous conversation revolved around food. They continued to perform well at intellectual and academic tasks but developed intrusive and interrupting obsessions about food. They began to salt, pepper, and season their food in excessive ways; they began to use so much coffee, tea, and chewing gum that these substances had to be limited by the researchers conducting the study. This group of conscientous objectors were mostly Quaker men. As a group they were friendly and sociable. But as chronic undernutrition set in, they became irritable, quarrelsome, and socially isolated. They did not sleep well. At times they had no energy, and at other times they were agitated, nervous, and anxious. They had mood swings, at times nearly euphoric, but eventually depressed. Interest in sex decreased. They developed odd eating habits, cutting their food into small pieces and arranging the food in patterns; they ate with chewing and swallowing rituals. In many ways they looked and acted just as anorexic girls do—except that the male volunteers never believed they were fat. Selected from more than 1,000 volunteers, the 32 Quaker men had been carefully chosen because they were normal. In spite of their normality, starvation, alone, made these men behave as very disturbed individuals.

To summarize, the psychological symptoms of starvation seen in the 1944 study included:

- Preoccupation with food (dreaming and talking about food, collecting recipes)
- Odd food-handling behaviors and rituals (overseasoning of food, cutting food into small pieces)
- Ahedonia (an inability to be happy)
- Poor judgment, dishonesty
- Excessive use of nonfood pacifiers (gum, coffee, teas)
- Moodiness (irritability, euphoria, depression)
- Difficulty sleeping
- Disturbed energy (agitated or apathetic)
- Decreased interest in sex

PHYSICAL RESPONSES TO STARVATION

The physical changes observed among the men in the study were also interesting. All had gastrointestinal problems—bloating, belching and constipation. All lost muscle mass despite consuming protein meals calculated to prevent muscle loss and despite participating in daily exercise and marches. One highly visible area of muscle wasting was the temporal area just above the cheekbones. Heart size also decreased. The men had muscle cramps and weakness, and became dehydrated. Scalp hair thinned, and fine body hair, called lanugo, covered the body. Body temperature decreased, and the men felt cold all the time. The most prominent effect was the decrease in basal metabolic rate by 40 percent. Basal metabolic rate refers to the rate at which energy is used to run the body at its "base" or resting state. Resting state, or basal, work of the body includes keeping the heart beating, keeping the body warm, keeping all the various organs and involuntary work of the body going, and keeping all the cellular chemical systems running. Faced with inadequate food, drought, famine, or during diets, the body's metabolic rate falls, a phenomenon called hibernation metabolism.

In sum, the physical sequelae or aftereffects of starvation are:

- Gastrointestinal symptoms—bloating, constipation
- Muscle mass loss
- Temporal muscle wasting
- Decreased heart size
- Muscle weakness and cramping
- Slowed heart rate, decreased blood pressure

- Dehydration
- Hair loss
- Lanugo
- Decreased metabolic rate, coldness
- Decreased brain size

HIBERNATION METABOLISM

When caloric intake falls too low (below approximately 25 kcal per kilogram of body weight per day), the body shifts to conserve energy. The best example of this hibernation metabolism is in animals that sleep all or part of the winter. Bears, squirrels, and chipmunks eat very little in the cold winter months, and they sleep a lot. The kidneys and bowels become inactive. The heart beats slowly. Hair does not grow. Body temperature falls. Some animals do not even lose much weight because the body is so efficient at slowing down—doing less work to "get by" on less fuel, fewer calories.

The more a person diets, the more the body shifts to metabolically use fewer calories and to maintain body weight. The body fights weight loss. Not only is excessive dieting futile, the dieting-nondieting cycle is very dangerous. After a person stops dieting, and while the metabolic rate is still low, it will be very easy for him or her to regain previously lost weight. Furthermore, with each subsequent diet, the weight will be lost more slowly and after ending each subsequent diet, the regain will occur even more rapidly. This type of dieting and weight loss, followed by normal eating and weight gain, is called yo-yo dieting. Yo-yo dieting is associated with ever-increasing levels of body fat over time.

TRANSITIONS

Dieting and maintaining chronic undernutrition are not successful behaviors. Most people who diet and lose weight will regain the lost weight. Many young adolescent females want to weigh less than is biologically reasonable. For instance, to support menstrual periods, most women need 17 percent to 25 percent body fat. Elite female athletes who achieve very low body fat percentages usually do not have periods and are infertile until they regain lost body fat.

The brain is mostly fat. When starvation occurs, brain size diminishes. When starved people are finally fed, brain size does not fully return to its prestarvation level. Body fat helps keep the body warm and cushions various organs from trauma with ordinary body motion. Appropriate amounts of body fat are necessary and healthful.

People who undereat usually remain hungry. Frustration of appetite satiation serves to further increase appetite with an eventual outcome of eating at a fast pace and in large volume. In animal model experiments among underfed animals given full access to food, vomiting commonly results, both with and without electroshock to mimic the anxiety stress for dieters who give in to their hunger. When humans diet and then have full access to food, they usually will eat and often overeat. Vomiting is a frequent response to even mild overeating following starvation. In fact, some of the Quaker men in the "Minnesota experiment" vomited after overeating at a celebration meal at the end of the experiment (Keyes et al. 1950). It is easy to understand one reason why the majority of anorexic girls end up becoming bulimics.

Chronic starvation states can be very dangerous. "Refeeding Syndrome" (Brooks & Malnik, 1995) refers to life-threatening blood, chemistry problems that can occur when a starving person begins to eat. There can be massive shifts in cal-cium, magnesium, and phosphorus. If refeeding syndrome occurs, various electrolyte and mineral levels can fall to such low levels that the person can experience muscle weakness, cardiac arrhythmias, seizures, and death.

SUMMARY

Restrained eating, chronic undernutrition, and extreme dieting for weight loss not only do not succeed but are detrimental to one's health. The dangers, both physical and psychological, are many (Lambe, 1997). The fertile soil of starvation during dieting may spawn the very serious illnesses of anorexia nervosa and bulimia nervosa.

REFERENCES

Brooks, Marta, & Malnik, George. (1995). The refeeding syndrome: An approach to understanding its complications and preventing its occurrence. *Pharmacotherapy 15*(6), 713–726.

Keyes, Ancel, et al. (1950). *The biology of human starvation.* Minneapolis: University of Minnesota Press.

Lambe, Evelyn. (1997, June). Cerebral gray matter volume deficits after weight recovery from anorexia nervosa. *Archives of General Psychiatry 54*, 537–542.

Serotonin and the Biology of Bingeing
by Matthew Keene, M.D.

By now, you must realize that there is no single gene, trauma, or environmental cue that triggers an eating disorder. Yet as we exit the 1990s, and what has been coined "the decade of the brain," our exploration into the origins and treatment of binge eating shifts emphatically toward the realm of neurochemistry.

To this end, the biology of bingeing undoubtedly involves an interplay of several neurochemicals, including dopamine, norepinephrine, and the endogenous opioid system. However, with the introduction of Prozac, and the catastro-phe of Redux, emphasis now shifts to the unique neurotransmitter that these two controversial medicines affect: serotonin.

SEROTONIN: THE FEEDING AND FEELING CHEMICAL

Serotonin is the body's calming chemical. It promotes a sense of well-being and keeps one's mood on an even keel. Experts believe that defects in serotonin production result in a spectrum of illnesses. Research indicates that the repeated behaviors of the obsessive-compulsive, the suicidal thoughts of the depressed, the panic felt by the anxious, and the alcoholic's urge to drink may all be related to deficiencies in production of this one powerful neurotransmitter (Keene, 1997).

Serotonin is stored in several parts of the body, including the gastrointestinal tract, blood cells, and most importantly, the brain. Although serotonin is distributed throughout the entire brain, higher concentrations exist in two crucial areas: the hypothalamus and the limbic system.

The hypothalamus is the "caveman" part of the brain, making sure all of our primitive needs are met (e.g., thirst, hunger, libido). In other words, the hypothalamus is the "feeding brain." It feeds our basic biologic instincts and drives. The limbic system, on the other hand, is the "feeling brain." It perceives and expresses our emotions. Surprisingly, and despite obvious structural and functional differences, the hypothalamus and limbic system communicate with each other through a vast net of neurons whose primary messenger is serotonin. In doing so, the processes of feeding and feeling become intimately connected.

Several recent studies suggest that serotonin levels are significantly lower in compulsive overeaters and bulimics than in non-binge eaters (Blum, 1993); (Fava, 1989). Conceivably, when serotonin production is disrupted, the limbic system (feeling brain) is functionally "weakened," creating feelings of depression, anxiety, or irritability (Wallins, 1994). The hypothalamus (feeding brain) senses this discomfort via its neuronal interconnections and offers this primitive solution: Binge! Yet as primitive and unhealthy as this solution may be, it works. Bingeing temporarily boosts serotonin and alters mood.

THE TRYPTOPHAN EXPRESS

The body manufactures serotonin from the amino acid tryptophan. Like all amino acids, tryptophan comes from protein. Intuitively, one might assume that eating a protein-rich meal would lead to an increase in brain serotonin. Instead, the opposite occurs. Here's why.

For tryptophan to reach the brain and be converted into serotonin, it must first hitch a ride on a carrier molecule. Protein meals, however, supply the body with several amino acids, not just tryptophan; and all of these amino acids are competing for a ride on the same carrier. Unfortunately, tryptophan is the least abundant amino acid. Other

amino acids outnumber tryptophan and "bully" their way onto the transport molecule. As a result, protein meals cause both tryptophan and serotonin levels to decline.

Paradoxically, carbohydrate meals (which don't contain any tryptophan) are capable of producing a rapid and considerable increase in serotonin levels. Research confirms that eating a carbohydrate meal of just two slices of bread with jam will yield a rise in serotonin by 447 percent; whereas, a protein-rich chicken breast actually decreases serotonin by 28 percent (Keene, 1997). Clearly the potential exists to manipulate serotonin levels through diet, especially with carbohydrates, but how?

OFFICER INSULIN

Carbohydrates' ability to influence tryptophan and serotonin levels actually makes perfect medical sense because even though protein is the source of these neurochemical wonders, carbohydrates help them reach the brain by stimulating the release of insulin. Once released, insulin acts as a transit cop, dispersing the other amino acids out of the bloodstream and clearing the way for tryptophan. Technically, insulin increases the ratio of available tryptophan, making the carrier molecule more accessible.

The amount of insulin the pancreas secretes depends on several factors. Two conditions, however, greatly increase the release of insulin:

Condition 1: a rapid rise in sugar concentration

Condition 2: consumption of many calories at once

The summation of conditions 1 and 2 equals the prototypical binge: several hundred calories' worth of processed, sugary, fatty foods capable of releasing a bolus of insulin to manipulate serotonin.

SEROTONIN, CARBOHYDRATE CRAVING, AND THE SELF-MEDICATION THEORY

Among the illnesses where abnormalities in serotonin play a role is premenstrual syndrome. Several recent studies have demonstrated that in the week prior to menses, women with premenstrual syndrome develop markedly lower levels of serotonin than women without PMS. With this reduction in serotonin comes much of the discomfort and moodiness that typifies PMS (Halbreich, 1993).

Although the symptoms of PMS vary widely from woman to woman, carbohydrate craving seems to be universal. Controlled studies show that women with PMS increase their carbohydrate intake by as much as 500 calories in the three to four days prior to their period. These same women report feeling less depressed and less anxious after eating a meal loaded with carbohydrates. Researchers believe this finding proves the effectiveness of self-medicating with certain foods to manipulate serotonin (Wurtman, 1993).

Many nutritionists advise PMS sufferers to eat extra bread, pasta, and sweets in the days prior to menses. Doing so can relieve the transient emotional symptoms of menstrually related serotonin deficiencies. But can you imagine having to eat like that every day just to feel normal? That is in fact the basis for the self-medication theory of binge eating.

Conceivably, binge eaters and bulimics inherit a particularly fragile and persistent serotonin deficiency. Unlike PMS sufferers, they must compensate for this deficiency by continuously overeating. Because their serotonin systems are always disrupted, they are constantly driven to binge.

Support for this theory is found within the study of alcohol dependence. There appears to be a sizable group of alcoholics who, when sober, are deficient in serotonin. In other words, their nonintoxicated level of this calming chemical is low. Yet when they binge on alcohol, their serotonin levels markedly increase. That's really no surprise, considering alcohol is often described as "liquid sugar with a kick."

Scientists now believe that alcohol's ability to boost serotonin, like that of carbohydrates, can markedly improve one's sense of well-being. In fact, from a chemical standpoint, some alcoholics may feel normal only when intoxicated. Sound familiar? It should. These alcoholics seem to self-medicate with booze in the same way binge eaters and bulimics use processed carbohydrates, sugar, and excess fat. It's the same serotonin production defect and the same behavior. The only difference is the vehicle used to alter serotonin levels.

WHY FOOD FAILS

Binge food offers the promise of an immediate increase in serotonin and a temporary sense of well-being. But the operative word here is *temporary*. Over the long run, recurrent bingeing may lead to an even greater deficiency in serotonin. Here's why.

Binge food appears to have a biphasic effect on serotonin. In the first phase (binge phase), serotonin levels climb higher and higher, creating a sense of well-being. Unfortunately, this is a transient state, inevitably followed by a second phase (crash phase) where serotonin levels plummet toward, or even below, baseline. Why this happens is not entirely clear. However, one likely candidate is a process called the negative feedback loop.

To visualize this process, imagine that your job is to place widgets on thingamabobs as they roll along a conveyer belt. Suppose one day, a gazillion thingamabobs come barreling down the assembly line at once. You think to yourself, "This must be some kind of horrible mistake. If a gazillion thingamabobs and widgets were to fall into the wrong hands, it would upset the very balance of world power." So being the quick thinker that you are, you hit the factory's emergency stop button, halt production, and save humanity.

The body is a pretty sophisticated factory and works in a similar fashion. Emergency stop buttons exist for several metabolic activities. Of course, now that we are talking about the body, we have to start using unnecessarily complicated words. So the emergency stop button becomes a negative feedback loop. The principle is the same. The body halts production of a chemical once it senses that enough already exists.

Bingeing may fool the binge eater's or bulimic's system by producing a burst of serotonin that mistakenly forewarns an excess level of serotonin and signals the body to shut down production. By the time the body realizes that it's just a false alarm, it's too late. Again, the end result is another decrease in serotonin, another worsening of mood, and another reason to binge.

SEROTONIN STABILIZATION: THE TREATMENT OF BINGEING

As evidence of the role of serotonin dysfunction in the development of binge eating and bulimia mounts, there grows even greater evidence to support the role of "serotonin stabilization" as a vital component in the treatment of these disorders. Thousands of anecdotal reports from the annals of Overeaters Anonymous attest to the benefits of behaviorally eliminating, that is, "abstaining" from, sugary and highly processed carbohydrates. In theory, the substitution of whole, complex carbohydrates allows for a steady release of insulin and serotonin, as opposed to the peak and valley levels of serotonin production that accompany binge food. Furthermore, whole, complex carbohydrates take longer to digest, thereby improving satiety while reducing cravings and subsequent binges

Exercise represents another form of behavioral modification that improves serotonergic function. A recent study from Brazil demonstrated that regular exercisers have brain serotonin levels that are 50 percent higher than their nonexercising counterparts (Soares, 1994). Other reports suggest that 20 minutes of aerobic exercise can greatly curtail the desire to binge. However, given the propensity of some eating-disordered patients to compulsively exercise as a means of purging, a cautious inquiry must be made before recommending exercise as an integral component of treatment.

Cognitive psychotherapy is also known to effectively increase serotonin and stabilize serotonergic function (Neziroglu, 1994). The process of reversing negative self-thought and improving coping and communication skills has definite medicinal value and is currently considered the gold standard "talk therapy" for bulimic and binge eating-disordered patients.

Next is pharmacology. In 1987, Prozac was introduced in the United States. It is the only medication that is FDA approved for the treatment of bulimia, and it represents the first of a new generation of medicines known as selective serotonin reuptake inhibitors (SSRIs). Clinically, Prozac inhibits the metabolism of this single neurochemical, increasing serotonin in the "feeding" and "feeling" parts of the brain. Whereas binge food accomplishes this effect only briefly (and carries the risk of excess weight), Prozac achieves more enduring results without unwanted calories. In fact, several dozen double-blind studies demonstrate a reduction in the binge or binge/purge cycle by 50 percent or more when SSRIs are prescribed to the right patient at the proper dose (Mareus, 1990; Hudson, 1996). The effects are even more dramatic when combined with cognitive behavioral therapy.

Finally, it is important to recognize that too much of a good thing is not necessarily good, as evidenced by the disastrous fallout from Redux (the "fen" in fen-phen). Like Prozac, Redux also delayed the body's breakdown of serotonin and significantly reduced binge episodes. Unfortunately, Redux also forced extra serotonin into brain synapses. It was this serotinergic overload that was credited with the toxic cardiopulmonary side effects of Redux that necessitated its removal from the market.

CONCLUSION

The road to overeating and bulimia does not begin and end with serotonin. Yet study after study demonstrates that medication, exercise, and even food can alter levels of this powerful neurochemical, serving to either help or hinder recovery. So, as the decade of the brain draws to a close, the definitive importance of serotonin in the biology of bingeing remains to be seen. Perhaps the answer lies ahead in the year 2000 and beyond, in what will undoubtedly be "the century of the brain."

REFERENCES

Blum, I., et al. (1993). Food preferences, body weight, and platelet-poor plasma serotonin and catecholamines. *American Journal of Clinical Nutrition 57*, 486–489.

Fava, M., et al. (1989). Neurochemical abnormalities of anorexia nervosa and bulimia nervosa. *American Journal of Psychiatry 146*, 963–971.

Halbreich, U., et al. (1993). Altered serotonergic activity in women with dysphoric premenstrual syndromes. *International Journal of Psychiatry in Medicine 23*, 1–27.

Hudson, J. I., et al. (1996). Antidepressant treatment of binge-eating disorder: Research findings and clinical guidelines. *Journal of Clinical Psychiatry 57*, 73–79.

Keene, M. S. (1997). *Chocolate is my kryptonite: Feeding your feelings/how to survive the forces of food*. Phoenix, AZ: Saguaro.

Marcus, M. D., et al. (1990). A double-blind, placebo-controlled trial of Fluoxetine plus behavior modification in the treatment of obese binge-eaters and non-binge-eaters. *American Journal of Psychiatry 14*(7), 876–881.

Neziroglu, F. (1994, January). Serotonin levels altered by behavior therapy in obsessive-compulsive disorder. *Psychiatric Times*, 14.

Soares, J., et al. (1994). Increased serotonin levels in physically trained men. *Brazilian J Med Biol Res 27*, 1635–1638.

Wallin, M. S., et al. (1994). Food and mood: Relationship between food, serotonin and affective disorders. *Acta Psychiatr Scand*, Suppl 377, 36-40.

Wurtman, J. J. (1993). Depression and weight gain: The serotonin connection. *Journal of Affective Disorders 29*, 183–192.

PART 3
Sociocultural Issues and Subgroups Affected by Eating Disorders

Are You Really "Too Fat"? The Role of Culture and Weight Stereotypes

by Nancy Ellis-Ordway, A.C.S.W.

Since the beginning of time, human beings have used food as more than just a source of nutrition. Food is used to celebrate special occasions, comfort in times of grief, provide a way to share within a common community, express love and affection, identify ethnic traditions, and express artistic creativity. Human beings are programmed from birth to enjoy food, especially sweet, salty, and rich food. What is unique to our culture is that, for the first time in history, attractiveness is equated with thinness rather than plumpness.

"Compulsive overeating" is widely identified in our culture as an eating disorder. Although there are some similarities in behavior, anorexia nervosa and bulimia nervosa are distinct illnesses that are different from compulsive overeating. However, it is impossible to understand any of these illnesses without understanding something about "society" attitudes toward obesity.

WEIGHT SET POINTS

Within each individual is a "set point," a genetically programmed desirable weight. If a person eats when hungry and stops when full, having access to a variety of foods, then that individual's weight will stay within a set range. The set point itself may change slightly with such variables as illness, age, or depression, but it is determined genetically. With few exceptions, if a person's parents are fat, the individual will be fat. If the parents are thin, the person will be thin. Little can be done to change this. Whether a person overeats or undereats, the body compensates by adjusting its metabolism, as well as the amount of hunger experienced, to try to keep the body at the same weight (Bennett & Gurin, 1982).

Research studies have shown for years that fat people, on average, do not eat more than thin people; that adopted children of thin biological parents who are placed with fat adoptive parents grow up to be thin, and vice versa; and that people who engage in restrictive eating (commonly known as "dieting") regain the weight they lose.

Studies that attempt to overfeed genetically thin people to make them fat have shown that it cannot be done (Ciliska, 1990).

SOCIETY AND WEIGHT CONTROL

Yet our society persists in believing that weight can be, and therefore should be, controlled. This belief is nurtured by a multibillion-dollar-a-year business that sells us products and services promising to make us thinner. As the fashionable ideal for attractiveness gets thinner and thinner, more and more people are vulnerable to the claims of advertisers that thinness is within the grasp of anyone who can find and afford their product or program. When the person fails to lose weight, or regains the lost weight, he or she is criticized for "not having enough willpower."

In fact, the body reacts to a diet the same way our cave-dweller ancestors reacted to famine. Faced with restricted food intake, the body's metabolism becomes more efficient to conserve fuel or calories. As the body learns to get by with less food, the dieter hits the proverbial "plateau." To lose more weight, eating must become more restrictive, and the dieter feels more deprived. When in the presence of food (even food presented in a magazine or television ad), the body reacts with increased hunger to try to ensure its own survival. Sooner or later the dieter, battling with the implacable demands of his or her own body, gives in and eats. The body continues to be ravenously hungry until the original, or set point, weight is achieved. However, now the body is afraid of another famine, so it stores up a little extra fuel, just in case. In addition, the metabolism has learned to be more efficient so that the body can actually weigh more on less food. Dieters, beset with feelings of failure and worthlessness, set out on other diets, hoping that this time they have found the magic solution. The cycle begins again.

REASONS FOR OVEREATING

Everyone occasionally eats for emotional reasons; thin people are not criticized for it. Everyone occasionally overeats; thin people are not criticized for this either. Only when a person is genetically programmed to be heavier than the current fashionable style do eating patterns come under scrutiny. Compulsive overeating is almost always a response to chronic dieting. Thus, treatment that focuses on food control and weight loss just reinforces the cycle. According to Ellyn Satter (1986), it's like giving a person with a hand-washing compulsion a basin and a towel, and saying, "Here, if you just get your hands clean enough, the problem will go away." Treatment that instead focuses on reestablishing normal eating habits and weight is becoming more available. Shifting one's attitude from dieting and intake to responses to hunger can be difficult but successful in the long run. People who get this kind of treatment may never be thin, but they can be thinner, eat more, and feel more relaxed and better about themselves.

Eighty to 90 percent of people on diets are women, in spite of research that shows most women have fewer health risks associated with being heavy than men do. In fact, many women engaged in dieting behavior are actually within or below "ideal body weight range" as defined by statistics compiled by life insurance companies. Yet studies show that dieting behaviors can be observed in as many as half of all fifth-grade girls studied and that children in early elementary grades perceive being fat as worse than being disabled.

SOCIETY'S CRITICISM OF OVERWEIGHT PEOPLE

It is no longer acceptable in our society to discriminate against people on the basis of color, gender, religion, or ethnic background. Fat people are exempt from this dictate. Fat people participate in their own persecution, believing that their failure to be thin is due to some flaw within themselves, some lack of willpower. Genetically thin people then feel smug about their own superior willpower.

This attitude has an insidious effect on everyone, including people who do not have a weight problem. Individuals who are at their set points and are content with their weight nevertheless feel compelled to watch their weight. Normal-weight people especially feel guilty when eating and feel they have to forgo or justify especially desirable foods. Historically, eating has been a source of great pleasure. It is increasingly a source of guilt. Advertisers recognize and capitalize on this with commercials promoting "guilt-free" foods.

It is not surprising, given the widespread societal disgust with people who are overweight, that some individuals choose to be anorexic or bulimic. Recovery is much more difficult when the person is surrounded by the cultural attitude that weight gain is shameful and a sign of weakness. Understanding the role of the news, entertainment, and advertising media is helpful, but the family members, friends, co-workers, and schoolmates of the recovering person are all still subjected to the same cultural message. After a long struggle in inpatient or intensive outpatient treatment, the client may return to a family with several members on diets, boyfriends or girlfriends who make cruel comments about overweight peers, and uninformed friends who compliment the client on his or her willpower when he or she does not eat.

Family members of people with eating disorders often confront them loaded with information about all the physical risks and side effects associated with the disorder, expecting them to change. The reason that scare tactics do not work is that often no threats of death, illness, or permanent physical impairment can be as terrifying as the thought of being fat.

The current preoccupation with weight loss now seems to be influenced by an emphasis on fitness as well as thinness. Unfortunately, for people who are vulnerable to eating disorders, this can translate into a dangerous exercise compulsion that can be just as disruptive as bulimia. Some social scientists predict that we have seen the extreme in the pursuit of thinness and that the pendulum will now swing back to more realistic standards. Only time will tell.

REFERENCES

Bennett, W., & Gurin, J. (1982). *The dieter's dilemma.* New York: Basic Books.

Ciliska, D. (1990). *Beyond dieting: Psychoeducational interventions for chronically obese women: A non-dieting approach.* New York: Brunner/Mazel.

Satter, E. (1986). *Child of mine: Feeding with love and good sense.* Menlo Park, CA: Bull.

Satter, E. (1987). *How to get your kid to eat . . . but not too much.* Menlo Park, CA: Bull.

SUGGESTED READING

Chernin, K. (1981). *The obsession: Reflections on the tyranny of slenderness.* New York: Harper & Row.

Chernin, K. (1986). *The hungry self: Women, eating and identity*. New York: Harper & Row.

Cooke, K. (1996). *Real gorgeous: The truth about body and beauty*. New York: W. W. Norton.

Freedman, R. (1986). *Beauty bound*. New York: Lexington Books.

Freedman, R. (1990). *Body love: Learning to like our looks and ourselves*. New York: Harper & Row.

Hirschmann, J., & Munter, C. (1988). *Overcoming overeating*. New York: Fawcett Columbine.

Hirschmann, J., & Munter, C. (1995). *When women stop hating their bodies: Freeing yourself from food and weight obsession*. New York: Fawcett Columbine.

Culture and Eating Disorders
by Cindy Davis, Ph.D., and Melanie Katzman, Ph.D.

Think about how you would answer the following questions:

- Are you happy with the way you look?
- Would you like to lose weight or gain weight?
- Do you ever think about dieting?
- Do you wish you were taller or shorter?
- What is the ideal body shape?
- If you could look like anyone, who would it be?

What factors influenced the way you answered these questions? Did television, movies, and magazines have any influence on your answers? Do you think people in other parts of the world would have answered the questions similarly? Do you think your grandmother or grandfather would have answered these questions differently when they were your age?

An important factor influencing the way we respond to these types of questions is culture. Culture can be defined as the environment in which we live and includes values, beliefs, practices, and assumptions. Culture influences what we eat, what clothes we wear, how we fix our hair, what music we listen to, and how we talk. The influence of culture becomes more obvious when meeting someone from a different culture or when traveling to a different culture.

WHAT DOES CULTURE HAVE TO DO WITH EATING DISORDERS?

Many people believe that culture is a very important aspect of eating disorders. From early childhood, we are influenced by culture, particularly when it comes to standards of beauty. In Western cultures, girls are influenced by the unrealistic "Barbie-doll" body shape and constantly told that thin is beautiful, whereas boys are influenced by muscular images and told that they should be big and strong. Television, movies, and magazines provide constant messages about the ideal standard of beauty and how we should look and behave. Unfortunately, these standards are unrealistic and impossible for most people to achieve. Culture, however, is not just about beauty but about the social and political organizations of family, power, and success.

As people move among different cultures or are exposed to different cultural values in their home countries, they experience what is known as *acculturation* or the blending of two or more cultures. Acculturation is a complex process requiring contact between at least two cultural groups that results in some type of change. Although reciprocal change can occur between groups, one group generally dominates the other. The domination of one group over another suggests that what happens between contact and change is likely to be difficult and conflictual rather than conciliatory and consensual (Berry,

1980). This transition from one culture to another is likely to affect one's physical and psychological functioning. Studies have found that as people from other cultures are exposed to Western values, they are more likely to develop symptoms associated with eating disorders (Davis & Katzman, 1998; Furnham & Alibhai, 1983; Furukawa, 1994). For example, research on Chinese girls living in the United States found that those girls who were more acculturated or "Westernized" were more likely to have symptoms of eating disorders, such as bulimic behavior and an obsession with thinness (Davis & Katzman, 1998, in press).

One does not have to live in a Western culture to be exposed to Western values or to develop an eating disorder. Research on Chinese students in Hong Kong found that students mirrored gendered patterns previously reported in Western cultures with respect to their bodies—boys wanted to be larger and girls wanted to be more petite, despite already being quite thin by Western standards. In addition, Chinese students in Hong Kong reported significant problems with self-esteem and depression (Davis & Katzman, 1998). One possible explanation for these findings in Hong Kong as well as other countries may be the stress experienced by the new generation in a rapidly developing country (Katzman & Lee, 1997). Hong Kong, like many other countries, has recently been heavily exposed to the values of modernization. In addition, the introduction and accessibility of the Internet now make it possible to easily experience Western culture. These new values and roles conflict with many traditional cultural values, especially for women in more traditional nations.

It has been suggested that in an effort to conform to new demands and pressures individuals may "overcorrect" real or imagined deficits (Root, 1990). For girls and boys the effort to perfect oneself may become focused on altering the body. This focus on body perfection, an ultimate, unobtainable goal, may further accentuate a sense of ineffectiveness and conflict rather than alleviate it (Davis & Katzman, in press). The development of attitudes and behaviors associated with disordered eating has been cited by many researchers as an indication of acculturation among individuals exposed to changing cultural images in their home country or those living in a new country (Katzman & Lee, 1997; Lee, 1995).

DO STANDARDS OF BEAUTY DIFFER AROUND THE WORLD?

Much research has examined differences in standards of beauty across various cultures as well as changes in beauty standards over time. Different cultures have different ideas of what makes a person attractive. In Western culture, the focus of ideal beauty for females is on thinness, and obesity is portrayed as a negative quality. Conversely, certain African tribes view obesity as a sign of beauty and wealth, and thinness as a sign of poverty. Men are considered good providers, and their status is enhanced if they marry a woman who is plump (Boskind-White & White, 1986).

Standards of beauty also change over time. In Western cultures, plumpness was once viewed as the ideal. However, cultural views have evolved to reflect the saying "Thin is in." Over the past 20 years, Miss America contestants have become both taller and thinner, reflecting changes in the cultural view of ideal beauty, and women's magazines have drastically increased the number of articles about diet and thinness (Garner et al., 1980).

Standards of beauty are also changing in other countries. For example, the Chinese traditionally regarded plumpness as a sign of beauty and wealth. Current trends now suggest that Chinese girls in Hong Kong have similar values to Western girls and desire a thinner body shape even though they are already generally thinner than most girls in Western countries. Chinese boys in Hong Kong are also dissatisfied with their bodies and would like a more muscular body shape resembling images portrayed in Western countries (Davis & Katzman, 1997).

DO PEOPLE ALL AROUND THE WORLD DEVELOP EATING DISORDERS?

Several years ago, eating disorders were generally thought to occur only in Caucasian women from Western continents, such as North America, Europe, and Australia. However, we now know that eating disorders affect women from all over the world, including Native Americans, Asians, Asian Americans, Africans, African Americans, and Middle Easterners (Davis & Yager, 1992). We can no longer simply ask about Western values, but more importantly, we must ask whether *West-*

ern values have now become *global* values. Eating disorders are no longer just a Western illness—they are a global illness.

The reasons for this increase in eating disorders around the world are uncertain. One possibility is the increased exposure to Western culture through television and magazines, and the increased exposure to Western foods such as McDonald's hamburgers. Another possibility is that doctors around the world are more aware of eating disorders and are more likely to recognize when a person has an eating disorder. Additional reasons may have less to do with food and more to do with the struggles women face with regard to their roles and status. Although we may not know the exact cause, we do know that the expression of distress through disordered eating and body discomfort is no longer bound to any geographic region (Katzman, 1996).

WHAT CAN BE DONE ABOUT THE INFLUENCE OF CULTURE?

Culture is an integral part of our lives. Culture is not only about beauty, but also about the social and political organizations of family, power, and success. It is important to understand how our own beliefs and values are influenced as well as how others' values and beliefs may differ from our own. What can we learn about cultures where women like their bodies, and what is unique about them? Also, what can we learn about cultures in which men are beginning to dislike their bodies, and what does this tell us about power (rather than gender) struggles and the development of eating disorders? (Katzman, 1997). We have much to learn from and about the role of cultural influences in the development of the attitudes and behaviors associated with eating disorders. The development of eating disorders is not simply about food or body—it is about culture, power, family, and self-esteem.

REFERENCES

Berry, J. (1980). Acculturation as varieties of adaptation. In Padilla (Ed.), *Acculturation: Theory, models and some new findings.* Boulder: Westview Press.

Boshkind-White, M., & White, W. C. (1986). Bulimarexia: A historical-sociocultural perspective. In K. K. Brownell & J. P. Foreyt (Eds.), *Handbook of eating disorders: Physiology, psychology and treatment of obesity, anorexia, and bulimia.* New York: Basic Books.

Davis, C., & Katzman, M. (1997). Charting new territory: Body esteem, weight satisfaction, depression and self-esteem among Chinese males and females in Hong Kong. *Sex Roles 36*(7/8), 447–457.

Davis, C., & Katzman, M. (1998). Chinese men and women in the USA and Hong Kong: Body and self esteem ratings as a prelude to dieting and exercise. *International Journal of Eating Disorders 23*(1), 99–102.

Davis, C., & Katzman, M. (in press). Perfection as acculturation: Psychological correlates of eating problems in Chinese male and female students living in the United States. *International Journal of Eating Disorders.*

Davis, C., & Yager, J. (1992). Transcultural aspects of eating disorders: A critical review of the literature. *Culture, Psychiatry and Medicine 16*, 377–394.

Furnham, A., & Alibhai, N. (1983). Cross-cultural differences in the perception of female body shape. *Psychological Medicine 13*, 829–837.

Furukawa, T. (1994). Weight changes and eating attitudes of Japanese adolescents under acculturative stresses: A prospective study. *International Journal of Eating Disorders 15*(1), 71–79.

Garner, D. M., Garfinkel, P. E., Schwartz, D., & Thompson, M. (1980). Cultural expectations of thinness in women. *Psychological Reports 47*, 483–491.

Katzman, M. (1996). Asia on my mind: Are eating disorders a problem in Hong Kong? Eating Disorders: Journal of Treatment and Prevention 3(4), 379–380.

Katzman, M. (1997). Getting the difference right: It's power not gender that matters. *European Eating Disorders Review 5*(2), 71–74.

Katzman, M., & Lee, S. (1997). Beyond body image: The integration of feminist and transcultural theories in the understanding of self starvation. *International Journal of Eating Disorders 22*, 385–394.

Lee, S. (1995). Self starvation in context: Towards a culturally sensitive understanding of anorexia nervosa. *Social Science Medicine 41*(1), 25–36.

Root, M. (1990). Disordered eating in women of color. *Sex Role 22*, 525–536.

The Truth About Dieting: A Feminist View

by Carol Bloom, C.S.W., Andrea Gitter, M.A., Susan Gutwill, C.S.W., Laura Kogel, A.C.S.W., and Lela Zaphiropoulos, A.C.S.W.

DIETING AS A SOLUTION

- You have a test, you're nervous. Do you find yourself thinking about food, your body, or dieting?
- You had a fight with your mother/father/boyfriend/girlfriend. A little while later do you find yourself thinking of dieting . . . or of eating the whole chocolate cake?
- You're shopping for clothes. You don't look like the models or the skinniest girl in the class. Do you start to think about dieting?
- A magazine article promises you can lose five pounds in seven days. Do you feel tempted to try, thinking, "Maybe this will work"?
- You're nervous about putting on a bathing suit . . . about a blind date . . . . Is dieting a solution?
- Your girlfriend asks you to go on a diet with her. Can you let her down?
- Your parents promise you a new wardrobe if you lose 20 pounds. Are you tempted to diet?
- Your girlfriends all seem more confident, more beautiful, more desirable than you. This time you'll stick to the diet.
- You wake up feeling lousy, begin your morning mirror routine, worrying about what you ate last night or yesterday. You resolve not to eat today . . . and the next day.
- You look at your thighs, your stomach in disgust, or you frequently say to yourself, "I hate my body." Is dieting the only way you feel you can get control?
- You feel depressed. It must be because you're too heavy, so you plan to diet.

DIETING AS A PROBLEM

Dieting may seem like a solution to all these moments—moments of tension, conflict, confusion, and unhappiness—but does it work? What does dieting really do for you?

Let's look at how diets work in society at large. Sixty-five million people and 85 percent of women in the United States are dieting at any given moment (Brumberg, 1989; Orbach, 1986; Schwartz, 1986). Ninety-five percent of all people who lose weight on a diet gain back more than they lost (Goode, 1990; Miller, 1989; Orbach, 1978). Hundreds of thousands of young women and increasing numbers of men suffer from anorexia and bulimia (Brumberg, 1989). Dieting often leads to bingeing, which reinforces the feeling of lack of control and the need to diet again. Because the diet feels so restricting and depriving, you end up bingeing again, creating a real yo-yo syndrome (Bennett & Gurin, 1982; Goode, 1990; Hirschmann & Munter, 1988; Polivy & Herman, 1983). In spite of the extent to which dieting fails people, it channels $35 billion a year into an industry that very successfully sells the same thing to the same people over and over again (Miller, 1989; Schwartz, 1986). The profits of the diet industry are made from the fact that diets fail, but because people have insecure and uncomfortable feelings about themselves, lack self-confidence, and can't find an alternative, they return to dieting as the solution.

Culture and the Female Body

It is no surprise that most girls and women (and some boys and men) in our society believe something is very wrong with their bodies (Brumberg, 1989; Jacoby, 1990). We wonder if we can ever be shapely enough, thin enough, or pretty enough.

We wonder if we can ever relax and be comfortable in our own skins. Much of our uncertainty stems from the fact that advertising seduces and frightens women—it threatens, "You are nothing," without your looks. Advertising feeds off of women's sense of inadequacy. Throughout history women have rarely had full ownership and control over their bodies. Sometimes women's bodies have been the property of men, other times women's bodies have been viewed as breeding machines, and, for the last few hundred years, women's bodies have been viewed as objects, objects for men to gaze upon, lust after, and conquer. Today, women's bodies have become objects even to themselves. We look in the mirror as if we were an object to scrutinize. We gaze at ourselves with critical eyes, as if we were outside ourselves as men looking at our reflection, sizing us up. And we ourselves believe that we have to be thin to feel good. Over the last few decades, the standard that women are supposed to attain has gotten thinner and thinner.

TV, magazines, and the news media bombard us constantly with their images of beauty—the sleek, lean look that can never be thin enough, rich enough, toned enough. The multibillion-dollar advertising industry uses its conception of the ideal female body to sell its products: lipsticks, cars, clothes, computers, cigarettes, and liquor. These sales pitches are intentionally directed at women to sell us not just the latest car but, just as importantly, this year's image of how we are supposed to look and feel. In the face of this image avalanche, women who don't conform experience their uniqueness, their individuality to be their failing rather than a gift.

Gender

Dieting encourages us to value only one aspect of ourselves and makes that aspect represent the whole self as if there were no other important parts of our being. Girls, in particular, need to learn to value themselves and be valued in additional and different ways. Many girls at ages 8, 9, and 10 develop their voice, speak up, say what they think, and sometimes take charge. But by adolescence, girls no longer speak as forthrightly. How come? Studies show that the ways in which girls (and women) tend to look at and solve problems are valued less in society. Girls are devalued even in the classroom, where they are called on less often than boys (Gilligan, 1990; Sakber, 1994).

The gender roles in society, although changing, still emphasize a woman's appearance over other qualities and her ability to attract a mate as primary. Mastery, achievement, and assertion are not as valued for women as for men and, hence, some girls begin (consciously or unconsciously) to inhibit their power, assertiveness, and even intelligence as they deal with becoming women. Feeling pleasure in one's developing body and sexuality is one way to feel powerful, but for many women it is the only way. But even that channel is frought with gender-biased complications. Girls still must navigate between the dangers of being thought of as a "slut" and the undermining confinement of behaving like a "good girl." No matter what, it is imperative to have the "right" body and the "right" look, which these days is very thin. But not all bodies were meant to be thin. Nevertheless, many girls heed this injunction, rejecting their own bodies and beginning to diet (if they haven't already done so) to fit the current cultural ideal.

The Family

Unfortunately, we can also get negative messages from our families. How we were seen and how we were cared for when we were small, vulnerable, dependent, and impressionable beings shapes our sense of self and how we care for ourselves. This is particularly true for mothers in relation to their daughters. As women, mothers are made to feel insecure about their own sense of self, body, and ability to take care of themselves. Parents, affected by their own parents as well as by social prejudices, in turn visit their anxieties on their children.

Sometimes mothers and/or fathers are overly involved with their daughters, particularly when it comes to their appearance. Others are emotionally absent. In neither case does a daughter feel supported, valued, or seen as an individual in her own right. Often these relationship difficulties manifest themselves through food: Food can be used inappropriately by the parent or child to assert power, to show love, to gain control, to reward, and to punish. Such behavior distorts the basic purpose of feeding and eating: to feed physiological hunger in a nurturing way.

Women's response to this pressure—from society and from their families—is to diet. The business of becoming a woman in our world is a complicated, bumpy road to navigate. Dieting seems like a way to get control over this difficult process.

The Real Effects of Dieting

But what happens when you chronically diet and chronically think about diets? As soon as you go on a diet, you find yourself wanting to binge. Have you ever noticed that when someone tells you not to have a certain food, that's the food you really want? It seems special; you can't stop thinking about it, and it practically calls to you. Dieting makes you worried, scared, anxious, and fearful of temptation of those forbidden foods. Over time, you stop listening to your body's hunger signals and you start fearing them instead. You stop feeling you have any power to know your own hunger and satiation. Although at the beginning of a diet you may feel excited and hopeful, by the end of it you feel defeated, inadequate, and out of control. You just don't trust yourself anymore. You buy magazines containing diet articles, make pacts with girlfriends, and pay the many diet clubs, all the while feeling less confident in your own abilities. Eventually, not only do you feel like a "failed" dieter, but you feel like a "bad" person, out of control and "messed up."

Your body has become so much your focus that every insecure feeling—envy, fear, hate, need, every conflict with a friend, every difficulty in school and at home, every confusing relationship—translates into insecurity about your body and a fear of food and eating.

This is not your fault!

THE NATURAL SOLUTION: WHAT YOU CAN DO

We believe there is a way you can both eat food and enjoy and maintain a body size that is comfortable for you. How? First and foremost, find, discover, listen to, and respect your physical hunger. This is your body's gift to you about when to feed yourself. Just as people are learning about the need to respect and care for our natural environment, your hunger is a major part of your natural inner environment. You must not violate it or you begin a process of bodily misattunement and, eventually, harm.

Next, offer yourself all foods. No foods must be considered off limits. Any food that is denied becomes "magical"—too special—and triggers the next binge. You must be thinking we are crazy! No dieting, and you can eat sweets, pizza, etc.! But, yes, we are very, very serious. Over time (and it might take a long time), as you allow yourself off-limit foods when you are physiologically hungry, they will lose their magical powers and take their place as foods you enjoy without bingeing. Furthermore, all foods will take their rightful place in your "diet" once you start to eat in a more balanced and, hence, healthy way.

Finally, there is a way to know when your body has had enough. It is the feeling of satiation. If you eat when you are hungry, you will know when you have had enough. Satiation is another aspect of your body's environment that you can learn to trust. But it is essential that you not yell at yourself when you can't follow each step of this process. The yelling only makes you feel bad, and it is these "bad" feelings that can make you reach for food when you're not physically hungry. In fact, it would help if you began paying attention to how much and when you critique and yell at yourself in general.

Learning to eat when you're hungry and to stop when you're satisfied will be new experiences which, like any other skills, need to be practiced to be developed. In other words, you may not be able to do this easily at first. But if you keep practicing, you will know just what to eat and when to stop. Slowly, you will find yourself in sync with your personal environment. You will feel better, in control, and more self-reliant and secure about food, eating, and body image. This, then, may generalize into other aspects of how you feel about and treat yourself.

WHAT ABOUT MY SIZE?

A body that eats in tune with hunger and satiation will eventually reach its natural weight. This may not be the weight the magazines say you should be but rather what your body naturally is meant to be. If you are overweight, eating with hunger and satiety means you will slowly lose weight. If you have been starving yourself and are very skinny, as you gain a few pounds you may feel anxious and uncomfortable, so much so that you might wish to get professional help. Eventually, however, you can feel healthier and more confident.

IS THIS A FORMIDABLE PROJECT?

Yes! But, many positive outcomes will accompany your effort! You can make your body a natural environment where food is what it's supposed to be—food—and not confuse it with feelings. Until now, food and feelings were entangled. You ate and dieted because you felt depressed, anxious, lonely, ugly, needy, shameful, and envious. Now, you can learn not to eat in response to your feelings and, instead, to tolerate and even respect them despite how intense, complicated, or uncomfortable they can be. Neither do you have to do this alone. You can share this approach to eating with friends, speak to a professional who understands this philosophy, or form a self-help group.

It is a courageous act to give up the false and destructive idea that being thin and viewing food as an enemy will solve life's problems as well as make you a more desirable, "perfect" female. To stand apart from the cultural madness is to challenge it while affirming your own unique value.

REFERENCES

Bennett, W., & Gurin, J. (1982). *The dieter's dilemma.* New York: Basic Books.

Brumberg, J. J. (1989). *Fasting girls: The history of anorexia nervosa.* New York: New American Library.

Goode, E. (1990). Getting Slim. *U.S. News and World Report,* May 14, p. 64.

Hirschmann, J., & Munter, C. (1988). *Overcoming overeating.* Reading, MA: Addison-Wesley.

Miller, A. (1989). Diets incorporated. *Newsweek,* September 11, pp. 56–60.

Orbach, S. (1978). *Fat is a feminist issue.* New York: Paddington Press.

Orbach, S. (1986). *Hunger strike.* New York: Basic Books.

Polivy, J., & Herman, C. P. (1983). *Breaking the diet habit.* New York: Basic Books.

Schwartz, H. (1986). *Never satisfied.* New York: Free Press.

SUGGESTED READING

Bordo, S. (1993). *Unbearable weight: Feminism, western culture and the body.* Los Angeles: University of California Press.

Bruch, H. (1979). *The golden cage.* New York: Vintage Press.

Brumberg, J. J. (1997). *The body project: An intimate history of American girls.* New York: Random House.

Gilligan, C. (1982). *In a different voice.* Cambridge, MA: Harvard University Press.

Gilligan, C. (1990). *Making connections: the relational worlds of adolescent girls at Emma Willard School.* Cambridge, MA: Harvard University Press.

Hirschmann, J., & Munter, C. (1995). *When women stop hating their bodies.* Reading, MA: Addison-Wesley.

Hirschmann, J., & Zaphiropoulos, L. (1993). *Preventing childhood eating problems.* Carlsbad, CA: Gurze Books.

Pipher, M. (1994). *Reviving Ophelia.* New York: Putnam.

Roth, G. (1984). *Breaking free from compulsive eating.* Indianapolis/New York: Bobbs-Merrill.

Sakber, M. and D. (1994). *Failing at fairness: How America's schools cheat girls.* New York: Charles Scribner's Sons.

Seligman, J. (1990). The losing formula. *Newsweek,* April 30, pp. 52–61.

Wolf, N. (1991). *The beauty myth.* New York: William Morrow.

Women's Therapy Centre Institute, Bloom, C., Gitter, A., Gutwill, S., Kogel, L., & Zaphiropoulos, L. (1994). *Eating problems: A feminist psychoanalytic treatment model.* New York: Basic Books.

Prevention of Eating Disorders, Eating Problems, and Negative Body Image
by Michael P. Levine, Ph.D.

PREVENTION OF EATING DISORDERS AND EATING PROBLEMS

This chapter provides an introductory overview of the "primary" prevention of severe eating disorders, including anorexia nervosa and bulimia nervosa, and less severe but still dangerous eating "problems." The latter category includes various combinations of unhealthy eating and weight-management behaviors (calorie-restrictive dieting, binge eating, punishing exercise to compensate for food eaten) in conjunction with attitudes that in the extreme constitute *nervosa*. These attitudes, which are so common as to be normative in Western, industrialized societies (Gordon, 1990), are listed in Table 1 (see page xx). Eating problems are often the focus of prevention because they increase the risk for full-blown eating disorders, and because they compromise physical health, create a good deal of misery, and otherwise reduce the personal and interpersonal quality of life (Neumark-Sztainer, 1995).[1]

"Primary" Prevention

"Primary" prevention (hereafter called, simply, prevention) refers to systematic efforts to reduce the number of new cases ("incidence") of a disorder or problem (Bloom, 1996). One way to accomplish this is to reduce "risk" factors such as sexual harassment by peers or dispensation of unhealthy "dieting" advice by physicians, whose presence increases the probability of the disorder. The second way is to increase factors (e.g., self-esteem, problem-solving skills, social support, or media promotion of multiple avenues of success for women) whose presence actively "protects" people from developing the disorder.

Ideally, prevention involves translating theory and research about the nature and causes of both disorder and optimal health into policies and programs designed to (1) keep large groups of people who are well from developing that disorder in the first place; and (2) systematically evaluate the success or failure of those efforts (Price, Cowen, Lorion, & Ramos-McKay, 1987). Prevention work is thus inherently exciting, challenging, perplexing, and controversial because it involves changes in one's own behavior at work and at home, as well as changes in education, mass media, public health, and politics (Levine, 1994). Readers seeking more information about prevention are referred to Albee and Gullotta (1997) and Bloom (1996).

Some psychologists and psychiatrists believe that "primary" prevention is unscientific and totally impractical. They argue forcefully that money and time should be devoted instead to treatment of those who are already suffering from the disorder (rehabilitation, sometimes called *tertiary prevention*) or of those who are evincing early signs of eating disorders and need intervention lest they fully develop the disorder (early identification, sometimes called *secondary prevention*). Given the serious, chronic, and even life-threatening nature of eating disorders, this argument commands attention.

However, the case for prevention is also very strong. A conservative estimate is that in the United States some two million females (5%) ages 14–34 have a full-blown or subthreshold eating disorder (Shisslak, Crago, & Estes, 1995). If we further assume that the total number of psychiatrists, psychologists, social workers, and dietitians in the United States is approximately 900,000 (Levine, 1996), it becomes clear that identification and rehabilitation are incomplete, inadequate (and expensive) solutions to the problem of eating disorders, and eating problems. Applying the same argument in parallel to the more prevalent problems of mood disorders, anxiety disorders, and substance abuse strengthens an inescapable conclusion: Prevention is neither a luxury nor a fantasy, but a necessity, and there is no theoretical or practical reason to wait until we fully understand the causes (Albee, 1987). Detailed descriptions of successful prevention programs for individuals, families, and communities can be found in Price et al. (1988), Bloom (1996), and Albee and Gullotta (1997).

Targets for Prevention

It is useful to think carefully about the general conceptual models that have guided selection of targets for preventive change. At the risk of oversimplifying, it appears that there are three such models, which in some instances are applied in combination.

---

[1] Detailed reviews of theory, programs, and outcome research can be found in Franko and Orosan-Weine (1998); Killen (chapter in Smolak, Levine, & Striegel-Moore, 1996); Shisslak and colleagues (chapter in Fallon, Katzman, & Wooley, 1994; and chapter in Smolak et al., 1996); Piran and Levine (1996); and Vandereyecken and Noordenbos (in press). Shisslak et al. (chapter in Smolak et al., 1996) offer especially useful prevention suggestions organized by developmental level of target audiences. See "Good Introductory Resources for Primary Prevention" at the end of this article for a list of readable and practical background material for prevention work with schools, families, and other important aspects of one's community.

The Disorder-Specific "Continuity" Model

Many prevention efforts attempt to eliminate the specific causes or components of (or pathways to) the continuum of disordered eating which ranges from weight and shape dissatisfaction to full-blown eating disorders. The focus here is on preventing negative body image, calorie-restrictive dieting, binge-eating, unhealthy weight management techniques (e.g., excessive exercising, cigarette smoking, or fasting), and the attitudes shown in Table 1. This model works from a psychosocial or social learning approach (Killen chapter in Smolak et al., 1996; Stice, 1994) to help teachers, coaches, peers, parents, physicians, and media decrease the presence of "noxious agents" (specific risk factors such as weight and shape-related teasing) and increase individual "resistance" to those agents, for example through promotion of critical thinking skills for evaluating media messages about weight and shape.

The continuity model emphasizes the many similarities between full-blown eating disorders, subthreshold eating problems, and normative weight and shape concerns (Shisslak et al., 1995; see Table 1). However, people at the most pathological end of the continuum also differ in some fundamental ways (Levine & Smolak, 1992). If one follows the logic of a disease-specific perspective, then it is unrealistic to expect that typical prevention efforts—in schools, for example—will have any impact on the development of genetic affective instability, personality disorders, high levels of depression and anxiety, and unhealthy family dynamics (including sexual abuse).

The Nonspecific Life Stress Model

Research has repeatedly shown there is a nonspecific relationship between life stress, coping, and mental disorder. Consequently, "effective prevention programs do not have to await the discovery of specific connections between identifiable causes and the appearance of specific emotional disturbances [such as eating disorders] because such specific connections will never be established" (Albee, 1987, p. 14). According to this model, prevention of many different types of emotional disorders will be facilitated by efforts to reduce stressors while increasing self-esteem, life skills (decision-making, communication, coping with stress), and social support (Albee, 1987; Bloom, 1996).

The life-skills component of this model has been combined with a problem-specific approach in successful school-based curricular programs for the prevention of cigarette smoking in young adolescent boys and girls (Schinke, Botvin, & Orlandi, 1991). In fact, building competencies is an important part of successful prevention programs because education and knowledge are necessary but far from sufficient to effect meaningful changes in attitudes and behavior (Price et al., 1988).

Feminist Model

Piran (1995; and in Piran & Levine, 1996) has described a promising approach to prevention which situates the targets and mechanisms for change primarily in the "lived experience," rela-

---

Table 1. The Continuum of "Nervosa": Attitudes Associated with Eating Disorders and Eating Problems

1. Glorification of slenderness and weight loss

2. Irrational fear of dietary and body fat

3. Prejudicial devaluing of fat people

4. Belief that body shape is the defining feature of one's self-concept and a moral statement about one's life

5. Dichotomous thinking about "good" vs. "bad" foods

6. Negative body image

7. Low self-esteem, often coupled with perfectionist standards

tionships, and potential "authority" of young girls and women, not in the power of experts delivering didactic lessons or making paternal/maternal changes in stressors. Thus, a fundamental target is the *process* of empowering girls and women to change (create) themselves and their environments.

Relational and systemic changes are accomplished by fostering respectful dialogue among girls and between girls and the adults intent on nurturing them. Piran helps girls to articulate issues of harassment, abuse, objectification, and power which are often missing (silenced) in traditional "lessons" designed to prevent eating disorders. Simultaneously, she actively works in her consultant role to ensure that the systems in which girls find themselves (e.g., schools, athletic teams, dance classes) are ready to take seriously the girls' concerns and to change in directions that favor the multidimensional development of young girls.

Based on her long-term work with a high-risk population of students in an elite ballet company, Piran has documented that this process of facilitating and respecting the personal and relational wisdom of young girls leads to (1) changes in specific factors related to eating disorders (e.g., drive for thinness, reduction in peer teasing); (2) dramatic changes in the environment (the reprimanding or firing of teachers who are disrespectful of developing bodies), and (3) improvements in communication skills, problem-solving, interpersonal relationships, and self-esteem (Piran, in press; and in Piran & Levine, 1996).

PRINCIPLES AND ASSUMPTIONS IN EATING DISORDERS PREVENTION

In my own work (see Levine, 1987 in "Good Introductory Resources" and Levine & Hill, 1991 in "Selected Circular Resources" at the end of the article; Levine & Maine, 1995; Smolak, Levine, & Schermer chapter in Vandereycken & Noordenbos, in press) I have found it extremely important for my colleagues and me to clarify the basic principles underlying our prevention efforts. Below is a partial list of the principles that represent our avowedly feminist-cultural perspective (Levine, 1994; Levine & Smolak, 1992). Readers are encouraged to use this list of principles primarily to initiate the important and ongoing *process* of dialogue with one's family, co-workers, and peers, as well as to foster self-awareness.

Five Key Principles

1. ***Beware of the distance created by the "ics"*** (medicalized terms like "anorexics" and "bulimics"). No matter where people are along the spectrum of disordered eating, they are *people,* not *"ics,"* struggling with fantasies, motives, anxieties, and coping mechanisms established and vigorously reinforced by our culture (Gordon, 1990; Silverstein & Perlick, 1995—see "Good Introductory Resources"). Prevention needs to acknowledge the ways in which eating disorders express issues (the meaning of femininity and of power, for example) and processes (the construction of body image, engagement with mass media) embedded in the culture(s) we all live in and create.

2. ***Resist oversimplification, expressed as the "justs."*** There is no scholarly or practical justification for the frequently heard statements that "Eating disorders are just an addiction" . . . "just a variation of depression" . . . "just dieting gone mad." Eating disorders and eating problems, like such other major disorders as depression, have multidimensional causes and complex, heterogeneous manifestations.

3. ***Eating disorders are not "just a woman's problem."*** Boys and men (as friends, lovers, fathers, professionals, politicians) play an important role in reducing risk factors and promoting female "resistance" to developing eating problems (Levine, 1994). Moreover, some groups of men, such as wrestlers, jockeys, gays, and weightlifters, are themselves at high risk for disordered eating.

4. ***Prevention is a social justice issue.*** Eating disorders thrive in the "soil" of prejudice against women and against fat people (Fallon et al., 1994; Levine, 1994). It is unlikely that significant progress in prevention will be made without addressing emotionally and politically charged topics such as fear of women's desires and hungers, sexual harassment and sexual abuse, and limitations in women's avenues for success apart from beauty and sexuality (Piran, 1995). People committed to prevention must consider carefully the implications of the facts that (a) 8–9 times as many females as males develop eating disorders; (b) the high-risk periods of early and late adolescence are those that highlight the meanings of femininity in terms of body

shape, sexuality, and achievement; and (c) eating disorders have proliferated during historical periods (like the present) in which there is marked tension between expanding opportunities for females and continued emphasis on domesticity and subservience to males (Levine, 1994; Levine & Smolak, 1992; Silverstein & Perlick, 1995).

5. ***Collaboration between various professionals and between men and women is essential.*** The factors that contribute to disordered eating are found within concentric circles of personal, familial, peer, media, educational, social, and cultural influences (Smolak et al., 1996; Stice, 1994). These specific causes reflect topics and factors that range from the nature of body fat to success in athletics to the impact of magazine advertisements. Consequently, the teaching and reinforcement of preventive knowledge and life skills requires collaboration between people with varying emphases and skills, including psychologists, physicians, social workers, dietitians, parents, coaches, media consultants, and concerned students, etc. (Levine, 1987; Neumark-Sztainer, 1996). Moreover, egalitarian, respectful, and effective collaboration between

men and women helps to provide young people with multiple models of Principles 3 and 4 listed above.

PREVENTION IN SCHOOLS

Lessons

The public school system is a logical setting for prevention via transmission of knowledge, promotion of healthy attitudes, and teaching of life skills to large numbers of children and adolescents who have not yet developed eating problems or eating disorders (Levine, 1987; Neumark-Sztainer, 1996). A list of available curricular resources follows this article and Table 2 offers a summary of the topics that these "lessons" tend to cover.

Outcome Research

The status of prevention outcome research has been reviewed in detail elsewhere (see, e.g., Franko & Orosan-Weine, 1998; Shisslak & Crago chapter in Fallon et al., 1994; see also Piran, 1995). Based on that work and on more recent developments, three conclusions are warranted. First, the most extensive, sophisticated, and carefully evalu-

---

Table 2. Summary of Topics in Curricular Lessons

1. Increase knowledge about, and promote acceptance of,
   a. physical changes associated with puberty
   b. body fat and fat people
   c. diversity and heritability of weight and shape
   d. regular physical exercise for fun, fitness, and friendship
   e. the nature and dangers of eating disorders, and what students can do to identify them and support friends in getting help
   f. set-point regulation and defense of body weight

2. Discourage calorie-restrictive dieting and promote, in accordance with the Food Guide Pyramid, eating of a wide variety of foods in moderation.

3. Reduce weight and shape-related teasing.

4. Increase knowledge of, and promote resistance to, negative media, peer, and family influences on eating and body image.

5. Promote self-acceptance and development of a positive body image.

6. Promote life skills and well-rounded development by teaching life skills for problem-solving, decision-making, interpersonal communication, and coping with stress.

7. Encourage students, teachers, and other school staff to work together to create a classroom and school environment which does not promote disordered eating.

ated lessons for adolescents (McVey & Davis, 1997; Killen chapter in Smolak et al., 1996; Paxton, 1993) have yielded disappointing results: moderate increases in knowledge but no meaningful prevention effects in terms of attitudes and behaviors.

Second, although these and other nonsignificant findings (Smolak et al. chapter in Vandereycken & Noordenbos, in press) are cause for concern, as is the possibility that lessons may inadvertently transmit disordered eating to those intent on weight loss (Mann et al., 1997), there is little reason for despair or defensiveness. Compared to the extensive theory and research in the field of preventing substance abuse (Schinke et al., 1991), relatively little systematic work has been done on the prevention of disordered eating in school settings. Moreover, recent curricular work by Neumark-Sztainer, Butler, and Palti (1995) with 10th grade Israeli girls, and by Kater (1997—see "Selected Curricular Resources") with fourth and sixth graders in the Minneapolis/St. Paul area, has shown significant increases in knowledge and some meaningful changes in eating behavior and exercising (Neumark-Sztainer et al., 1995) and in attitudes pertaining to body image, fat people, and dieting (Kater, 1997—see "Selected Curricular Resources"). Finally, as emphasized in the feminist-relational work of Piran (1995, in press) and Friedman (1994—see "Selected Curricular Resources"), it is distinctly possible that didactic lessons of the sort contained in standard curricular prevention programs can be only partially effective because neither manufactured knowledge, nor expert advice, nor basic life skills address the systemic basis of disordered eating and the need to empower young girls and women (see Principles 3 and 4 listed above).

Teachers as Models

It is also the case that most curricular prevention programs are limited to classroom lessons and thus do little to change the school environment, including teacher attitudes and behavior. School-based prevention programs are likely to be most successful when the lessons are reinforced by the behavior of teachers, administrators, parents, coaches, and the food service (Neumark-Sztainer, 1996). In their capacity as classroom instructors, coaches, and supervisors of cheerleaders and clubs, teachers in particular can play an important role in reducing risk factors such as the glorification of slen-

derness, prejudice against fat and fat people, and discrimination against women. Here is a partial list of some things teachers can do to help prevent eating disorders (Levine, 1987, 1994; Neumark-Sztainer, 1996):

1. Establish a classroom atmosphere (rules, pictures, practices) that empowers girls and women to feel safe, respected, and encouraged to achieve in ways unrelated to their body shapes and sexuality. Practice listening to and otherwise taking girls and women seriously for who they are—their substance—not for their body shape.

2. Establish rules for the classroom and for one's own behavior that prohibit teasing and other forms of harassment related to weight and shape.

3. Collaborate with other teachers and school staff to resist any practices which glorify slenderness, denigrate fat people, and promote unhealthy weight management behavior. Work to eliminate, for example, diet contests and implicit rules for the size and shape of cheerleaders or dancers.

4. Educate yourself and students about the destructive ways in which media, peers, and other social influences manipulate our attitudes about gender, body shape, sexuality, security, morality, and power. This is an especially important step for male teachers; learning and teaching about gender-related issues and body image is not the sole responsibility of women.

5. As often as possible, incorporate information (lessons) about the following into the teaching of history, social studies, mathematics, science, etc.: genetic determinants of weight and shape; physiological and psychological resistance to weight loss; critical thinking about media messages; and healthy physical changes (including fat accumulation) associated with maturity.

Coaches

Coaches are influential people in the lives of children and adolescents. Moreover, some groups of athletes (gymnasts, swimmers, dancers, and wrestlers, for example) are at high risk for disordered eating (Thompson & Sherman, 1993). In addition to the recommendations for teachers, there are two important things coaches can do (Katrina, pp. 375-376, in Piran & Levine, 1996). First, if possible, provide athletes with nutritional counseling from a professional who knows about the prevention of disordered eating in athletes. Emphasize the importance, especially for growing bodies, of a balanced diet to meet the high energy demands (Clark, 1990). Counseling should also cover myths about performance ("weight loss, fat loss, and becoming thinner is always better"), while highlighting the physical and psychosocial dangers of low weight and rapid, dramatic forms of weight loss.

Second, coaches, trainers, and other staff must avoid teasing, criticizing, and off-the-cuff comments or advice about weight, shape, and weight loss. They should also eliminate weigh-ins, weight-loss contests, and other arrangements (e.g., "weight cutting" in wrestling), which are likely to fuel the bases of disordered eating (see Table 1). Emphasis should be on strength, stamina, and the mental and emotional aspects of better performance.

Parents

Research and everyday observations strongly suggest that parents play an important role in the increasing or reducing risk for disordered eating in children and adolescents (Graber & Brooks-Gunn, in Piran and Levine, 1996; Maine, 1991—see "Good Introductory Resources"). As indicated in Body Image Task Force (undated), Slade (1995), Smolak & Levine (1994), and Maine (1991), to contribute to prevention, parents should reinforce the recommended practices for teachers and coaches. Parents, including fathers, should also:

1. Avoid making critical comments about their own eating, weight, and shape, comments which imply they would be better people if they were thinner.

2. Insist on the right to enjoy swimming, dancing, sunbathing, sexy clothing, etc., regardless of one's size or shape or weight.

3. Help children understand that weight and fat gain are normal, healthy aspects of development, especially during puberty.

4. Interpret "fat talk" as being about "what's eating you?" not "what are you eating?" Help children articulate feelings, understand the negative consequences of dieting, and learn about effective coping.

5. Teach themselves and their children to exercise in moderation for the three F's—fun, fitness, and friendship—not for weight management or compensate for "being bad" in your eating.

6. Work with schools, churches, the YMCA, and other community organizations to expose youth to multiple models of girls and women who are successful in ways related to intellect, artistic creativity, athletic accomplishment, caring, business, etc.

7. Via shopping and relaxed, criticism-free family meals, provide a variety of nutritious foods and refuse to dichotomize foods into "good/safe/low-fat vs. bad/dangerous/fattening."

8. Watch TV and read magazines with children and adolescents and discuss with them the nature and impact of media images of females and males.

9. Work with children to help them "develop interests and skills which will lead to success, personal expression, and fulfillment without emphasis on appearance" (Smolak & Levine, 1994, p. 3).

EATING DISORDER ORGANIZATIONS

Functions

In the United States and Canada there are a number of nonprofit organizations committed to helping professionals and the public understand, identify, treat, and prevent eating disorders. Some are national in scope (e.g., Eating Disorders Awareness & Prevention, Inc. [EDAP], and the National Association of Anorexia Nervosa and Associated Disorders [ANAD]), some are regional (e.g., Massachusetts Eating Disorder Association [MEDA]), and one prominent organization has a university affiliation (Harvard Eating Disorder Center [HEDC]). In the area of prevention these organizations (1) provide resource lists, informative newsletters, videos, and programmatic materials; (2) sponsor regional and national conferences for professionals; (3) facilitate networking between professionals and lay volunteers (Prevention Principle 5); (4) engage in many forms of political activism, including working with the United States government in the areas of public health and funding of prevention research (Prevention Principle 4); and (5) promote concentrated, multidimensional programs such as Eating Disorders Awareness Week (sponsored by EDAP). A selected list of eating disorders organizations appears in Section 7 of this book.

Activism

One area of special interest to eating disorder organizations is the role of mass media in the promotion and reinforcement of many of the components of disordered eating (see Table 1; Levine & Smolak, in Smolak et al., 1996; and in Vandereycken & Noordenbos, in press). ANAD in particular, and more recently EDAP, has been successful in protesting, and facilitating the removal of, advertisements such as the 1988 Hershey Chocolate's "You Can Never Be Too Rich or Too Thin" marketing campaign. Protest, coupled with praise and awards for companies who promote positive, sensible images of women and girls, helps to educate companies about ways they can contribute to prevention.

Activism is also one important way that people committed to prevention can model and otherwise facilitate respect and empowerment ("voice") for adolescent girls (Piran, 1995; Steiner-Adair chapter in Fallon et al., 1994). As I am writing this chapter, EDAP is developing a prevention research project called "GoGIRLS." This program gives adolescent girls the opportunity to (1) participate in feminist-relational discussion groups (Piran, 1995); (2) learn about mass media influences on body image, eating behavior, etc.; and (3) actively engage in working with adults and with one another to protest or praise magazine advertisements, television programs, etc.

CONCLUSIONS

No one exactly knows how to prevent eating disorders. Theory and speculation (including my own) abound, but as of August 1998 less than 20 formal programs have been implemented and systematically evaluated in schools and/or communities. Those programs that have been constructed and evaluated by sophisticated prevention researchers (e.g., Killen, Paxton, & Neumark-Sztainer) have generally been unsuccessful or otherwise limited in their effects. Nevertheless, prevention of eating disorders remains a commitment for those of us—professionals, parents, citizens—who have carefully read the literature on primary prevention (Albee & Gullotta, 1997), who have seen dramatic changes in our own philosophies and

behaviors concerning weight, shape, and gender, and who have witnessed dramatic changes during the latter half of the 20th century when it comes to domestic violence, women in athletics, drunk driving, seat belt use, and, of course, cigarette smoking. This commitment and conviction is succinctly expressed by George Albee (1987, p. 11), for over 30 years a leader in the field of prevention:

> Public health wisdom states that mass disorders afflicting humankind rarely or never have been brought under control or eliminated by attempts at treating each afflicted individual, nor by efforts at increasing the number of professional individual treatment providers. Rather, successes have come through public health methods that have stressed (a) finding the noxious agent and eliminating or neutralizing it, and/or (b) strengthening the host's resistance to the noxious agent, and/or (c) preventing transmission of the noxious agent to the host.

REFERENCES

Albee, G. (1987). The rationale and need for primary prevention. In S. E. Goldston (Ed.), *Concepts of primary prevention: A framework for program development* (pp. 7-19). California Department of Mental Health, Office of Prevention.

Albee, G., & Gullotta, T. (Eds.). (1997). *Primary prevention works.* Thousand Oaks, CA: Sage.

Bloom, M. (1996). *Primary prevention practices.* Thousand Oaks, CA: Sage.

Body Image Task Force/M. Griffin. (undated). *Building blocks for children's body image.* Pamphlet available from BITF, P. O. Box 934, Santa Cruz, CA 95061-0934.

Clark, N. (1990). *Nancy Clark's sports nutrition guidebook.* Champaign, IL: Leisure Press.

Fallon, P., Katzman, M., & Wooley, S. C. (Eds.). (1994). *Feminist perspectives on eating disorders.* New York: Guilford.

Franko, D. L., & Orosan-Weine, P. (1998). The prevention of eating disorders: Empirical, methodological and conceptual considerations. *Clinical Psychology: Science and Practice, 5*(4), 459–477.

Gordon, R. A. (1990). *Anorexia and bulimia: Anatomy of a social epidemic.* Cambridge, MA: Basil Blackwell.

Levine, M. P. (1987). *Student eating disorders: Anorexia nervosa and bulimia.* Washington, D.C.: National Education Association.

Levine, M. P. (1994). Beauty myth and the beast: What men can do and be to help prevent eating disorders. *Eating Disorders: The Journal of Treatment & Prevention, 2*(2), 101-113.

Levine, M. P. (1996). Researching the future of primary prevention. *The Renfrew Perspective, 2*(1; Spring; Prevention Issue), 6-7. Call 1-800-RENFREW.

Levine, M. P., & Maine, M. (1995). *A guide to the primary prevention of eating disorders.* Pamphlet available from EDAP, Inc., 603 Stewart Street, Suite 803, Seattle, WA 98101.

Levine, M. P., & Smolak, L. (1992). Toward a model of the developmental psychopathology of eating disorders: The example of early adolescence. In J. H. Crowther, D. L. Tennenbaum, S. E. Hobfoll, & M. A. P. Stephens (Eds.), *The etiology of bulimia nervosa: The individual and familial context* (pp. 59-80). Washington, D. C.: Taylor & Francis.

Mann, T., Nolen-Hoeksema, S., Huang, K., Burgard, D., Wright, A., & Hanson, K. (1997). Are two interventions worse than none? Joint primary and secondary prevention of eating disorders in college females. *Health Psychology, 16*(3), 1-11.

McVey, G. & Davis, R. (1997). *A program to promote positive body image in young adolescent females: A 1-year follow-up.* Unpublished manuscript, available from Dr. McVey, The Hospital for Sick Children, 555 University Avenue, Toronto, Ontario, Canada M5G 1X8.

Neumark-Sztainer, D. (1995). Excessive weight preoccupation: Normative but not harmless. *Nutrition Today, 30*(2), 68-74.

Neumark-Sztainer, D. (1996). School-based programs for preventing eating disturbances. *Journal of School Health, 66*(2), 64-71.

Neumark-Sztainer, D., Butler, R., & Palti, H. (1995). Eating disturbances among adolescent girls: Evaluation of a school-based primary prevention program. *Journal of Nutrition Education, 27*(1), 24-30.

Paxton, S. J. (1993). A prevention program for disturbed eating and body dissatisfaction in adolescent girls: a 1 year follow-up. *Health Education Research: Theory & Practice, 8,* 43-51.

Piran, N. (1995). Prevention: Can early lessons lead to a delineation of an alternative model? A critical look at prevention with schoolchildren. *Eating Disorders: The Journal of Treatment & Prevention, 3*(1), 28-36.

Piran, N. (in press). A trial of prevention in a high risk school setting. *Journal of Primary Prevention.*

Piran, N., & Levine, M. P., (Eds.). (1996). Special prevention issue. *Eating Disorders: Journal of Treatment & Prevention, 4*(4), 291-384.

Price, R. H., Cowen, E. L., Lorion, R. P., & Ramos-McKay, J. (Eds.). (1988). *14 ounces of prevention: A casebook for practitioners.* Washington, D.C.: American Psychological Association.

Schinke, S. P., Botvin, G. J., & Orlandi, M. A. (1991). *Substance abuse in children and adolescents: Evaluation and interventions.* Newbury Park, CA: Sage.

Shisslak, C. M., Crago, M., & Estes, L. S. (1995). The spectrum of eating disorders. *International Journal of Eating Disorders, 18*(3), 209-219.

Slade, P. (1995). Prospects for prevention. In G. Szmukler, C. Dare, & J. Treasure (Eds.), *Handbook of eating disorders. Theory, treatment and research* (pp. 385-398). Chicester: Wiley.

Smolak, L., & Levine, M. P. (1994). The role of parents in the prevention of disordered eating. *Newsletter of the National Eating Disorder Organization, 17*(3), 1-4, 9. (See appendixes for address information for NEDO.)

Smolak, L., Levine, M. P., & Striegel-Moore, R. (Eds.). (1996). *The developmental psychopathology of eating disorders.* Mahwah, NJ: Lawrence Erlbaum Associates.

Stice, E. (1994). Review of the evidence for a sociocultural model of bulimia nervosa and an exploration of the mechanisms of action. *Clinical Psychology Review, 14*(7), 633-661.

Thompson, R. A., & Sherman, R. (1993). *Helping athletes with eating disorders.* Champaign, IL: Human Kinetics.

Vandereycken, W., & Noordenbos, G., (Eds.). (in press). *Prevention of eating disorders.* London: Athlone.

Good Introductory Resources for Primary Prevention

Costin, C. (1996). *The eating disorder sourcebook: A comprehensive guide to the causes, treatments, and prevention of eating disorders.* Los Angeles: Lowell House.

Costin, C. (1996). *Your dieting daughter: Is she dying for attention?* New York: Brunner/Mazel.

Freedman, R. J. (1988). *BodyLove.* New York: Harper & Row.

Friedman, S. S. (1997). *When girls feel fat: Helping girls through adolescence.* Toronto: HarperCollins.

Hall, L. (Ed.). (1993). *Full lives: Women who have freed themselves from food & weight obsession.* Carlsbad, CA: Gurze Books.

Ikeda, J., & Naworski, P. (1992). *Am I fat? Helping young children accept differences in body size.* Santa Cruz, CA: ETR Associates.

Levine, M. P. (1987). *Student eating disorders: Anorexia nervosa and bulimia.* Washington, D.C.: National Education Association.

Maine, M. (1991). *Father hunger: Fathers, daughters & food.* Carlsbad, CA: Gurze Books.

Silverstein, B., & Perlick, D. (1995). *The cost of competence: Why inequality causes depression, eating disorders, and illness in women.* New York: Oxford University Press.

Valette, B. (1988). *A parent's guide to eating disorders: Prevention and treatment of anorexia nervosa and bulimia.* New York: Walker.

Selected Curricular Resources for the Prevention of Eating Disorders

Late Elementary School

Department of Food Science. (undated). *Healthy growth: Nutrition lessons for 9- to 12-year-old children.* Available from Dr. R. D. Terry, Human Nutrition, Iowa State University, Ames, IA 50011. [contains lessons on body image, growth, and nutrition]

Kater, K. J. (1997). *Teaching kids to eat, and love their bodies too!* [grades 4–6]. Available from the author, Franklin Center, Suite 109, 2497 Seventh Avenue East, North St. Paul, MN 55109. (Available from EDAP, Inc., see p. 235, Nonprofit Eating Disorders Organizations)

National Eating Disorder Information Centre. (1989). *Teacher's resource kit: A teacher's lesson plan kit for the prevention of eating disorders.* Available from NEDIC, 200 Elizabeth Street, CW 1-328, Toronto, Ontario M5G 2C4.

Adolescence

Carney, B. (1986). *Preventive curriculum for anorexia nervosa and bulimia.* Windsor, Ontario: Bulimia and Anorexia Nervosa Association (BANA)—Can/Am. Available from BANA, University of Windsor, 401 Sunset Avenue, Ontario, Canada N9B 3P4.

Friedman, S. (1994). *Girls in the 90's facilitator's manual.* Vancouver: Salal Books (Salal Communications, Ltd., 101-1184 Denman St., #309, Vancouver, B.C. V6G 2M9.

Levine, M. P., & Hill, L. (1991). *A five-day lesson plan book on eating disorders: Grades 7-12.* Available from the National Eating Disorder Organization, 6655 South Yale Avenue, Tulsa, OK 74136.

Neumark-Sztainer, D. (1992). *The weight to eat! A program for the prevention of eating disturbances among adolescents.* Contact the author at Division of Epidemiology, School of Public Health, 1300 South Second Street, Suite 300, University of Minnesota, Minneapolis, MN 55454.

Eating Disorders in Males: Critical Questions

by Arnold E. Andersen, M.D.

Eating disorders in males makes up a fascinating, sometimes neglected, area of clinical and research interest, of increasing importance currently as pressures on males to change their weight and shape increase.

Eating disorders, usually associated with females, have historically existed in men as well. For example, in 1694 Dr. Richard Morton, physician to the King of England, first described anorexia nervosa in a study of two patients, one of whom was male. The outcome of treatment for the male was good, while the female died. These two points remain important to any discussion of the subject of eating disorders in males today: Males do develop eating disorders, and maleness is not a negative risk factor.

Sir William Gull, in his detailed study of anorexia nervosa in the mid-19th century, also described males suffering from this disorder. So why has there been so little mention of eating-disordered males since then? First, some psychodynamically based theories of anorexia nervosa required the presence of a "fear of oral impregnation" or the presence of amenorrhea (abnormal absence of menstruation), both of which would exclude males.

On a less theoretical level, males with eating disorders may have sought professional help so infrequently that they became a statistical rarity. Finally, socioculturally determined stereotypes held by both patients and clinicians that males do not develop eating disorders often result in this diagnosis being overlooked, whereas similar symptoms in a female would prompt a correct identification.

Beginning in the 1960s, Crisp and others noted the occurrence of anorexia nervosa in male subjects, and interest among researchers has been increasing since. Unlike anorexia nervosa, bulimia nervosa was not defined as a clinical syndrome until the late 1970s. Bulimia in males is still being studied for prevalence, treatment response, and long-term outcome, but appears similar in most ways to the disorder in females.

CRITICAL QUESTIONS

The following are some provocative questions and tentative answers related to the occurrence of eating disorders in males, based on currently available information.

1. Do Males Develop Eating Disorders?

The answer is a definite "yes." The three essential requirements for the diagnosis of anorexia nervosa pertain equally well to males and females: (1) self-induced weight loss of a substantial degree; (2) a morbid fear of becoming fat; and (3) an abnormality of reproductive hormone functioning.

The diagnosis of bulimia nervosa likewise can be applied equally to males and females. The essential diagnostic features are compulsive binge eating, followed by remorse and/or physical distress, excessive fear of fatness as with anorexia nervosa, and a variety of compensating behaviors to avoid weight gain from the binge episodes—purging by vomiting, laxatives, or diuretics in 80 percent of cases, and other means (compensating, fasting, over-exercising) in 20 percent. Binge eating disorder, still being studied as a possibly distinct new syndrome, requires binge eating with *no* compensation. Only males appear to develop "reverse anorexia" in which no degree of bigness is adequate for them.

2. How Many Males Suffer from Eating Disorders?

Ten percent of cases presenting to Johns Hopkins Hospital Eating and Weight Disorders Clinic and the University of Iowa were males (Andersen,

1992). A recent community-based study from Sweden found an almost identical incidence of 10 females to 1 male having an eating disorder (Rastam, Gillberg, & Gorton, 1989), confirmed by studies in Denmark (Nielsen, 1990). The number of individuals with an eating disorder in the 75 million young people aged 5 to 25 in the United States ranges from 2 percent to 5 percent, depending on the criteria used, with at least one-tenth of these being male.

3. Why Do So Few Males Develop Eating Disorders?

Four factors have been suggested as biological reasons why males are less likely to develop eating disorders.

First, some recent studies have suggested that males may respond differently to intravenous doses of L-tryptophan, an amino acid precursor to the neurotransmitter serotonin, when compared with females. While not proven to relate to weight gain or site or fat deposition, serotonin affects mood and hunger/satiety cues. Second, the male hypothalamus from early in fetal life produces a steady-state rather than a cyclical, "pulsed" pattern of sex hormones. Third, the presence of a high testosterone to estrogen ratio in the developing male contributes to an increased ratio of lean muscle mass to body fat. Fourth, men have a substantially lower percentage of body fat than women, the fat tissue serving as an important organ in metabolizing hormones.

Having recognized the presence of these four biological differences between males and females, the conclusion is that they probably are insignificant with regard to the development of eating disorders. Current evidence weighs heavily in favor of psychological and social rather than biological reasons for the differential rate of eating disorders in males and females. Hsu (1989) has examined the gender gap in eating disorders and concludes that "eating disorders are more prevalent in the female because more of them are dieting to lose or control weight." Other support in this direction comes from studies by Andersen and DiDomenico (1990). When the 10 popular magazines most frequently read by men were compared with the 10 most often read by women, they found a ratio of 10.5 to 1 in women's versus men's magazines for articles and advertisements concerning weight loss. This ratio duplicates almost exactly the ratio of eating-disordered women to

men. Men, however, are disproportionately influenced toward changing body *shape*, especially to achieve a hyper-masculine, V-shaped upper-body appearance.

The hypothesis that females are encouraged more strongly by society and culture to lose weight is well supported. Every significant difference in gender-related frequency of behaviors related to body weight or shape change can be correlated with intensity of existing sociocultural values. Where a sociocultural norm is equally distributed between the sexes, the behavioral response is roughly equal in both sexes. These behavioral disorders, it appears, are primarily triggered by society and culture, not caused by biomedical problems, although there undoubtedly are important secondary biological mechanisms responsible for the perpetuation of illness. It may help to conceptually divide the illness process into predisposing features, precipitating factors, and sustaining mechanisms.

4. Why Do Certain Males Develop Eating Disorders?

The major risk factors that have been associated in general with the development of an eating disorder are:

a. Living in an industrialized country whose sociocultural norms promote slimness and the avoidance of fatness.

b. An increased incidence of affective (mood) disorders in the family of the patient.

c. The presence of a vulnerable personality, either from Cluster B of the *Diagnostic and Statistical Manual* (*DSM-IV*) of the American Psychiatric Association (narcissistic-histrionic-borderline, predisposing to bulimia) or Cluster C (sensitive-avoidant-obsessional, predisposing to anorexia, restricting).

d. Dieting behavior, especially during the critical adolescent and early adult years.

e. Dysfunctional family patterns in which an eating disorder produces a stabilizing effect.

f. Membership in a vulnerable sports or interest subgroup where weight loss is required, such as wrestling.

g. A history of sexual abuse, the emergence of "sex disgust" during adolescence, or the presence of other issues in sexuality that are made more tolerable by patterns of weight loss and strict self-denial.

In addition, males, compared with females, diet for four major reasons:

a. In contrast with women who, in general, *felt* fat before they dieted but were actually at normal weight, males who went on to develop eating disorders *were*, generally, mildly to moderately obese at some time, especially if the eating disorder included any bulimic features. They were especially sensitive as boys to being teased about their weight (Andersen & Holman, 1997).

b. Men, more often than women, dieted either to attain certain goals in sports or to avoid the possible weight-gaining effects of a sports-related injury that forced them to decrease temporarily their physical activity (Garner & Rosen, 1991).

c. More men than women diet to avoid potential medical complications, especially ones they had seen develop in their fathers. No young women dieted to avoid future medical illness, and only one older woman in her 40s did so.

d. Occasionally males dieted to be more attractive to a gay partner.

These four specific factors were statistically much more likely to occur in males ($p < .01$) than in females (Andersen & Holman, 1997).

5. Do Differences Exist in the Natural History of Males and Females in the Development of Eating Disorders?

Tables 1 and 2 suggest a series of stages through which anorexia nervosa and bulimia nervosa progress in both males and females. The process of development from relatively normal behavior (dieting) to a clinically recognizable eating disorder occurs in a predictable, sequential fashion, but the mechanisms to explain this transition are not yet well understood.

6. What Is the Nature of Sexuality in Males with Eating Disorders?

In teenaged males, issues concerning sexual identity seem to trigger eating disorders, while later life issues, such as marital and work-related conflicts, may be primary triggers in older men. Herzog, Bradburn, and Newman (1990) have noted that "anorexic males display a considerable degree of anxiety with regard to sexual activities and relationships" (p. 41). Low levels of sexual activity before and during the onset have been noted among anorexic males by Fichter and Daser (1987).

Bulimic males, as with bulimic females, are generally more sexually active both before the onset of bulimia and at the time of their illness. Burns and Crisp (1990) have associated the outcome of anorexia nervosa in males with the fre-

---

Table 1. Stages of Development of Anorexia Nervosa

Stage 1: **A Normal Behavior**
Normal, voluntary dieting behavior.

Stage 2: **A Diagnosable Clinical Disorder**
Dieting not under personal control, with serious medical, social, psychological consequences. Characterized by morbid fear of fatness. *DSM-IV* criteria met.

Stage 3A: **Autonomous Behavior: Illness Becomes Fixed**
The disorder does not resolve itself even if conditions stimulating its origin improve. Behavior is not responsive to any degree of personal control. Secondary mechanisms frequently present.

Stage 3B: **Illness Becomes an Identity**
The patient identifies with being the illness, not only having the illness (I *am* anorexic). Prospect of loss of illness leads to existential fears of nothingness.

Table 2. Stages of Development of Bulimia Nervosa

Stage 1A: **Normal Dieting Behavior**

Similar to anorexia nervosa, Stage 1.

Stage 1B: **Involuntary Binge Behavior**

Dieting behavior and weight loss lead to bingeing, based on response to hunger.

Stage 2: **A Diagnosable Disorder**

The trigger for binge behavior generalizes from hunger to a variety of painful mood states. Marked fear of fatness is present. Meets *DSM-IV* criteria. May have serious medical, social, psychological consequences.

Stage 3A: **Autonomous Behavior**

Binges are autonomous, frequent, large. Secondary mechanisms often present.

Stage 3B: **Illness Becomes an Identity**

The thought of living without bulimic behavior provokes great fear, leading to an existential lack of identity and fear of inability to cope with mood changes, stress, relationship difficulties.

quency of pre-eating disorder sexual activity. The worst outcome occurred in those with the least pre-eating disorder sexual activity. Gay males represent about 20 percent of eating-disordered males, several times the baseline prevalence, but still a minority. The increased occurrence in gay males is most likely related to the higher valuation placed on slimness in the gay community, not on biological factors (Siever, 1994).

Several studies have documented that anorexia nervosa in males is associated with a decrease in plasma testosterone. In contrast to the "on-off" phenomenon of amenorrhea in females, the decreased testosterone in males is more linearly proportional to the decrease in the male's weight, suggesting it may be one parameter to monitor to establish return to healthy weight during treatment of anorexic males.

7. What Are the Psychological Characteristics of Males with Eating Disorders?

Both males and females with eating disorders appear more likely to have other co-morbid major psychiatric disorders as well as companion personality disorders. The most common diagnoses are mood disorders, drug and alcohol abuse, anxiety syndromes, obsessive-compulsive disorders, and personality disorders.

What is the reason for the increased incidence of eating disorders in patients from families with diagnosed mood disorders? It can be argued

(Andersen, 1990) that since mood disorders are heritable, when a young person experiences depressive illness, the low mood appears to make them more self-critical especially toward body fat. Also, self-starving and/or binge-purge behaviors temporarily improve mood, somewhat like a drug fix.

Numerous studies have documented an increase in the frequency of personality disorders with eating disorders. There is also some differential frequency of the type of personality disorders with subtype of eating disorder. Piran et al. (1988) have found that bulimic patients, compared with anorexic patients, have a higher probability of having abnormal personality features from Cluster B, the narcissistic-histrionic-borderline category. In contrast, food-restricting anorexics have a higher probability of deriving their personality disorder, when present, from Cluster C, with the characteristic obsessional, sensitive, perfectionistic, and obsessive-compulsive features.

Although males share with females many of the predisposing factors of eating disorders, they also experience some important separate issues reflecting male vulnerabilities and societal pressures. First, males who are actually obese in either childhood or adulthood, versus perceiving themselves to be, are more apt to have lasting sensitivity to being criticized. This is true especially in males with high sensitivity during critical phases of development.

Second, low self-esteem, whether from personality vulnerabilities or crucial family inter-

---

Table 3. Stages in Treatment of Eating Disorders with Male Focus

Stage 1: Decision regarding inpatient versus outpatient treatment, or day hospital (partial hospital).

Stage 2: Accurate diagnosis and exclusion of differential diagnoses (e.g., swallowing disorders, primary medical illness, primary mood disorder).

Stage 3: Medical evaluation and stabilization.

Stage 4: Diagnosis of Axis I and Axis II co-morbidities with comprehensive treatment plan.

Stage 5: Nutritional rehabilitation to restore healthy body weight, including even modest underweight.

Stage 6: Interruption of binge-purge behavior and identification of triggers.

Stage 7: Psychological testing to assess quantitatively the eating disorders and general psychopathology.

Stage 8: Appropriate psychopharmacology to treat persistent depression and obsessive-compulsive disorder if weight restoration and normalized eating do not suffice.

Stage 9: Sequence of psychotherapy according to patient needs, emphasizing cognitive-behavioral psychotherapy (CBT) and integrating family therapy, especially for patients under 18.

Stage 10: Identification and treatment plan for unique male issues, including relationship with father, sexual identity, body shape, and emotional expressivity.

Stage 11: Behavioral practice in choosing meals, purchasing clothing, and planning everyday activities without eating-disordered behaviors.

Stage 12: Extended follow-up, generally for two to five years. The evidence is accumulating that intensive definitive early care costs more in the beginning but soon becomes cheaper and much more enduring than a "revolving door" approach (Kaye, Kaplan, & Zucker, 1996).

---

actions, can lead males to attempt to attain through dieting a stereotypical, mesomorphic shape, which they fantasize will make them feel more masculine, in greater control of themselves, and more commanding of respect from those around them. Males generally wish to change their bodies from the waist up, while females usually dislike their bodies from the waist down. Use of steroids to change body shape and size may lead to physical and psychological dependence (Brower et al., 1990).

8. Treatment of Males with Eating Disorders: How Are They Similar, How Are They Different?

Table 3 summarizes the essential steps of treatment for males with eating disorders. Treatment involves working with a series of interactive methods, appreciating both the shared and the unique features of males and females; recognizing the biological, psychological, and sociocultural contributions to the illness; and addressing the need for individual, group, and family methods.

With some exceptions, most males with bulimia nervosa can be treated as outpatients,

while most patients meeting the criteria for anorexia nervosa need to be treated in the hospital. Medical assessment should be followed by prompt medical stabilization, especially of vital signs, laboratory abnormalities, and cardiac rate and rhythm. The most pressing initial issues are usually treatment of severe starvation, with its associated medical dangers, and treatment of the systemic effects of hypokalemia (potassium deficiency in the blood) and other metabolic disorders that are secondary to vomiting and/or purging behavior.

A variety of approaches to nutritional rehabilitation have been tried, but no definitive studies can confirm that one particular method is clearly superior. In general, I favor the approach of "normal food eaten normally," supervised by nurses or other trained staff. A weight restoration of two and one-half to three and one-half pounds a week can usually be safely accomplished without significant refeeding syndrome (peripheral edema hypophosphatemia, gastrointestinal bloating).

Closely supervising patients during the vulnerable phase after admission to inpatient care will promptly interrupt bingeing and purg-

Table 4. Sequence of Psychotherapy Methods for Most Eating-Disordered Males[a]

Method	Comment
Supportive and psychoeducational work	To restore morale, reintegrate existing defenses, and educate concerning nature of illness. (First two weeks)
Cognitive-behavioral methods, including body image work, challenging core beliefs and schemas	To identify and replace abnormal beliefs, attitudes, and behaviors leading to the eating disorder's patterns. This is the core of treatment. (Several weeks to months)
Psychodynamic psychotherapy	To make "connections" and resolve central dynamic conflicts. Often done on an outpatient basis during relapse prevention continuing care. Focus on readapting to male role. (Several months to one to two years)
Existential psychotherapy	To explore issues in meaning, values, and suffering. To develop purpose and spiritual dimensions. (Several months to one year)

a: All forms of psychotherapy can be implemented in an individual, group, or family context.

havior or out-of-control exercise. The next and considerably more difficult goal is to translate this external supervision into the patient's own will so that normal eating and avoidance of binge-purge behavior becomes a self-governed, rather than other-governed, practice. For many patients, this transition requires identifying clearly the triggers for binge behavior and learning to choose alternative healthy behaviors. All-or-none reasoning tends to lead patients to think that any relapse, such as an occasional binge, is a sign of failure and, therefore, an excuse to give up. We encourage the outpatient approach of "shaping" binge-related behaviors toward decreased frequency, recognizing that progress often occurs gradually, rather than the less achievable "gone for good" goal that leads to demoralization if relapse occurs. In the inpatient program, all abnormal behaviors are immediately interrupted.

Patients with personality disorders generally benefit less from medication than from an approach that helps them increase their strengths and decrease their weaknesses. Identifying and working with those aspects of personality that are functioning effectively to deal with those features that are not remains the essence of treatment of a personality disorder. Borderline personality is generally the greatest challenge.

The fundamental core of treatment of eating disorders is psychotherapeutic work—persuading people to understand the origin and course of their eating disorder; the purpose it serves; how to

"trade in and trade up"; how to act sanely in a weight- and shape-preoccupied culture of narcissism and densely packed calories; how to deal in a healthy way with their own life development issues and relationships; and how to decrease their overvalued ideas and misbeliefs about the benefits of thinness. To arrive at the point of beginning effective psychotherapeutic work, however, many hurdles must be overcome. Starvation needs to be treated so that thinking is clear and focused. Metabolic abnormalities must be corrected. Co-morbidities that interfere with psychotherapy, such as mood disorders, anxiety states, obsessive-compulsive disorder, and alcohol and drug abuse, must be treated. Table 4 suggests a four-stage approach to psychological treatment, with an emphasis on males.

In particular, male athletes may benefit from specific limits on weight loss such as those successfully implemented in Wisconsin for wrestlers (Oppliger et al., 1995). Males may have as much of a problem with the medical complications of osteopenia as females.

CONCLUSION

More questions than answers exist regarding males with eating disorders. Nonetheless, adequate information is available to allow clinicians to diagnose accurately eating disorders in males and to organize comprehensive, multidimensional treatment. A practical approach to males with eating disorders will address those aspects of illness that are shared with women as well as those that are unique to males. Maleness is not an adverse factor for short-term or long-term wellness. There is no evidence that males with eating disorders have a worse prognosis or outcome than females. The goal is cure—cultural normality—not simply improvement. Virtually every aspect of these illnesses is treatable. A stance of optimism tempered with realism, knowledge, and experience will guide current practice until well-designed research inquiries into causes, mechanism, and treatment lead to more fundamental understanding for the future.

REFERENCES

Andersen, A. E. (1990). A proposed mechanism underlying eating disorders and other disorders of motivated behavior. In A. E. Andersen (Ed.), *Males with eating disorders* (pp. 221–254). New York: Brunner/Mazel.

Andersen, A. E. (1992). Analysis of treatment experience and outcome from the Johns Hopkins Eating Disorders Program: 1975-1990. In K. H. (Ed.), *Psychobiology and Treatment of Anorexia Nervosa and Bulimia Nervosa* (pp. 93–124). Washington, D.C.: American Psychiatric Association Press.

Andersen, A. E., & DiDomenico, L. (1992). Diet vs. shape content of popular male and female magazines: A dose-response relationship to the incidence of eating disorders? *International Journal of Eating Disorders* 11(3), 283–287.

Andersen, A. E., & Holman, J. E. (1997). Males with eating disorders: Challenges for treatment and research. *Psychopharmacology Bulletin* 3, 391-397.

Brower, K. J., Eliopulos, G. A., Blow, F. C., Catlin, D. H., & Beresford, T. P. (1990). Evidence for physical and psychological dependence on anabolic androgenic steroids in eight weight lifters. *American Journal of Psychiatry* 147(4), 510–512.

Burns, T., & Crisp, A. H. (1990). Outcome of anorexia nervosa in males. In A. E. Andersen (Ed.), *Males with eating disorders* (pp. 163–186). New York: Brunner/Mazel.

Fichter, M. M., & Daser, C. C. (1987). Symptomatology, psychosexual development, and gender identity in 42 anorexic males. *Psychological Medicine 17*, 409–418.

Garner, D. M., & Rosen, L. W. (1991). Eating disorders among athletes: Research and recommendations. *Journal of Applied Sports Science Research 5*(2), 100–107.

Herzog, D. B., Bradburn, I. S., & Newman, K. (1990). Sexuality in males with eating disorders. In A. E. Andersen (Ed.), *Males with eating disorders* (pp. 40–53). New York: Brunner/Mazel.

Hsu, L. K. G. (1989). The gender gap in eating disorders: Why are the eating disorders more common among women? *Clinical Psychology Review 9*, 393–407.

Kaye, W. H., Kaplan, A. S., & Zucker, M. L. (1996). Treating eating-disorder patients in a managed care environment: Contemporary American issues and a Canadian response. In J. Yager (Ed.), *The psychiatric clinics of North America* (pp. 793-810). Philadelphia: W.B. Saunders.

Nielsen, S. (1990). The epidemiology of anorexia nervosa in Denmark from 1973 to 1987: A nationwide register study of psychiatric admission. *Acta Psychiatrica Scandinavica 81*, 507–14.

Oppliger, R. A., Harms, R. D., Hermann, D. E., Streich, C. M., & Clark, R. R. (1995). Grappling with weight cutting: The Wisconsin wrestling minimum weight project. *The Physician and Sportsmedicine 23*(3), 69-78.

Piran, N., Lerner, P., Garfinkel, P. E., et al. (1988). Personality disorders in anorexic patients. *International Journal of Eating Disorders 7*, 589–599.

Rastam, M., Gillbert, D., & Garton, M. (1989). Anorexia nervosa in a Swedish urban region: a population-based study. *British Journal of Psychiatry 155*, 642–646.

Siever, M. D. (1994). Sexual orientation and gender as factors in socioculturally acquired vulnerability to body dissatisfaction and eating disorders. *Journal of Consulting and Clinical Psychology 62*(2), 252–260.

Eating Disorders Among Athletes

by Catherine M. Shisslak, Ph.D., and Marjorie Crago, Ph.D.

Eating disorders exist in all subgroups of the general population. Among females the prevalence of anorexia nervosa is estimated to range from 0.5 percent to 1.0 percent; bulimia nervosa is estimated to range from 1 percent to 3 percent (Leon, 1991; Shisslak, Crago, & Estes, 1995).

Subclinical or partial syndrome eating disorders are estimated to occur in an additional 3 percent to 5 percent of females (Shisslak et al., 1995). Marked gender differences characterize eating disorder rates: Only 5 percent to 10 percent of eating disorder cases occur among males in the general population (Wilmore, 1991).

Prevalence rates for eating disorders are considerably higher, however, in certain subgroups of the population. Rates tend to be higher among athletes who participate in sports that emphasize thinness for performance and/or appearance, such as gymnastics, ballet, figure skating, swimming, and running (Brownell, 1995; Leon, 1991; Yates, 1991). Rates also tend to be higher among female than male athletes. For example, in a study of more than 4,000 runners, 24 percent of the females had high scores on a screening measure for eating disorders, compared with only 8 percent of the males (Kiernan, Rodin, Brownell, Wilmore, & Crandall, 1992). Wrestling and body building are the two sports in which the greatest number of eating disorder cases among male athletes have been reported (Dick, 1991; Pope, Katz, & Hudson, 1993).

To attain and maintain a low body weight, many athletes resort to using the same unhealthy weight-loss methods employed by eating-disordered patients. These include restrictive dieting; ingesting laxatives, diet pills, and diuretics; and self-induced vomiting. Across a variety of studies, 15 percent to 62 percent of female athletes reported using one or more of these methods at some time in their athletic career (Brownell & Rodin, 1992; Leon, 1991; Wilmore, 1991). However, only a subset of these athletes go on to develop a full-syndrome eating disorder. Most discontinue such behaviors when the athletic season ends or when they retire from competitive sports. It should be noted, however, that even athletes who develop a partial- rather than full-syndrome eating disorder may experience impaired athletic performance, an increased risk of injury, and medical complications due to their disordered eating or use of unhealthy weight loss methods (Beals & Manore, 1994). Also, individuals with a partial-syndrome eating disorder may go on to develop a full-syndrome eating disorder later on (Beals & Manore, 1994; Shisslak et al., 1995).

Thus far, no large-scale studies have examined the prevalence of eating disorders in both male and female athletes across a variety of sports. Those studies reported to date are likely to underestimate the actual prevalence of eating disorders among athletes as several studies acknowledge that athletes tended to underreport eating disorder symptoms (e.g., Brownell & Rodin, 1992; Sundgot-Borgen, 1993; Wilmore, 1991). Large-scale longitudinal research is needed to provide a more accurate estimate of the prevalence of eating disorders among athletes participating in different sports and to identify those factors that increase the likelihood that an athlete will develop an eating disorder.

RISK FACTOR

One of the most obvious risk factors for eating disorders among athletes is participation in sports that emphasize thinness for performance and/or appearance. However, some investigators have raised the question of whether participation in these sports causes eating disorders or whether individuals with eating disorders are drawn to these sports (Brownell, 1995). The possible link between sports, exercise, and eating disorders has been explored in a number of studies (for reviews, see Eisler & le Grange, 1990, and Yates, Shisslak, Crago, & Allender, 1994). In a series of well-controlled animal studies, Epling and Pierce (1992) demonstrated that food restriction can lead to excessive exercise, which, in turn, leads to further restricted food intake by the animal. Approximately 80 percent of food-deprived rats who were allowed to engage in high levels of physical activity reduced their food intake even further, resulting in death from starvation in some cases. Davis and colleagues (1994) found evidence of exercise-induced anorexia nervosa in a study of 45 eating-disordered patients. Sixty percent of the patients reported being competitive athletes before the onset of their disorder, and 75 percent reported that their physical activity levels increased as their food intake decreased, just as Epling and Pierce (1992) found in their animal studies.

Another avenue of research that has yielded a number of studies focuses on the similarities of certain personality traits in athletes and eating-disordered patients. Among these are high achievement motivation, perfectionism, obsessive-compulsive tendencies, and persistence in accomplishing one's goals despite discomfort or pain (Beals & Manore, 1994; Hauck & Blumenthal, 1992; Johnson, 1994; Yates, 1991). Pruitt, Kappius, and Imm (1991) hypothesize that, despite these similarities, a major difference is that athletes tend to have higher self-esteem than eating-disordered patients, which may offer them protection against eating disorders.

Other risk factors for the development of eating disorders were identified by Sundgot-Borgen (1994) in a study of 603 elite female athletes in

Norway. Based on their responses to a screening measure for eating disorders, 22.4 percent of the athletes were classified as at risk. Interviews with 103 of the at-risk athletes revealed that the trigger factors associated with the onset of their eating disorder were prolonged periods of dieting or frequent weight fluctuations (41 percent), traumatic events such as illness, injury, a new coach, relationship problems, or failure at school or work (48 percent), and a significant increase in training volume (11 percent). Lopiano and Zotos (1992) contend that participation in athletics involves a number of pressures and responsibilities that are likely to increase the risk of eating disorders in athletes. These include performance pressures, pressure exerted by coaches, time demands, social isolation, fatigue-related stress, and injury.

Williamson and colleagues (1995) studied risk factors for the development of eating disorder symptoms in 98 female college athletes recruited from eight different sports. The risk factors significantly associated with eating disorder symptoms were pressure from teammates and coaches to be thin, athletic performance anxiety, and a negative self-appraisal of one's athletic achievement. It is important to note that these risk factors were strongly predictive of eating disorder symptoms only when accompanied by a preoccupation with body shape and size.

MEDICAL COMPLICATIONS

Caloric restriction, binge eating, and the use of unhealthy means of losing weight, such as laxatives, diuretics, and diet pills, can have a negative effect on athletic performance by decreasing endurance, strength, reaction time, speed, and ability to concentrate (Johnson, 1994). A form of anorexia nervosa, referred to as anorexia athletica, is characterized by caloric restriction, an intense fear of gaining weight, excessive exercise, and sometimes the use of laxatives, diuretics, or self-induced vomiting for weight control (Beals & Manore, 1994; Sundgot-Borgen, 1993). The female athlete eating disorder triad, consisting of disordered eating, amenorrhea, and osteoporosis, has been described by a number of researchers and clinicians (e.g., Stephenson, 1991; Wilmore, 1991; Yeager, Agostini, Nattiv, & Drinkwater, 1993). The long-term consequence of amenorrhea is a decrease in bone density, which can lead to fractures of the hip, pelvis, and spine. The spinal density of some

young female athletes is similar to that of women in their 70s and 80s (Yeager et al., 1993).

Other medical complications that can occur among athletes with eating disorders include electrolyte imbalances, irregular heartbeat, gastrointestinal problems, thyroid dysfunction, cold intolerance, kidney stones, edema, dehydration, elevated blood pressure, and muscle weakness (Johnson, 1994; Pomeroy & Mitchell, 1992; Stephenson, 1991). Many of the resulting deaths are due to electrolyte abnormalities, especially low potassium levels (Pomeroy & Mitchell, 1992). Individuals with low potassium levels are often asymptomatic, making it impossible to predict when a potentially life-threatening cardiac arrhythmia may occur.

DIAGNOSIS

A number of potential barriers hinder identification of eating disorders among athletes. Athletic participation may legitimize an eating disorder because of the norms and expectations that exist within the athletic community (Ryan, 1992; Thompson & Sherman, 1993). For example, a lower than average weight is likely to go unnoticed in an athletic environment that rewards thinness. Also, excessive exercise patterns may be difficult to detect in an environment that expects athletes to train hard. Coaches may avoid approaching an athlete about an eating problem if the athlete is performing well and the coach does not want to interfere with the athlete's success. Teammates may be reluctant to report an eating problem as they may recognize some of the same behaviors in themselves. Athletic administrators may not want to deal with eating problems because of legal issues and public relations concerns.

No single, accurate method exists for identifying eating disorders in athletes. Various screening measures for eating disorders exist, but athletes may not respond truthfully because of denial, fear of reprisal, or shame (Ryan, 1992). Even if a screening measure is used, an individual interview is essential for diagnosis of an eating disorder. The best time to screen for eating disorders is during the medical examination required prior to the athlete's admittance to the sports program. Van De Loo and Johnson (1995) have devised a short screening questionnaire for female athletes that can be used in the physician's office. Responses to the questionnaire can alert the physician to inquire further if eating disorder symptoms are present. Yates and colleagues (1997) are in the process of developing a questionnaire aimed at differentiating athletes at risk for eating disorders from healthy athletes, based on their exercise attitudes and behaviors.

TREATMENT

Once an athlete has been diagnosed with an eating disorder, treatment should begin as soon as possible as eating disorders not only impair athletic performance but can be life-threatening. The longer an eating disorder is allowed to progress, the more difficult it becomes to treat. Ideally, the treatment team should consist of a physician, nutritionist, and mental-health practitioner experienced in treating eating disorders. Severe cases involving extreme weight loss, electrolyte abnormalities, cardiac arrhythmias, or suicidal behavior may require hospitalization (Johnson, 1994; Tobin, Johnson, & Franke, 1992). Less severe cases can be treated in an outpatient setting through individual and/or group therapy. The treatment team must monitor the athlete's progress and devise relapse prevention strategies once treatment is completed. Beaumont and colleagues (1994) have developed a supervised exercise program for eating-disordered patients who are also compulsive exercisers. In this program, patients are educated about what constitutes healthy levels of exercise, are taught to pay attention to pain and fatigue rather than ignoring them, and are encouraged to abandon unrealistic notions of physical perfection.

One of the first issues likely to arise in treating athletes with eating disorders is how the treatment plan will affect the athlete's training and performance schedule (Brownell, 1995; Tobin et al., 1992). In addition, clinicians treating eating disorders in an athletic population must be sensitive to the athlete's desire to keep the disorder secret so as not to incur disapproval from coaches and teammates or risk the loss of an athletic scholarship (Brownell, 1995). Also, the athlete's self-esteem may be seriously threatened if the treatment plan includes curtailment of the athlete's training and performance schedule. In such a scenario, the treatment team must help the athlete see that temporarily limiting training or competition will be beneficial to his or her athletic career in the long run.

No published reports detail long-term follow-up of athletes with eating disorders. Thus, it is not known how often eating disorder symptoms subside when athletic training and competition are cut short. Based on their clinical experience, Johnson (1994) and Yates (1991) report that some athletes continue to struggle with weight concerns and problematic eating behaviors even after their athletic careers are over.

PREVENTION

Several reputable sports and medical organizations, including the U.S. Olympic Committee, the U.S. National Collegiate Athletic Association (NCAA), USA Gymnastics, and the American College of Sports Medicine, have expressed serious concern about eating disorders in athletes (Brownell, 1995; Powers & Johnson, 1996). Due to these concerns, primary prevention efforts within the athletic community have increased dramatically in the past five years. It is generally agreed that education is a necessary first step in the prevention of eating disorders. USA Gymnastics, the national governing board for gymnastics in the United States, has organized educational programs for athletes, parents, and coaches and prepared videos on the subject. A video series on eating disorders in athletes was also developed by the NCAA.

The athletic department at the University of Texas was one of the first to establish a combined eating disorder prevention and intervention program for female athletes (Ryan, 1992). In a one-year evaluation of the program, 120 female athletes from seven different sports had their body composition (but not their weight) assessed four to six times during the year by a sports medicine specialist (Brownell, 1995); coaches were not allowed to weigh the athletes, set weight goals, or discuss the athletes' body weight with them as had been done previously. At the end of the year, the athletes were leaner and more fit, and they reported feeling healthier and happier than they had been in the previous year. These results suggest that weight monitoring by coaches is unnecessary and perhaps even detrimental to the fitness of athletes. Thompson and Sherman (1993) also emphasize the importance of not weighing athletes (especially in group weigh-ins) and recommend that athletes diet only under the supervision of a nutritionist.

Prevention efforts in the athletic community have only recently begun. It is important that the governing bodies of various sports take a strong stand against unhealthy demands for thinness and unhealthy weight loss methods, and emphasize the importance of health and fitness over thinness. Developing prevention programs such as the one at the University of Texas may also help to decrease the prevalence of eating disorders among athletes.

In addition to interventions that focus on nutrition and unhealthy weight-loss methods, other types of interventions focus on strengthening defenses against eating disorders. Self-esteem enhancement involves experiencing success and mastery in different areas of one's life (Shisslak, Crago, Renger, & Clark-Wagner, 1997). Although athletes may experience success in sports, if this is the primary or only area in their life in which they feel successful, then their self-esteem can suffer if for some reason they are unable to achieve. Williamson et al. (1995), for example, found that a negative self-appraisal of one's athletic achievement can increase the risk for eating disorders when combined with other risk factors. Efforts to promote positive self-esteem in athletes may not only reduce their risk for eating disorders but could prove beneficial for their athletic performance as well.

REFERENCES

Beals, K. A., & Manore, M. M. (1994). The prevalence and consequences of subclinical eating disorders in female athletes. *International Journal of Sport Nutrition 4*, 175–195.

Beaumont, P. J. V., Arthur, B., Russell, J. D., & Touyz, S. W. (1994). Excessive physical activity in dieting disorder patients: Proposals for a supervised exercise program. *International Journal of Eating Disorders 15*, 21–36.

Brownell, K. D. (1995). Eating disorders in athletes. In K. D. Brownell & C. G. Fairburn (Eds.), *Eating disorders and obesity* (pp. 191–196). New York: Guilford.

Brownell, K. D., & Rodin, J. (1992). Prevalence of eating disorders in athletes. In K. D. Brownell, J. Rodin, & J. H. Wilmore (Eds.), *Eating, body weight and performance in athletes* (pp. 128–145). Philadelphia: Lea & Febiger.

Davis, C., Kennedy, S. H., Ravelski, E., & Dionne, M. (1994). The role of physical activity in the development and maintenance of the eating disorders. *Psychological Medicine 24*, 957–967.

Dick, R. W. (1991). Eating disorders in NCAA athletic programs. *Athletic Training 26*, 136–140.

Eisler, I., & le Grange, D. (1990). Excessive exercise and anorexia nervosa. *International Journal of Eating Disorders 9*, 377–386.

Epling, W. F., & Pierce, W. D. (1992). *Solving the anorexia puzzle.* Toronto: Hogrefe & Huber.

Hauck, E. R., & Blumenthal, J. A. (1992). Obsessive and compulsive traits in athletes. *Sports Medicine 14*, 215–227.

Johnson, M. D. (1994). Disordered eating in active and athletic women. *Clinics in Sports Medicine 13*, 355–369.

Kiernan, M., Rodin, J., Brownell, K. D., Wilmore, J. H., & Crandall, C. (1992). Relation of level of exercise, age, and weight-cycling history to weight and eating concerns in male and female runners. *Health Psychology* 11, 418–421.

Leon, G. R. (1991). Eating disorders in female athletes. *Sports Medicine* 12, 219–227.

Lopiano, D. A., & Zotos, C. (1992). Modern athletics: The pressure to perform. In K. D. Brownell, J. Rodin, & J. H. Wilmore (Eds.), *Eating, body weight, and performance in athletes* (pp. 275–292). Philadelpia: Lea & Febiger.

Pomeroy, C., & Mitchell, J. E. (1992). Medical issues in the eating disorders. In K. D. Brownell, J. Rodin, & J. H. Wilmore (Eds.), *Eating, body weight, and performance in athletes* (pp. 202–221). Philadelphia: Lea & Febiger.

Pope, H. G., Jr., Katz, D. L., & Hudson, J. I. (1993). Anorexia nervosa and "reverse anorexia" among 108 body builders. *Comprehensive Psychiatry* 34, 406–409.

Powers, P. S., & Johnson, C. (1996). Small victories: Prevention of eating disorders among athletes. *Eating Disorders* 4, 364–377.

Pruitt, J. A., Kappius, R. V., & Imm, P. S. (1991). Sports, exercise, and eating disorders. In L. Diamant (Ed.), *Psychology of sports, exercise, and fitness* (pp. 139–151). New York: Hemisphere.

Ryan, R. (1992). Management of eating problems in athletic settings. In K. D. Brownell, J. Rodin, & Wilmore, J. H. (Eds.), *Eating, body weight, and performance in athletes* (pp. 344–362). Philadelphia: Lea & Febiger.

Shisslak, C. M., Crago, M., & Estes, L. S. (1995). The spectrum of eating disturbances. *International Journal of Eating Disorders* 18, 209–219.

Shisslak, C. M., Crago, M., Renger, R., & Clark-Wagner, A. (1997). *Self-esteem and the prevention of eating disorders.* Manuscript submitted for publication.

Stephenson, J. N. (1991). Medical consequences and complications of anorexia nervosa and bulimia nervosa in female athletes. *Athletic Training 26*, 130–135.

Sundgot-Borgen, J. (1993). Prevalence of eating disorders in elite female athletes. *International Journal of Sport Nutrition 3*, 29–40.

Sundgot-Borgen, J. (1994). Risk and trigger factors for the development of eating disorders in female elite athletes. *Medicine and Science in Sports and Exercise 26*, 414–19.

Thompson, R. A., & Sherman, R. T. (1993). *Helping athletes with eating disorders.* Champaign, IL: Human Kinetics.

Tobin, D. L., Johnson, C. L., & Franke, K. (1992). Clinical treatment of eating disorders. In K. D. Brownell, J. Rodin, & J. H. Wilmore (Eds.), *Eating, body weight, and performance in athletes* (pp. 330–43). Philadelphia: Lea & Febiger.

Van De Loo, D. A., & Johnson, M. D. (1995). The young female athlete. *Clinics in Sports Medicine 14*, 687–707.

Williamson, D. A., Netemeyer, R. G., Jackman, L. P., Anderson, D. A., Funsch, C. L., & Rabalais, J. Y. (1995). Structural equation modeling of risk factors for the development of eating disorder symptoms in female athletes. *International Journal of Eating Disorders 17*, 387–93.

Wilmore, J. H. (1991). Eating and weight disorders in the female athlete. *International Journal of Sport Nutrition 1*, 104-117.

Yates, A. (1991). *Compulsive exercise and the eating disorders: Toward an integrated theory of activity.* New York: Brunner/Mazel.

Yates, A., Edman, J. D., Crago, M., Crowell, D., & Zimmermen, R. (1997). *Measurement of exercise orientation in normal subjects: Gender and age differences.* Manuscript submitted for publication.

Yates, A., Shisslak, C. M., Crago, M., & Allender, J. (1994). Overcommitment to sport: Is there a relationship to the eating disorders? *Clinical Journal of Sport Medicine 4*, 39–46.

Yeager, K. K., Agostini, R., Nattiv, A., & Drinkwater, B. (1993). The female athlete triad: Disordered eating, amenorrhea, osteoporosis. *Medicine and Science in Sports and Exercise 25*, 775–77.

Eating for Two: Unique Challenges for Pregnant Women with Eating Disorders

by Erika Neuberg, Ph.D.

Contrary to romantic perceptions, pregnancy is often associated with significant physical and emotional stress. The realities of pregnancy include moodiness (9 percent experience a major depression; 84 percent "the blues"), anxiety (50 percent report significant sleep disturbances), tearfulness (68 percent report unexplained crying), increased vulnerability, and body-image disturbances (Lederman, 1996). These problems are only exacerbated for women with eating disorders, given their predispositions for mood disorders, identity disturbances, and body-image problems. It is critical that this unique subset of eating-disordered women receive attention, not only to safeguard their health but that of the fetus as well. Understanding these women's unique concerns and experiences, as well as how the eating disorder and pregnancy affect each other, is the first step in providing effective and safe medical and psychological treatment.[1]

UNIQUE CONCERNS AND FEARS

Not surprisingly, most concerns for pregnant women with eating disorders center around food and weight. Eighty-eight percent of these women worry that their past or current eating habits will hurt the baby, and 86 percent fear losing control of their eating. Almost three-fourths of the women fear that they will not be able to return to their previous weight, and about half worry that their child will grow up with an eating or weight problem. Finally, how one resolves the typical conflicts and concerns regarding impending motherhood closely relates to flexibility and self-esteem, areas of difficulty for women with eating disorders (Bailey & Hailey, 1987; Hollifield & Hobdy, 1990; Lemberg & Phillips, 1989).

PREGNANCY'S EFFECT ON SYMPTOMATOLOGY

The literature on pregnancy's effect on symptomatology is somewhat mixed, likely due to differences and limitations in the studies' designs (e.g., different inclusion criteria, limited samples, different assessment tools). The largest surveys, however, suggest a decrease in eating pathology due to a desire to eat well for the baby. Generally, about 70 to 75 percent of women with bulimia report significant improvement in symptomatology during their pregnancies, with one study even showing a 75 percent remission rate in the third trimester. Despite the improved eating behavior, disturbances in body image remain at a high level. Approximately 20 percent of women with bulimia experience a worsening of symptoms during pregnancy, likely due to stress and fears associated with approaching motherhood and the accompanying weight gain (Franko & Walton, 1993; Lacey & Smith, 1987; Lemberg & Phillips, 1989; Stewart, Raskin, Garfinkel, MacDonald, & Robinson, 1987).

The data on anorexia are even more inconsistent. Several case studies report inadequate weight gain due to restricted eating, vigorous exercise, and hyperemesis, while two more recent studies document the opposite (Ho, 1985; Namir, Melman, & Yager, 1986; Rand, Willis, & Kuldau, 1987; Strimling, 1984; Treasure & Russell, 1988). This inconsistency may be due to a large percentage of the subjects in the latter studies being in treatment, suggestive of the importance of diagnosing and treating an eating disorder during pregnancy.

---

[1] The research on pregnant women with eating disorders is extremely sparse. The few empirical studies that do exist are limited, comprising mostly retrospective or case studies with few controls. Conclusions from these studies must be interpreted with caution.

MEDICAL COMPLICATIONS FOR MOTHER AND BABY

Pregnant women with eating disorders may be at greater risk to both maternal and birth complications, although again the data are mixed. One of the largest surveys to date did not reveal a higher incidence of birth defects, although the mixed sample (women with both restricting and purging behaviors) reported a slightly higher than average weight gain during their pregnancies (Lemberg & Phillips, 1989). In contrast, some studies documented a higher than expected occurrence of obstetrical complications and fetal abnormalities, including miscarriage, breech or forcep delivery, hypertension, premature delivery, low birth weights, fetal bradycardia, and lower birth Apgar scores (see Franko & Walton, 1993, for a review). There is some concern that severe eating pathology with significant hyperemesis may increase the risk of congenital malformations, although this concern is unsubstantiated. The strongest and most consistent results suggest that poor maternal weight gain is associated with lower birth weights (a potential risk factor for complications), and normal maternal weight gain is associated with positive results.

POSTPARTUM EXPERIENCES

We know very little about the postpartum experiences of women with eating disorders. Unfortunately, it appears that the majority who experienced symptomatic improvement relapse, with only about 25 percent retaining some benefit (Lacey & Smith, 1987; Lemberg & Phillips, 1989). Women attribute their relapse to a fear of being fat and a desire to lose weight. A more underlying cause, however, likely relates to the pressures and concerns of mothering, which no doubt lead to greater perceptions of stress and feelings of being out of control, and subsequent maladaptive eating. Although no current data exist, women with eating disorders are likely more vulnerable to experience postpartum depression and/or anxiety given their predisposition for mood disorders in general.

TREATMENT

There are steps that professionals can take to help these women. First, it is imperative that primary care physicians and/or OB-GYNs assess eating behaviors to identify women with eating disorders either before or early on in their pregnancies; fewer than half of such women will report eating problems spontaneously (Lemberg, Phillips, & Fischer, 1992; Levine, in press). Once an eating disorder is diagnosed, the physician must respond with empathy, honesty, and direction. The issue of weight gain needs to be addressed in a non-judgmental and direct fashion, with medical language that cannot be misinterpreted as suggesting one is "good" or "bad." Although it is important to empathize with the fear of weight gain to support a strong patient-doctor bond, the physician must convey optimism and expectation that the patient will be able to comply with necessary dietary requirements. It is crucial not to reinforce a desire to be thin. Unfortunately, about half of those who do confide in their physicians report negative experiences, often due to a perception that their desire for minimal weight gain is supported (Lemberg et al., 1992). Women with a more serious eating pathology should be considered high risk and should receive more frequent weigh-ins and examinations. (Such women often experience weigh-ins as stressful, and they often respond better if given the option to face away from the scale.) Finally, these women need to be referred to an experienced counselor as soon as possible to receive the specialized psychological treatment they require.

Psychologically, a therapy agenda should emphasize pregnancy education, including fetal development, nutritional needs for both mother and fetus, expected concerns and fears, medical risks of disordered eating, and signs of postpartum adjustment problems. Social support can buffer many of pregnancy's stresses and should be bolstered; pregnancy adjustment support groups when available are ideal. A therapist can increase the pregnant woman's sense of responsibility by making the fetus real and concrete, although this approach needs to be handled delicately to avoid excessive guilt and fear, which could potentially increase disordered eating. Imagery techniques can be helpful in improving body image, associating the rounded belly with fertility, health, beauty, and nurturance. When possible, a nutritionist can help build a stable and healthy diet that creatively incorporates foods that are more comfortable for the patient.

Regular consultations between the obstetrician, nutritionist, and therapist are necessary to provide a consistent and comprehensive treatment. Finally, these women should not be forgotten during the postpartum period, given their likely vulnerabilities to depression and anxiety.

CONCLUSION

Researchers have not examined the pregnancies and postpartum experiences of women with eating disorders sufficiently. The few empirical studies that do exist suggest unique concerns and fears that require empathy. Pregnancy may be an ideal time to appeal to these women to seek treatment. The help they receive cannot end with the pregnancy, however, as they are vulnerable to relapse and likely to experience a highly stressful postpartum period. Both researchers and clinicians need to focus more attention on this unique subset of women to improve our understanding of how pregnancy and eating disorders affect each other.

REFERENCES

Bailey, L. A., & Hailey, B. J. (1987). The psychological experience of pregnancy. *International Journal of Psychiatry in Medicine 16*, 263–74.

Franko, D. L., & Walton, B. E. (1993). Pregnancy and eating disorders: A review and clinical implications. *International Journal of Eating Disorders 13*, 41–48.

Ho, E. (1985). Anorexia nervosa in pregnancy. *Nursing Mirror 160*, 40–42.

Hollifield, J., & Hobdy, J. (1990). The course of pregnancy complicated by bulimia. *Psychotherapy 27*, 249–55.

Lacey, J. H., & Smith, G. (1987). Bulimia nervosa: The impact on mother and baby. *British Journal of Psychiatry 150*, 777–81.

Lederman, Regina P. (1996). *Psychosocial adaptation in pregnancy: Assessment of seven dimensions of maternal development.* New York: Springer.

Lemberg, R., & Phillips, J. (1989). The impact of pregnancy on anorexia nervosa and bulimia. *International Journal of Eating Disorders 8*, 285–95.

Lemberg, R., Phillips, J., & Fischer, J. E. (1992). The obstetric experience in primigravidia anorexic and bulimic women—some preliminary observations. *British Review of Bulimia and Anorexia Nervosa 6*, 31–38.

Levine, M. P. (in press). Bulimia nervosa (binge-purge syndrome; bulimia). In E. J. Quilligan and F. P. Zuspan (Eds.), *Current therapy in obstetrics and gynecology* (5th ed.) Philadelphia: W. B. Saunders.

Namir, S., Melman, K. N., & Yager, J. (1986). Pregnancy in restricter-type anorexia nervosa: A study of six women. *International Journal of Eating Disorders 5*, 837–45.

Rand, C. S. W., Willis, D. C., & Kuldau, J. M. (1987). Pregnancy after anorexia nervosa. *International Journal of Eating Disorders 6*, 671–74.

Stewart, D. E., Raskin, J., Garfinkel, P. E., MacDonald, O. L., & Robinson, G. E. (1987). Anorexia nervosa, bulimia, and pregnancy. *American Journal of Obstetrics and Gynecology 157*, 1194-98.

Strimling, B. S. (1984). Infant of a pregnancy complicated by anorexia nervosa. *American Journal of Diseases of Children 138*, 68–69.

Treasure, J. L., & Russell, G. F. M. (1988). Intrauterine growth and neonatal weight gain in babies of women with anorexia nervosa. *British Medical Journal 296*, 1038.

PART 4
Dieting and the Obesities

Obesity: Causes and Management

by Sharon A. Alger, M.D.

The prevalence of obesity has increased dramatically in the Western world over the past 50 years. In the United States, obesity affects one-third of the adult population and is a risk factor for the development of other health problems such as diabetes, hypertension, heart disease, and stroke. Genetic, psychological, emotional, and environmental factors are all believed to play a role in the development of obesity, and attempts at long-term treatment or prevention have met with limited success.

This chapter will focus on defining the factors associated with the development of obesity: the various types of obesity, their causes, and strategies for long-term management.

WHAT IS OBESITY?

Obesity exists when adipose (fat) tissue makes up a greater than normal percentage of total body weight: greater than 30 percent for women and greater than 25 percent for men. However, accurate methods to measure body fat such as underwater weighing or impedance, a technique using electric current to determine body composition, are not readily available in many health centers. Therefore, obesity is often measured by means of the body mass index (BMI), which is an individual's weight in kilograms divided by the square of his or her height in meters. The BMI is easy to calculate and correlates well with more direct measures of body fatness. According to this index, values of BMI between 20 to 25 represent acceptable weight; those between 25 and 29, mild obesity; those between 30 and 39, moderate obesity; and those over 40, severe obesity. A BMI greater than 28 is associated with a three to four times greater risk for the development of stroke, heart disease, or diabetes mellitus (Rosenbaum, Leibel, & Hirsch, 1997).

The distribution of body fat is genetically determined, and it, too, is an important factor in establishing obesity-related health risk. Central obesity, in which a large proportion of excess fat is stored in the abdominal area, occurs more commonly in males and is associated with the development of hypertension, diabetes, and heart disease. Peripheral obesity, in which excess body fat is stored in the hip and thigh areas, is more common among females and is less likely to lead to the development of serious health problems. Central obesity is defined as a waist-to-hip ratio greater than 0.9 in women and greater than 1.0 in men.

WHAT CAUSES OBESITY?

Obesity represents a positive energy balance in which excess nutrients (from food) are stored as body fat. It requires an intake of calories in excess of energy expenditure. However, the balance between energy intake and expenditure is widely variable among individuals and is influenced by a variety of genetic, environmental, and psychological factors. Studies of twins, adoptees, and families indicate that genetic factors determine as much as 80 percent of the differences in BMI between different individuals (Bouchard, 1994).

Energy Intake

No good evidence exists to suggest that overweight people consistently eat more or eat faster than lean individuals. Studies on taste preference suggest that the obese may prefer foods with a higher fat content than normal-weight people (Drewnowski, Brunzell, Sande, et al., 1985). This finding, however, may relate to the diet status of the individual rather than to body weight, because restrictive dieting is known to increase the preference for highly palatable "forbidden foods." The increased appetite and craving for high-calorie, high-fat foods, which occurs as a result of dieting and weight loss, is mediated by very potent neuropeptides acting in the hypothalamus and other areas of the brain. The brain receives signals from many areas of the body, including the gastrointestinal tract, endocrine system, peripheral nervous system, and even adipose tissue itself. It has recently been discovered that adipose tissue (fat) is not an inactive substance but has the ability to produce the protein leptin, which is released from fat tissue and travels to the brain through the bloodstream. Leptin works as a "satiety hormone" in the brain. When an individual diets and loses body fat, the amount of leptin produced decreases. This decrease in leptin within the brain allows for increased activation of other brain peptides such as neuropeptide Y, melanocortin-stimulating hormone (MSH), and neurotensin. These peptides are potent stimulators of appetite, working to increase food intake and restore the lost body fat (Rosenbaum, Leibel, & Hirsch, 1997).

Diet-induced cravings for high-calorie foods may also contribute to the development of binge eating in a subset of the obese population. Between 25 percent to 46 percent of overweight individuals have been reported to engage in binge eating at least twice weekly (Marcus & Wing, 1987). These obese binge eaters have food attitudes, personality traits, and depressive symptoms similar to normal-weight bulimics and quite different from non-bingeing obese individuals. Diagnostic criteria for binge eating disorder are included as an appendix in the *DSM-IV* (*Diagnostic and Statistical Manual*, 4th edition, of the American Psychiatric Association).

Frequency of meals and snacks also seems to influence body weight. Many obese individuals limit their food intake to one meal per day in an effort to restrict calories. The meal is often in the evening, after completion of daily activities. This pattern of eating may actually hinder weight loss because the amount of energy burned off as heat is reduced, and therefore, the body becomes more efficient at storing energy as fat. In addition, this eating pattern is more likely to be associated with a higher fat intake. Individuals who are starved during the day are less able to control their appetite and tend to choose faster, less healthy meals at night.

Energy Expenditure

The second half of the energy balance equation involves the way the body uses food. The basal metabolic rate accounts for the majority of daily energy expenditure (60 percent to 70 percent in a sedentary individual). This rate represents the energy burned by the body under resting conditions and in a fasted state; it is the "idling" speed of the body. The thermic (or heat) effect of food accounts for an additional 10 percent to 15 percent of daily energy expenditure, which is energy used by the body for the metabolic processing of ingested nutrients (food). The thermic effect of food increases with a high carbohydrate intake and with increased meal frequency. The energy used by voluntary

physical exercise is the most variable and adjustable component of daily energy expenditure and is dependent on the intensity and duration of the exercise as well as on the individual's body weight. Exercise can account for between 15 percent and 30 percent of the daily energy expenditure.

Basal metabolic rate varies greatly and is largely determined by the fat-free mass, fat mass, age, and sex of the individual (Ravussin, Zurlo, Ferraro, & Bogardus, 1991). However, basal metabolic rate is at least partially genetically determined (Bogardus, Lillioja, Ravussin, et al., 1986). Individuals with a low basal metabolic rate are at increased risk for weight gain. Genetic factors, therefore, influence the rate at which food is burned as energy or stored as body fat. Metabolic rates may relate to differences in sympathetic nervous system activity (Peterson, Rothschild, Weinberg, et al., 1988) or possibly to genetically determined differences in muscle fiber types (Wade, Marbut, & Round, 1990).

A reduction in body weight through dieting will result in a lower daily energy expenditure. Studies have shown that a formerly obese person requires approximately 15 percent fewer calories to maintain his or her weight than a person of similar body composition who has never been obese (Leibel, Rosenbaum, & Hirsch, 1995). This is due to a reduction in basal metabolic rate and a greater efficiency of skeletal muscle in converting chemical energy into mechanical work (Krotkiewski, Grimby, Holm, et al., 1990).

In summary, differences in daily food intake patterns and energy expenditure result in wide variations in the energy balance equation between individuals. For example, a 20-year-old male, 5'10", with no family history of obesity may consume 3,000 kcal/day (calories per day) to maintain his usual body weight of 160 pounds. In contrast, his next-door neighbor, a 45-year-old woman of the same height but with a strong family history of obesity maintains her weight of 210 pounds with a dietary intake of only 1,700 kcal/day! Several possible explanations can account for the apparent contradiction in the weight maintenance of these two individuals.

1. They ate different kinds of food. (High-fat foodstuffs may increase the risk of weight gain.)

2. They had different eating patterns (one meal a day vs. multiple meals throughout the day).

3. They had different rates at which ingested nutrients—food—are burned as fuel. (Their basal metabolic rate and thermogenesis were dissimilar.)

4. They had different levels of voluntary physical activity.

5. The 210-pound woman may be a "reduced obese" individual with an adaptive response to weight loss including a lower daily energy expenditure and decreased energy output with physical activity.

MANAGEMENT STRATEGIES FOR WEIGHT LOSS

In planning an appropriate weight-loss program, it is important to assess the severity of obesity and the potential for development of obesity-related health problems. The risk of hypertension, cardiovascular disease, and diabetes is much greater in individuals with a BMI greater than 30 and with a central distribution of body fat. Individuals in this category may significantly reduce their risk of long-term health problems through weight reduction. Individuals with a peripheral distribution of body fat or a BMI of less than 27 may benefit from instruction in healthful eating and exercise patterns, but should be discouraged from severely restrictive weight-loss regimens. Because the health risks associated with this degree of obesity are less significant, greater emphasis should be placed on helping the individual maintain a healthy lifestyle and accept his or her body shape.

A history of binge eating, multiple fad diets, or abuse of diet pills or laxatives is a warning signal for the development of a serious eating disorder. Severely restrictive diets should be discouraged in these individuals. A careful screening of the individual by a multidisciplinary team before beginning a weight-loss program can determine an appropriate combination of nutritional, psychological, and behavioral interventions.

Dietary Modifications

The composition of the ideal or most healthful diet is not known. However, diets should contain adequate protein, vitamins, minerals, and essential fatty acids. A diet low in total and saturated fat will reduce the severity of cardiovascular risk factors. A high-carbohydrate, low-fat (20 percent fat) diet may facilitate weight loss. Carbohydrate is less calorically dense than fat (4 kcal/gm for carbohydrate vs. 9 kcal/gm for fat) and therefore can be consumed in greater quantities. A high-carbohydrate diet will also burn off more calories as heat (increased dietary-induced thermogenesis) than a high-fat diet. Meals should be eaten at regular intervals throughout the day, and periods of fasting should be avoided. Fasting may result in a reduction in metabolic rate, with fewer calories burned off as heat. Eating more meals a day increases dietary-induced thermogenesis. The level of caloric restriction recommended is variable, depending on the individual's body weight, activity level, and pattern of food intake.

Exercise

Exercise should be strongly encouraged (after medical approval, if indicated). Regular exercise enhances weight loss and increases the capacity of the muscle to use fat as a fuel, hence decreasing the likelihood of fat accumulation. Physical exercise, because it increases energy expenditure, helps to offset any decline in energy expenditure that may result from a weight-reducing diet. Increased physical activity not only increases caloric expenditure but also promotes dietary compliance. Exercise may increase the desire for foods that are high in carbohydrates and reduce the desire for foods that are high in fat (Tremblay & Buemann, 1995). Individuals who successfully incorporate regular physical activity into their lifestyle are more likely to achieve long-term success with weight reduction.

Behavioral and Psychological Treatment

Obesity is a complex disorder with multiple contributing factors. In some individuals, environmental and psychological factors and attitudes about food and eating patterns may be the primary factors associated with weight gain, whereas, in others, genetics and a decreased level of energy expenditure may be the primary causes or etiologic factors.

The psychologist, as part of the multidisciplinary treatment team, can determine the psychological factors involved in the development or maintenance of obesity. Binge eaters, for example, are at increased risk for depression, food phobias, and anxiety disorders. Binge-eating behavior may be associated with a family history of alcohol abuse, drug abuse, or sexual and/

or physical abuse. Early detection and initiation of psychological counseling in these individuals is critical to long-term recovery and weight control.

Cognitive-behavioral techniques, which attempt to modify psychological and environmental factors associated with obesity, have shown positive results in achieving short-term weight loss. Individuals involved in a behavioral group program may benefit from the supportive nature of the group and increased sense of control over their lives (Rodin, Schank, & Striegel-Moore, 1989). Behavioral interventions, such as eating in only one place, learning to control the rate of eating, and avoiding "buffet-style" meals, are also effective in controlling the enhanced response to food cues noted in some individuals. Binge eaters may respond well in behavioral programs but tend to regain weight more rapidly than non-bingers once the treatment is completed (Marcus & Wing, 1987). This may reflect a return to the old habits of dietary restriction, followed by binge eating.

Drug Therapy

Recognition of the strong genetic and physiologic components involved in body weight regulation has made the treatment of obesity an area of active research investigation. Medications that work to increase energy expenditure, increase satiety (fullness), reduce cravings for high-calorie foods, and inhibit the absorption of fat from the gastrointestinal tract are under investigation.

Dexfenfluramine, a serotonin-reuptake inhibitor and releasing agent, was approved for use by the Food and Drug Administration (FDA) in 1996. This drug facilitates weight reduction primarily through suppressing hunger signals in the brain. However, the drug was voluntarily withdrawn from the market worldwide after reports of an increased risk of valvular heart disease associated with its use.

Sibutramine, a drug that increases both serotonin and norepinephrine, was recently approved by the FDA. This drug reduces the appetite and increases slightly energy expenditure. It has been shown to produce a 5 percent to 10 percent weight loss sustained over a two-year period.

Orlistat is another drug currently being developed for the treatment of obesity. This lipase inhibitor inhibits the absorption of approximately 30 percent of ingested fat. It is associated with a 5 percent to 10 percent weight reduction.

Drug therapy should be administered as part of a comprehensive lifestyle modification program with recommendations for dietary modification and exercise.

Surgical Therapy

Individuals with severe obesity (BMI > 40) who have been unable to sustain weight reduction with diet and exercise regimens are candidates for surgical intervention. The gastric bypass procedure is believed to provide the greatest long-term weight and risk-factor reduction. This procedure involves the creation of a small gastric pouch with a capacity of approximately two ounces. The pouch is anastomosed (connected) to the jejunum (a portion of the small intestine). The efficacy of this procedure relates to the increased feeling of fullness upon consumption of small volumes of food. Individuals who binge on high-calorie foods may experience an unpleasant sensation of nausea, referred to as "dumping"; those who consume large volumes of food or liquids at one time will vomit. Individuals undergoing gastric bypass surgery lose an average of 30 percent of their highest weight and improve significantly blood pressure, glucose, and cholesterol levels.

SUMMARY

The development of obesity may be due to a variety of factors, including genetic, environmental, psychological, and neurochemical mediators. The management of obesity should address each of these factors. Dietary modification and an active lifestyle should be advocated in all individuals. Individuals with a BMI greater than 30 and health problems related to excess body weight may be candidates for drug therapy if they are unable to achieve or maintain weight loss with diet and exercise alone. Surgical intervention is an option for those individuals with severe obesity (BMI > 40).

REFERENCES

Bogardus, C., Lillioja, S., Ravussin, E., et al. (1986). Familial dependence of the resting metabolic rate. *New England Journal of Medicine 315*, 96–100.

Bouchard, C. (Ed.). (1994). *Genetics of obesity*. Boca Raton, FL: CRC Press.

Drewnowski, A., Brunzell, J. D., Sande, K., et al. (1985). Sweet tooth reconsidered; Taste responsiveness in human obesity. *Physiological Behavior 35*, 617–622.

Krotkiewski, M., Grimby, G., Holm, G., et al. (1990). Increased muscle dynamic endurance associated with weight reduction on a very-low-calorie diet. *American Journal of Clinical Nutrition 51*, 321–330.

Leibel, R. L., Rosenbaum, M., & Hirsch, J. (1995). Changes in energy expenditure resulting from altered body weight. *New England Journal of Medicine 332*, 621–628.

Marcus, M. D., & Wing, R. R. (1987). Binge eating among the obese. *Annals of Behavioral Medicine 9*(4), 23–27.

Peterson, H. R., Rothschild, M., Weihberg, C. R., et al. (1988). Body fat and the activity of the autonomic nervous system. *New England Journal of Medicine 318*(17), 1077–1083.

Ravussin, E., Zurlo, F., Ferraro, R., & Bogardus, C. (1991). Energy expenditure in man: Determinants and risk factors for body weight gain. In *Recent Advances in Obesity Research: Proceedings of the 6th International Congress on Obesity*. London: J. Libbey.

Rodin, J., Schank, D., & Striegel-Moore, R. (1989). Psychological features of obesity. *Medical Clinics of North America 73*(1), 47–66.

Rosenbaum, M., Leibel, R. R., & Hirsch, J. (1997). Obesity. *New England Journal of Medicine 337*(6), 396–407.

Tremblay, A., & Buemann, B. (1995). Exercise-training, macronutrient balance and body weight control. *International Journal of Obesity and Related Metabolic Disorders 19*, 79–86.

Wade, A. J., Marbut, M. M., & Round, J. M. (1990). Muscle fibre type and etiology of obesity. *Lancet 335*, 805–808.

Out of Balance, Out of Bounds: Obesity from Compulsive Eating

by Bonnie Marx, R.N.

There are times when all of us overeat and gain weight. There are times when we all wish we were thinner, shorter, taller, huskier, more shapely, less shapely, whatever. Experiences like these are pretty normal and usually come and go without much ado. They need not signal danger and vary greatly from the experiences of compulsive eaters.

Six women meet to form a self-help group. They are concerned about their weight and their inability to manage dieting. They have several things in common. They all describe themselves as compulsive eaters. They all dislike their bodies and disassociate from them in some way. They feel off-balance, buffeted about between a compulsion to eat and a command to diet. They feel anxious and out of control around food. They all confess to some form of overeating followed by feelings of shame, guilt, and self-hate. They have all dieted and lost weight many times only to regain it. They all engage in secret eating.

As the women work together, it is apparent that they are eager to find out "why" and "from where" their problems arise. They look at family and social attitudes, messages and patterns that may have contributed to their uneasiness about their bodies, their weight, and the significance of food in their lives. These excursions into the past lend a new meaning and understanding to the present problem. However, after a number of weeks of self-study, a disturbing new question arises: "What now?" Their expanded awareness has not altered the fact that they still feel hopeless and powerless to control their behaviors around food.

The experiences of these women are not unique. Countless people in our society struggle to lose weight to perfect their bodies. In their attempts to do so they have tried the latest diets, frequented the nation's weight-loss and exercise centers, talked with physicians and therapists, read every book on the subject, and joined Overeaters Anonymous (OA) or other support groups. In doing so, some have succeeded in breaking the cycle of events associated with compulsive eating. Many others, however, have tried it all, failed, and, like the women in the story, are asking, "What now?"

What a hard question! What makes change so difficult for these people is the complexity of a disorder that is still too often defined simply as a "chronic weight problem" and treated as such. (Consider the overwhelming enthusiasm of physicians and compulsive eaters alike for using the prescription antiobesity drugs of the mid-'90s as testimony to the continued popularity of this theory.) This treatment track dismisses the painful experiences of those who are compulsive eaters. It traps treatment in a straitjacket, confining movement toward intervention to the old and ineffective "diet and exercise" routine. So, if not a "weight problem," what is obesity from compulsive eating?

COMPULSIVE EATING DEFINED

As an entity distinct from anorexia and bulimia, obesity resulting from compulsive eating is now being more precisely described, though it shares some features of both. Like anorexia and bulimia, it is characterized by patterns of suffering and shame, endless love-hate conflicts with self and food, inordinate amounts of time and energy spent thinking about the problem, and gross disturbances in eating behaviors. It is a complex system of beliefs, thoughts, feelings, and behaviors developed around self-image and body image that is played out in relationship with food. Compulsive eaters are often not even aware of some of these beliefs, thoughts, and feelings, so entrenched are they in the behavioral outcomes generated because of them. What they are acutely aware of, however, and what they present when they come into treatment, is a history dense with most or all of the following:

- Sustained, often daily overeating or highly irregular, inattentive, impulsive eating resulting in chronic overweight.
- Difficulty identifying physiological hunger and fullness.
- A strong desire to eat unrelated to any sense of physical hunger.
- Frequent attempts to lose weight by fasting or dieting without the ability to sustain motivation over time.
- Self-image and self-esteem based on body weight accompanied by an ongoing underlying fear and sadness about their adequacy as a person.

- Awareness of "feeling fat for as long as I can remember" even when in a healthy weight range.
- Feeling empty and using food to fill a void.
- Feeling addicted to food and helpless to change.
- Being obsessed with thoughts of food, weight, and dieting, yet feeling out of control and compelled to eat.
- Feeling driven into these activities by forces outside of themselves.
- Feeling big, out of place, left out, unacceptable, and unable to fit in.
- Taking in food that may be wanted, but considered unacceptable, then cycling into shame, guilt, depression, self-condemnation, and self-hatred.
- Using rigid, perfectionistic mechanisms to control the drive toward food. (Arenson, 1984; Marx, 1989)

It is obvious that obesity from compulsive eating is a serious, debilitating problem and one much too complicated in structure and manifestation to be treated only as a weight problem.

WHAT CAUSES COMPULSIVE EATING?

The "causes" of compulsive eating vary according to the views of those who have studied the problem. Obesity from compulsive eating has been linked theoretically to a number of interesting etiological possibilities, including obsessive-compulsive disorders (Mount, Neziroglu, & Taylor, 1991), addiction (Peele, 1989), even late 20th-century consumer society (Bloom, 1994). That the condition exists as more than a medical problem and as an entity separate from the major eating disorders may still be debated in some sectors. However, its reality is clear to the many clinicians who have described the thousands of people they see who are searching for release from this battle with themselves over food. These thousands are distinguished from the population of compulsive eaters who are not obese and from the population of obese who are not compulsive eaters.

Knowing that it exists and speculating about the causes does not tell much about obesity from compulsive eating. To fully explore the nature of this disorder demands a different question: What is it about?

The experiences of people who eat compulsively give clues as to the nature of compulsive eating and to issues central to its development. Sequences in these experiences may highlight and reflect stages in that development. It makes sense then to look first to the earliest remembered experiences reported by compulsive eaters, for example, dissatisfaction and embarrassment with their bodies and body image (i.e., body-image disturbances).

Most compulsive eaters have developed distorted views about themselves in relationship to their bodies, often as a response to early parental or peer messages regarding the inadequacy of some aspect of their size or shape or self. They begin to hate their bodies and see their bodies as fat and ugly and the cause of the growing sense of separation and anxiety they feel. They begin to disassociate from their bodies in some way, hoping this will make a difference in their relationships with parents or peers, hoping that they will feel safer. Some believe that they are their bodies and that they will not be acceptable and worthwhile until their bodies carry less weight. Others believe that their true and happy self lives locked inside a tomb of fat and will resurrect only when the fat is eliminated. As they do not belong with, take ownership of, or feel lovingly and responsibly connected with their bodies, it is no wonder that compulsive eaters feel no sense of control over this aspect of themselves.

Boundary and Control Issues

The splitting of the body from the self and subsequent boundary and control problems make up one of the core issues confronting compulsive eaters. The critical issue, of course, is one of control. Compulsive eaters feel powerless and out of control about food, their bodies, themselves, and their potential to change. Such a disturbance of body image then interferes with the development of the self-concept and the capacity to accept oneself as a whole, integrated person in charge of self and environment (Hardy, 1982). Without the body there are no physical boundaries, and without physical boundaries there is no place to live and "be" in the world, no place to experience oneself as separate from others, no place to "feel" in, and consequently no sense of authority over what happens. What creates this disruption?

In nearly every case, compulsive eaters come to believe that their bodies and their experiences are somehow not their own, that they belong to someone else or are too insignificant to attend to.

The belief (most often unconscious) develops over time after receipt of many "messages," spoken and unspoken, to support it. Some receive these messages when their bodies are used and abused for incest or other forms of sexual trauma. Some receive the messages through beatings or other kinds of physical abuse and neglect. Some receive messages in subtler, more insidious ways so "natural" to the context of their lives that they go unnoticed. What becomes noticeable, though, are the effects of these messages: never feeling good enough, smart enough, responsible enough, perfect enough; feeling pressure to take on roles and responsibilities in the family that the adults in the system have failed to perform; feeling responsible for everything and everybody; feeling discounted, unworthy, ashamed, alone, unlovable, abandoned. Simply, never feeling safe and sound in the world.

It is impossible for anyone to feel safe and competent when the foundation of their early experiences in the world has been built on harshness or confusion. When people have not been well taken care of, uncertainty surrounding self-worth (and in some cases even their right to exist) develops. It is very difficult for these people to learn how to take good care of themselves and their needs, to learn to make choices for their own well-being. In their attempts to take care of themselves, they often develop systems that seem to help them feel safe and in control at the time but fail to provide safekeeping in the long run. Obesity from compulsive eating is one such self-care system. For these compulsive eaters, focusing on weight and food and constantly looking for the perfect diet is an attempt to treat what ails them. Their treatment focus, however, can be seen as way off the mark once the whole picture of their problems comes into view.

TREATMENT OF COMPULSIVE EATING

What comprises adequate treatment for obesity from compulsive eating? Historically, treatment approaches that viewed compulsive eating as a "weight problem" or "medical problem" were all that were available to compulsive eaters. These therapies focused on the presenting problem—being "overweight"—and preached self-control and stimulus control. Many weight and diet programs, as well as physicians working with their obese patients, continue to ascribe to this method of treatment. (It must also be said here that numerous compulsive eaters repeatedly seek this method of treatment. They remain embedded in the belief that they should be able to handle this challenge alone and that the way to do it is to diet and lose the weight.)

Other treatment approaches for obesity from compulsive eating have developed as clinical interest in the disorder has deepened. The desire of the more informed clinician is to help people find relief from the cycle of blame and shame associated with obesity from compulsive eating. As many treatment modalities as there are theories about the causes and course of the disorder are now available.

Those looking for the underlying causes of their distress can go into some form of psychotherapy or counseling. Other interventions include hypnosis, cognitive-behavioral management, exercise programs, psychoeducational programs, addiction counseling or the OA systems, psychopharmaceutical programs (physician-prescribed medications that assist with the management of cravings, obsessive-compulsive tendencies, and depression), and even surgical procedures.

Treatment can start anywhere, but to promote long-lasting results it must eventually address the major psychological issues associated with obesity from compulsive eating and support development of a healthier system of self-care. Inherent in treatment must be the idea of ownership, of reclaiming and reparenting the body and reacquainting with it as part of the self. The recovery process requires it.

Compulsive eaters, often seekers of the "quick fix," must accept that *recovery is a process*. It is not a quicky diet plan guaranteed to take off 50 pounds in two weeks! It is not a magic pill to swallow that will forever halt the need to eat. For compulsive eaters, it is a movement out of fear, helplessness, and victimization supported by a willingness to learn how to "reparent" themselves, to learn to take good care of their physical, emotional, and mental needs. The treatment of choice for recovery may vary, but the treatment path must always lead compulsive eaters to develop healthy responses to questions such as:

- Who am I?
- What are my *own* thoughts, ideas, values, feelings?
- What are my *own* wants and needs?
- What scares me, angers me, pleases me, saddens me?
- What can I do when I feel fear, anger, joy, or sorrow besides eat?
- How can I stop obsessive thoughts and compulsions to eat?
- What stresses me and makes me tense?
- What can I do when I feel tense and stressed besides eat?
- How can I ask for what I need and want?
- How can I learn to accept that I have a right to ask for what I need and want?
- How can I learn not to abandon myself all the time for the sake of others?
- How can I learn to accept myself and be patient and harmless with myself while I heal?
- How can I learn to forgive myself?

Good treatment by professionals provides the safety, instruction, guidance, and atmosphere necessary to do this kind of work. The compulsive eaters, in turn, must provide the will and the courage to persevere. It is hard work, but it is freeing and fulfilling. It is like coming home.

REFERENCES

Arenson, G. (1984). *Binge eating.* New York: Rawson Associates.

Bloom, Carol. (1994). *Eating problems: A feminist psychoanalytic treatment model.* New York: Basic Books.

Hardy, G. E. (1982). Body image disturbances in dysmorphophobia. *British Journal of Psychiatry 141*, 181–185.

Marx, B. K. (1989). *Obese patient population analysis for N.I.M.H. survey.* Phoenix, AZ: St. Luke's Medical Center. 1–4.

Mount, D. R, Neziroglu, F., & Taylor, C. (1991). An obsessive-compulsive view of obesity and its treatment. *Journal of Clinical Psychology 46*(1).

Peele, Stanton. (1989). *Diseasing of America: Addiction treatment out of control.* Lexington, MA: D. C. Heath.

Obesity and the Link to Glucose Intolerance and Diabetes

by Donald S. Robertson, M.D.

Although obesity is not considered an eating disorder, per se, some individuals who compulsively eat develop weight problems that result in a variety of medical conditions, including noninsulin-dependent diabetes mellitus. This chapter considers when weight loss may be medically appropriate, keeping in mind that a "dieting mentality" should nevertheless be avoided.   —Editor

Obesity has been linked to a number of serious, potentially fatal conditions including high blood pressure, cardiovascular disease, orthopedic problems and diabetes, to name a few. Obesity is also an important risk factor for type 2 diabetes, which typically occurs in middle-aged adults who are sedentary and overweight. Approximately 80 percent of patients with type 2 diabetes are obese.

The progression from obesity to type 2 diabetes can be followed clinically, from normal glucose tolerance through glucose intolerance, which is the hallmark of diabetes. Type 2 diabetes is a disease of insulin resistance rather than insulin deficiency, which characterizes type 1 diabetes, the more severe form. Fat tissue is known to increase insulin resistance. Losing even 10 percent of excess weight can increase insulin sensitivity, resulting in a reduction in glucose levels.

In 1986, in *The Snowbird Diet*, this author described the importance of a carefully balanced weight-loss diet that limits the intake of simple carbohydrates to lower the high blood insulin levels which occur in most obese persons (Robertson & Robertson, 1986). Obesity raises the level of blood insulin, a condition that can actually prevent weight loss by converting as much as 50 percent of consumed food to fat instead of energy.

SUMMARY

There is a clear link between obesity and glucose intolerance. Because glucose intolerance can lead to type 2 diabetes, it is extremely important for obese persons to lose weight in order to control existing early glucose intolerance or avoid the progression to more severe glucose intolerance. Weight loss increases insulin sensitivity and may eliminate the need for pharmaceutical treatment of the diabetes and reduce the risk of diabetes-related complications.

INSULIN AND GLUCOSE METABOLISM: MECHANISM OF ACTION AND DIAGNOSIS

Insulin is a hormone manufactured by tiny clusters of cells, the islets of Langerhans, scattered throughout the pancreas. Within these clusters are beta cells which secrete insulin and alpha cells which secrete glucagon. Together, these two hormones regulate the amount of glucose (sugar) in the blood. After a meal, when glucose rises in the bloodstream, insulin is released, prompting body tissues to convert the glucose into fuel. When glucose levels drop, the alpha cells release glucagon which stimulates the liver to release stored glycogen, which is converted back to glucose. This hormonal check and balance system is critical. If correct blood glucose levels are not maintained, hyperglycemia (excess blood sugar) and glycosuria (sugar in the urine) can result.

IMPAIRED GLUCOSE TOLERANCE AND DIABETES

Impaired glucose tolerance (IGT) is defined as blood glucose levels that are higher than normal, but not high enough to be called diabetes. People with IGT may or may not develop diabetes. In the past, IGT was called borderline, subclinical, chemical, or latent diabetes, but these terms are no longer used.

Impaired glucose tolerance (IGT) and glucose intolerance can be diagnosed by any of the following tests:

- Fasting blood glucose (after no caloric intake for at least eight hours)
- Casual blood glucose (without regard to the time of the last meal)
- Oral glucose tolerance test (OGTT)

Fasting Blood Glucose Test

The fasting blood glucose test is used to determine how much sugar is in the blood. A blood sample is taken in a laboratory or doctor's office before the patient has eaten—usually in the morning. The normal, non-diabetic blood glucose range is 70 mg/dl to 110 mg/dl. In general, a blood glucose reading over 140 mg/dl indicates diabetes, except in newborns and some pregnant women. An international diabetes panel recommended in 1997 that this level be changed to 126 mg/dl. If results of the fasting glucose test are equivocal, the oral glucose tolerance test may be prescribed.

Casual Blood Glucose Test

The casual blood glucose test is similar to the fasting glucose test, except the test can be performed at any time, regardless of when the subject may have eaten. This test is typically used by individuals required to perform regular self-testing of blood glucose levels.

Oral Glucose Tolerance Test

An oral glucose tolerance test is performed to evaluate the ability to metabolize glucose. The test is started in the morning, before the patient has eaten, when an initial blood sample is drawn. The patient then drinks a concentrated glucose solution. Additional blood samples are drawn after one hour and two hour intervals. An oral glucose tolerance test value of 200 mg/dl in the two-hour sample indicates type 1 diabetes.

Blood Glucose Test Criteria

In June 1997, an international panel recommending changes in the definition of diabetes and other treatment practices also quantified impaired glucose tolerance. The panel recommended that IGT be diagnosed when oral glucose tolerance test results are 140 milligrams per deciliter (mg/dl) but less than 200 mg/dl in the two-hour sample. The panel recommended a new category, impaired fasting glucose (IFG), or a fasting blood glucose level of 110 mg/ml, but greater than 126 mg/dl.

The panel recommended lowering the level of blood glucose that defines diabetes from 140 mg/dl to 126 mg/dl when measured with the fasting blood glucose test. Casual blood glucose test results of at least 200 mg/dl, accompanied by symptoms of increased urination, increased thirst, and unexplained weight loss would meet the stricter criteria for diabetes, as would an oral glucose tolerance test value of at least 200 mg/dl in the two-hour sample. With these new criteria, more patients will be diagnosed as having diabetes rather than simply impaired glucose tolerance.

TYPES OF DIABETES AND INSULIN RESPONSE

In addition to lowering the levels for a diabetes diagnosis, the panel recommended changing the terminology for the two types of diabetes: insulin-dependent diabetes mellitus (IDDM), or type I diabetes, and noninsulin-dependent diabetes mellitus, or type II diabetes. The panel recommended changing the terms to type 1 diabetes and type 2 diabetes, respectively. This would alleviate outdated treatment references and avoid confusion caused by use of Roman numerals.

Insulin-dependent diabetes mellitus, henceforth referred to here as type 1 diabetes, is characterized by malfunction of the insulin-producing pancreatic beta cells. This condition generally progresses to total failure to produce insulin. There are two forms: idiopathic, which is rare and has no known cause, and immune-mediated diabetes mellitus, resulting from autoimmune destruction of the beta cells, a process that commonly starts in children or young adults.

Type 2 diabetes usually arises because of insulin resistance, in which the body fails to use insulin correctly, and is combined with relative (rather than absolute) insulin deficiency. A third type of diabetes, gestational diabetes, develops during pregnancy. While gestational diabetes generally disappears at the end of pregnancy, women who have had this condition run a greater risk of developing the type 2 form later in life.

PREVALENCE OF DIABETES

It is estimated that 16 million Americans have diabetes, but only about half have been diagnosed. About 700,000 Americans have type 1 diabetes. Nearly 22 times as many—15.3 million—have type 2 diabetes, and this form of diabetes is rising dramatically. In 1998 the American Diabetes Association reported a 9 percent per year increase in type 2 diabetes from 1986–1996. Gestational diabetes affects about 4 percent of U.S. pregnancies.

Type 2 diabetes is more common among older people, especially overweight women. It is also more common among African Americans, Hispanics, and Native Americans. Diabetes rates are 60 percent higher among African Americans than non-Hispanic whites, and 110 to 120 percent higher among Mexican-Americans and Puerto Ricans. Native Americans have the highest rates of diabetes in the world. Half of all adult Pima Indians in the Unites States have type 2 diabetes. Since minority groups and the elderly constitute the fastest-growing segments of the U.S. population, the prevalence of this condition is likely to increase.

A study of three American Indian populations found that the high rate of diabetes was more prevalent among women than men and was positively associated with age, level of obesity, amount of Indian ancestry, and parental diabetes status (Lee, et al., 1995). Even though the rates of diabetes were several times higher than those reported for the U.S. population, the rates of impaired glucose tolerance among the three populations were similar to those of the total U.S. population.

RISK FACTORS

Risk factors for impaired glucose tolerance and diabetes are:

- Obesity
- Having a first-degree relative with diabetes
- Being a member of a high-risk ethnic group (Asian Americans, African Americans, Hispanic Americans, Native Americans, Pacific Islanders)
- Being age 45 or over
- Delivering a baby weighing more than nine pounds or experiencing gestational diabetes
- Hypertension (blood pressure at least 140/90)
- A high-density lipoprotein cholesterol level of 35 mg/dl or lower, a triglyceride level of 250 mg/dl or higher, or both
- Impaired fasting glucose or impaired glucose tolerance
- Physical inactivity

OBESITY DEFINITION

In simplistic terms, obesity means weighing 20 percent more than the maximum desirable weight for one's height. It is technically defined as having more than 25 percent body fat for men or more than 30 percent body fat for women. Body fat is difficult to measure accurately, requiring underwater weighing in specialized laboratories for accurate readings. Skinfold thickness and bioelectrical impedance analysis (BIA) are general measures of body fat. Body mass index (BMI), waist circumference and body fat percentage are all needed for an accurate measure of the degree of obesity in an individual.

Skinfold Thickness

When using the skinfold thickness method, the thickness of skin and subcutaneous fat are measured using calipers at targeted sites, such as the triceps, for one. The degree of obesity is determined according to a table of values. The skinfold thickness method is highly variable; its accuracy depends on the skill of the examiner.

Bioelectrical Impedance

In bioelectrical impedance analysis, a harmless amount of electrical current is passed through the body, yielding an estimate of total body water. Mathematical equations are used to translate the percentage of body water into an indirect estimate of body fat and lean body mass. A higher water percentage generally indicates a larger amount of muscle and lean tissue. Bioelectrical impedance analysis is not accurate in severely obese patients, but it is quite accurate in persons with moderate obesity.

Body Mass Index

Body mass index (BMI) is the most commonly used measure of obesity. Body mass index is calculated by dividing the subject's weight in kilograms by height in meters squared. A male subject is deemed obese if his BMI is more than 27.8 kg/m2. For a female, the value is 27.3 kg/m2. The severity of obesity is determined by the following BMI measures (National Academy of Sciences, Institute of Medicine, 1995).

- Mild obesity— values near 27
- Moderate—near 30
- Severe—35
- Very severe—40+

Obesity may be further characterized by waist-to-hip ratio (WHR), which quantifies the distribution of body fat, or by waist circumference alone.

OBESITY VS. OVERWEIGHT

The terms obesity and overweight, while often used interchangeably, are not the same. Overweight means having an excess amount of body weight, including muscle, bone, fat, and water. Obesity is excess accumulation of body fat. A bodybuilder may be be overweight but not obese. However, most people who are overweight are also obese.

Prevalence of Overweight and Obesity

Approximately one-third of Americans age 20 to 74, or 58 million, are considered obese. The frequency (rate of occurrence) of overweight Americans increased from 25 percent in 1985 to 35 percent in 1995. Approximately 32 million adult females and 26 million adult males were overweight in 1990 (Kuczmarski, 1994). More than half of American adults have a BMI greater than 25 kg/m², and 20–25 percent of the adult population has moderate obesity (BMI greater than 30 kg/m²). In late 1997, new guidelines were being developed by the National Institutes of Health. These guidelines would lower the minimum levels for which an individual is considered obese.

An estimated 20 to 25 percent of children under age 18 are overweight (Troiano, et al., 1995). For children, overweight is defined as having a body mass index in the 95th percentile or higher for their age.

Central Obesity

Central or abdominal obesity is the distribution of excess body fat deep in the abdominal-visceral region. The waist-to-hip ratio may be used to measure body fat distribution, but it is not always the most effective measure. A ratio of 1.0 in women and .8 in men usually indicates abdominal fat. A circumference of 30 inches in women and 40 inches in men is associated with abdominal obesity. Abdominal obesity is an effective predictor of glucose intolerance and type 2 diabetes, high blood fats, coronary artery disease and high blood pressure.

Investigators in the recent Insulin Resistance and Atherosclerosis Study examined the link between abdominal obesity and insulin resistance and found that a minimum waist circumference was associated with insulin resistance after adjusting for age, sex, height, BMI, glucose tolerance status and ethnicity (Edelstein, et al., 1997). Waist circumference was also found to be related to fasting insulin which is an indirect measure of insulin sensitivity.

Obesity as a Risk Factor

It is estimated that obesity contributes to much of the $11.3 billion spent annually in the United States on diagnosing, treating and managing type 2 diabetes and related conditions. The total amount attributed to diagnosing and treating obesity and related disorders in the U.S. is $100 billion annually.

Obesity—especially abdominal obesity—is a major independent risk factor for coronary artery disease, high blood fats and hypertension as well as insulin resistance, hyperinsulinemia, impaired glucose tolerance and overt diabetes. Progressive insulin resistance may be associated with a type 1 diabetes. Weight loss results in improved glucose storage and an increase in insulin sensitivity.

All measures of obesity (BMI, waist-to-hip ratio and waist circumference) have been positively associated with the incidence of type 2 diabetes when the progression from impaired glucose tolerance to type 2 diabetes is examined (Karter, et al., 1996).

GESTATIONAL DIABETES

Researchers have found that central fat distribution, as measured by waist-to-hip ratio and waist circumference, is an independent predictor of gestational glucose intolerance (Branchtein, et al., 1997).

DIET AND EXERCISE

Diet, exercise, and glucose blood testing are used to manage type 2 diabetes. Some patients may also use oral drugs or insulin to keep their glucose levels in the normal range. However, drug therapy should be used only when diet and exercise fail to control blood glucose levels. Seventy to 80 percent of obese patients can lower blood sugar levels simply by losing weight, allowing them to reduce or eliminate the need for medication completely. In addition, studies have shown that implementing a diet and exercise program can significantly slow the progression from impaired glucose tolerance to type 2 diabetes (Pon, et al., 1997).

An investigation of methods used to promote weight loss in people with type 2 diabetes—behavioral therapy, exercise, diet, anorectic drugs, surgery or a combination of these—showed that dietary strategies are the most effective method for promoting short-term weight loss (Brown, et al., 1996). In the study, obese patients on a medically monitored, multi-disciplinary, formula-based weight-loss program were evaluated for increased glucose, blood pressure and cholesterol levels, since these conditions are often associated with obesity (Drawert, Bedford, & Largent, 1997). In all subjects who followed the weight-loss program, glucose, blood pressure, and cholesterol were significantly reduced from baseline levels.

It is imperative that a patient with diabetes keep blood glucose levels within the normal range, as this slows the onset and progression of eye, kidney, and nerve diseases caused by diabetes. This reduction in complications was demonstrated by the Diabetes Control and Complications Trial conducted from 1983 to 1993 by the National Institute of Diabetes and Digestive and Kidney Diseases.

PHARMACEUTICAL THERAPY

If diet and exercise are not enough to promote weight loss and bring blood glucose levels down to normal range, drug therapy is necessary. Oral antidiabetic drugs are generally sufficient, although severe cases of type 2 diabetes may require insulin administration.

Four classes of oral diabetes drugs are available:

- Sulfonylureas
- Biguanides
- Alpha-glucosidase inhibitors
- Insulin sensitizers

Sulfonylureas, the oldest class of oral antidiabetic drug, act on pancreatic tissue to produce insulin. The newest sulfonylurea, Amaryl (glimepiride, Hoechst Marion Roussel), was approved by the U.S. Food and Drug Administration (FDA) in 1995. Sulfonylureas can become less effective after 10 years of use or more, so alternative drug therapies are often needed. In addition, some sulfonylureas have been associated with increased risk of death from cardiovascular disease.

Biguanides act to lower cell resistance to insulin, a common problem with type 2 diabetes. The biguanides class includes Glucophage (metformin, Bristol-Myers Squibb), approved by the FDA in 1994.

Alpha-glucosidase inhibitors slow the digestion of carbohydrates, thus delaying absorption of glucose from the intestines. Alpha-glucosidase inhibitors include Precose (acarbose, Bayer), approved by the FDA in 1995, and Glyset (miglitol, Bayer), approved in 1996.

The newest class of oral antidiabetic drugs is insulin sensitizers. The first of these, Rezulin (troglitazone, Parke-Davis), was approved in 1997. This class of drugs resensitize tissues to insulin, thus helping patients make better use of their own insulin.

REFERENCES

Branchtein, L., Schmidt, M.I., Mengue, S.S., Reichelt, A.J., Matos, M.C.G., & Duncan, B.B. (1997). Waist circumference and waist-to-hip ratio as related to gestational glucose tolerance. *Diabetes Care, 20,* 509.

Brown, S.A., Upchurch, S., Anding, R., Winter, M., & Ramirez, G. (1996). Promoting weight loss in type II diabetes. *Diabetes Care, 19,* 613.

Drawert, S., Bedford, K., Largent, D. (1997). Change in glucose, blood pressure, and cholesterol with weight loss in medically obese patients, *Obesity Research. 4,* 678.

Edelstein, S.L., Knowler, W.C., Bain, R.P., Andres, R., Barrett-Connor E.L., Dowse, G.K., Haffner, S.M., Pettitt, D.J., Sorkin, J.D., Muller, D.C., Collins, V.R., & Hamman, R.F. (1997). Predictors of progression from impaired glucose tolerance to type 2 diabetes: An analysis of six prospective studies. *Diabetes, 46,* 701.

Karter, A.J., Mayer-Davis, E.J., Selby, J.V., D'Agostino, Jr., R.B., Haffner, S.M., Sholinsky, P., Bergman, R., Saad, M.F., & Hamman, R.F. (1996). Insulin sensitivity and abdominal obesity in African-American, Hispanic, and non-Hispanic white men and women *Diabetes, 45,* 1547.

Kuczmarski, R.J., Johnson, C.L., Flegal, & K.M., Campbell, S.M. (1994). Increasing Prevalence of Overweight Among U.S. Adults. *Journal of the American Medical Association, 272,* 205–211.

Lee, E.T., Howard, B.V., Savage, P.J., Cowan, L.D., Fabsitz, R.R., Oopik, A.J., Yeh, J., Go, O., Robbins, D.D., & Welty, T.K. (1995). Diabetes and impaired glucose tolerance in three American Indian populations aged 45-74 years. *Diabetes Care*, 18, 599-610.

National Academy of Sciences, Institute of Medicine. (1995). *Weighing the Options: Criteria for Evaluating Weight-Management Programs*, 50–51. Washington, DC.

Pan, X., Li, G., Hu, Y., Wang, J., Yang, W., An, Z., Hu, Z., Lin, J., Xiao, J., Cao, H., Liu, P., Jiang, X., Jiang, Y., Wang, J., Zheng, H., Zhang, H., Bennet, P.H., & Howard, B.V. (1997). Effects of diet and exercise in preventing type 2 diabetes in people with impaired glucose tolerance. *Diabetes Care*, 20, 537.

Robertson, D.S., & Robertson, C.P. (1986). *The Snowbird Diet*. New York: Warner Books, Inc.

Troiano, R.P., Kuczmarski, R.J., Johnson, C.L., Flegal, K.M., & Campbell, S.M. (1995). Overweight Prevalence and Trends for Children and Adolescents: The National Health ad Nutrition Statistics Related to Overweight and Obesity Examination Surveys, 1963 to 1991. *Archives of Pediatrics and Adolescent Medicine*, 149.

Diet Pill Controversy: Dangers, Promises, and Legitimate Applications

by Vicki L. Berkus, M.D.

It is no surprise with the media emphasis on body image and sexuality that more and more people are looking for a quick and easy way to lose weight and keep it off. The recent controversy surrounding the use of phen/fen and its subsequent recall demonstrate that the public still turns to medications as the most viable means of losing weight. Diets and weight loss have been topics of magazine articles and talk shows for years. Most people follow the struggles of celebrities to lose weight and empathize with friends and family members who have tried various programs and medications without success. More than 18 million prescriptions were written for phen/fen (phenteramine/ fenfluramine) or Redux (dexfenfluramine) in 1996. Already, the search for an alternative to phen/fen is well under way.

Americans spent nearly $500 million on prescription and over-the counter diet drugs in 1996 and $30 billion annually on diet programs and products (Grinfeld, 1997). The fact that so many people are taking pills while unaware of potential risks demonstrates the need for education and for safer alternatives to weight-loss medications.

Each of us holds a perception—accurate or inaccurate—of his or her body image. Often it is a distorted image resulting from society's view of the ideal body. Fashion is geared toward the tall and lean. Many members of ballet companies and gymnastics teams suffer from anorexia nervosa. Conversely, the percentage of Americans who are overweight continues to increase, and the health problems related to obesity are a source of financial and emotional concern. This concern channels the search for the "cure" in the form of a pill.

DIET PILL PROMISES

The medical profession's view of obesity has changed over time. Many now define obesity as greater than 25 percent of ideal body weight for a male (35 percent for females) or a Body Mass Index (BMI; a height/weight calculation) greater than $27kg/m^2$. The average person rarely considers such a measure when deciding to lose weight. Instead, perceptions such as " I feel fat" are the driving force behind reaching for a pill with less thought about the long-term effects of taking that pill. Change can take time and most people do not want to hear that message. Doctors are now looking at obesity as a chronic disease rather than a symbol of weakness or lack of willpower, and are encouraging patients to approach weight loss by setting and achieving small goals first. A 10 percent to 15 percent reduction in weight can lower blood pressure, cholesterol, and blood sugar levels. It seems logical for the medical profession to help people lose 10 to 15 pounds rather than set a long-term goal of 25 to 50 pounds. Rather than establish an ongoing relationship with a health care provider, however, most people obtain the pills after a brief in-office visit. Thus, there is little opportunity for the health care professional to delve deeper into the patient's behaviors as they relate to food. Looking at the symptom (excess weight) rather than the disease as a whole may set the person up for failure. Most overweight people can tell you about their multiple attempts at losing weight and share their immense knowledge of the nutritional components of the various food groups. It is the inability to keep the weight off that keeps the frustrating battle an ongoing one. Their eating behaviors may be their solution to other problems such as feeling insecure, lonely and unattractive. All of us have comfort foods—or foods we enjoy when we're feeling down. The relationship with food can become more important than other relationships and can take a lot of energy to maintain. We may not understand why we eat in a certain way and instead focus on how we look. The yo-yo effect of losing and gaining is all too common, which is why the behavioral aspects of the disease of obesity are now a part of the treatment. More emphasis is being placed on how people respond to a medication and how the medication affects sleep, productivity and mood.

The preferred characteristics of a diet pill include producing an anorectic effect (decreasing appetite), having low abuse potential, working better than a placebo, and being safe, with few side effects. People respond in many different ways to medications, and it is difficult to predict the wide range of responses. Safety is a key consideration, particularly for a population that already has health risks, which is why few medications are available. Currently, diet pills are also held to higher standards than other drugs and are only approved for short-term use. Limiting the time a diet pill is made available sets a patient up to regain the lost weight. Legislative changes are needed to allow for longer medication trials.

The effectiveness of medications for weight loss is uncertain. Some studies demonstrate that diet pills are effective in short-term weight loss and may even lead to long-term loss in some patients (Goldstein & Porvin, 1994). Other studies show only a pound or less loss per week (Atkinson

& Hubbard, 1994). Weight loss usually plateaus after five to six months because consumption of fewer calories over time lowers the resting metabolic rate, resulting in the body burning calories at a slower pace. When people stop taking weight-loss medications, their intake of calories increases because the anorectic effects of the drugs are no longer controlling cravings. This sets the patient up to revert to old eating behaviors as a way of dealing with the cravings and this regains weight. More physicians and health care workers agree that diet pills need to be combined with a healthy food plan and exercise program; the pills can help someone stick to a food plan and exercise program until they become part of the patient's daily routine.

THE DANGERS OF DIET PILLS

The recent associations of heart valve problems and lung problems (primary pulmonary hypertension) with fenfluramine and dexfenfluramine were not the first complications seen with diet pills (Manson & Faich, 1996; *Medical Sciences Bulletin,* 1996). In 1973, 582 cases of primary pulmonary hypertension were reported in patients using Menocil (aminorex fumarate). Side effects such as diarrhea and insomnia were reported in those taking phenteramine. Although structural manipulations of the amphetamines have reduced such central nervous stimulation effects as anxiety, insomnia, and diarrhea, these medications including Benzphetamine (Didrex), Phendimetrazine (Anorex), Manzindol (Sanorex, Mazanor), Phenylpropanolamine (Dexatrim), Diehylproprion (Tenuate, Tepanol) and Phenteramine (Fastin, Ionamine, Adipex-P, Phentrol) still have an abuse potential if not monitored carefully. More and more patients are being seen at drug treatment centers for abuse of amphetamines and cocaine, two drugs they started using to "lose weight." Serotonergic drugs such as fluoxetine (Prozac) work by increasing the amount of serotonin in the brain, which can result in decreased food intake. Normal adverse effects associated with the serotonergic drugs include diarrhea, increased thirst, dry mouth, and sleep disturbances. There can also be a rebound depression if the user stops taking the drugs, and a withdrawal syndrome if he or she stops taking them suddenly. Serotonin syndrome can occur if the user combines a selective serotonin reuptake inhibitor (SSRI) like Paxil, Prozac, Zoloft, or Luvox with alcohol or other antidepressants. Symptoms include an altered mental state, impaired coordination, muscle contractions, agitation, fever, and shivering. There is no simple way to predict who may be prone to side effects from medication. It is up to the person taking the medication to report any problems to his or her health professional.

Recently, attention has turned to the use of natural compounds for weight loss. "Diet Phen" is a combination of St. John's Wort and ephedra with additional vitamins and minerals (Momo,1997). Studies are now under way to determine the effectiveness of these herbal alternatives. A concern for many physicians with any over-the-counter treatment is the lack of medical supervision. The effects of combining herbal remedies with other prescription medications have not been established.

One consequence of using pills without proper medical supervision is the tendency to move from a healthy concern about one's weight to a level of focus that starts to become harmful to the patient. The shift from a healthy desire to lose weight to a full eating disorder can be subtle or rapid. Most people are aware when they have been overeating, especially during the holidays. That's the reason so many people make New Year's resolutions to lose weight. What transforms "dieting" into an eating disorder is the pervasiveness of the intensity and rigidity that spill over from eating habits into other areas of the patient's life, such as relationships, job performance, and self-esteem. The awareness of what is healthy and what is not is lost, and what started out as the use of diet pills to normalize weight becomes a quest for perfection and happiness. The ability to identify those people who are vulnerable to these changes is a challenge and rarely occurs early in the disease process. The move to a full eating disorder involves obsessive, unrelenting thoughts about the body and what goes into it. These thoughts can become all consuming.

As noted, people often use diet pills with little medical supervision and understanding of the possible risks involved in such use. They may borrow some pills from a friend or use some that they find in the medicine cabinet. Often, it is an impulse decision, motivated by a desire for a "quick fix." The person gets tired of restricting certain foods and following the rules for healthy eating. This may begin a cycle of restricting and bingeing (Fairburn, 1993). The desire to lose weight quickly becomes the goal. Weight is lost, but quickly regained once the pills are discontinued.

LEGITIMATE APPLICATIONS OF DIET PILLS

A number of medications are currently undergoing clinical trials. Sibutramine (Meridia) slows the reuptake of serotonin and noradrenalin. It has been effective in preliminary trials and will soon be available. Major side effects include headache and dry mouth. Orlistat works by inhibiting the absorption of fats; it too should be available soon. Other experimental drugs include RO-22-064, which stimulates fat breakdown; Cholorocitrate, which inhibits gastric emptying; and BRL 2380A, which increases energy.

Most doctors agree that they will dispense diet pills only to those patients who can cite a medical reason for using them. Patients who suffer with gallbladder disease, osteoarthritis, gout, sleep apnea, diabetes, or high blood pressure are among those for whom excess weight adds to their medical problems. The health risks brought on by these illnesses may outnumber the risks associated with weight-loss medications. This is different from taking pills to fit into a certain dress or to impress people at a high school reunion. The level of obesity that leads to recurrent doctor visits, limited physical activity, and deep-seated depression requires a much different focus. The medications listed above represent the increase in information and understanding of the biochemical aspects of obesity as well as the complexity of the problem. The goal shared by many is a pill that is a safe and effective means for permanent weight loss.

REFERENCES

Atkinson, Robert L., & Hubbard, Van S. (1994). Report on the NIH Workshop on Pharmacological Treatment of Obesity. *Am. J Clin. Nutr.* 60, 153–156.

Bray, George A. (1993). Use and abuse of appetite-suppressant drugs in the treatment of obesity. *Ann. Intern Med.*119(7 pt 2), 700–13.

Fairburn, Christopher G. (1995). Overcoming binge eating. New York: Guilford Press, p. 58.

Goldstein, D. E. Porvin. (1994). Long-term weight loss: The effects of pharmacological agents. *Am. J. Clin. Nutr. 60*, 647–57.

Manson, J., & Faich, G. (1996). Primary pulmonary hypertension. *NETM 335*, 659–60.

Momo, T. (1997). <www.tenzing.com/ec.html>. St. John's Wort; Diet.

National Task Force on the Prevention and Treatment of Obesity. (1996). *Long-term pharmacotherapy in the management of obesity 276*(23), 1907–11.

PART 5
Current Treatment Approaches

Eating Disorder Treatment Stories: Four Cases

by Susan Wagner, Ph.D.

The following case descriptions are taken from outpatient psychotherapy. Some of the details have been altered to protect the identities of the patients.

BULIMIA NERVOSA

Maria began therapy with me at age 24. She had made several failed attempts at psychotherapy but felt she was not ready to work on her problems. She had bulimia nervosa, with an eight-year history of bingeing and vomiting as often as three times a day. She had never gone longer than two weeks without doing this. Her physical exam and laboratory studies were normal, but she admitted to having lost some of her hair over the past year.

Maria was extremely attractive, intelligent, and witty, with a good figure on the slim side of normal. She was also moody, sensitive, and prone to temper tantrums. She had attended an Ivy League college, where she managed only moderately good grades. Her pattern of skipping classes and staying up all night to binge and vomit clearly interfered with her academic and social life. She had friends, but she never told them about her problem. Even her boyfriend, with whom she was "unofficially" living, had no idea she was in trouble.

When Maria was 16, she had felt deeply insecure. She was 10 or 15 pounds overweight. Boys were not interested in her, and her only friends were other "brainy" girls who were not socially successful. Her family life was stormy: Her sensitive, intelligent, irritable parents were often critical of Maria, her friends, each other, and anyone else who entered their lives. Her older sister coped with the parents by quietly withdrawing into her studies. Maria's response was the opposite: relentless arguments, screaming matches, and chronic frustration. Yet she wanted her parents' approval badly.

As part of a self-improvement campaign, Maria began to diet. She did well at first. Then she began to eliminate too many foods, which caused her to have intense food cravings. In this way, the binge/purge cycle began: The cravings led to binges; the binges led to a fear of becoming fat, which led to Maria making herself vomit after a binge. Maria also found that immersing herself in food and then throwing it up gave her a calm, serene sort of feeling. As her illness progressed Maria was bingeing and purging not only because her dieting was far too restrictive, but because she could soothe herself this way when life (her parents, school, boys) upset her. Although she knew in some way that the bingeing and purging were "wrong," it remained her secret way of "getting by."

When Maria entered therapy with me, she was tired, ashamed, and sick of being sick. She was willing to risk gaining a few pounds for the sake of getting well. To get her parents to pay for previous treatments, Maria had told them about her problem but had made it seem much milder than it really was. This time, she allowed me to tell them the details. At first, her parents became angry and very critical of Maria (and of me). As time passed, however, they settled down and were supportive of Maria's efforts to get well.

Maria and I met once a week. We worked out a program of slow but steady elimination of binge/purge behavior. The decision about how much to cut back on bingeing and purging from week to week was always hers. She made an effort to get three reasonable meals every day, and she sometimes kept a food diary, which she would share with me. She also went for brief nutritional counseling with a nutritionist who had years of experience counseling bulimics. Within a few months her bingeing and purging had stopped. She had gained five to 10 pounds, which bothered her, but she accepted this weight gain as a fair price for regaining her health. The remainder of the year's therapy sessions were spent on developing new ways of dealing with stress, which meant that Maria had to learn how to recognize what was bothering her. She had never had to do that, as her answer to every kind of discomfort had been the same: binge and vomit. Now Maria began to develop a healthy respect for some basic realities: her own needs and wishes, the needs of others, the limits of her ability to influence others, and the limits of others' abilities to respond to her needs. Maria learned to identify her needs and to think about ways of taking care of them. She also learned to evaluate whether particular people in her life were likely to help her meet those needs, or if they instead might interfere with her efforts to take care of herself. She learned that she did not have to sacrifice her preferences and beliefs to get approval.

Maria terminated psychotherapy with me after one year. She wanted to go back to school for an advanced degree, and she felt ready to apply what she had learned in treatment. We both assumed that she would return to therapy at some future point.

ANOREXIA NERVOSA

Tracy came to therapy at the age of 19, in her sophomore year of college, where she was getting good grades. She had a boyfriend from high school but had made few friends at college. Tracy stood 5'6" tall and weighed about 98 pounds. She had started losing weight deliberately about two years earlier, although she had been thin even then, weighing about 120 pounds. She just started eating less and less. Losing weight became the most important thing in her life, although she couldn't explain why. When she came to me Tracy was frankly unhappy about the prospect of gaining weight, but she was also frightened by feelings of fatigue, the loss of her period for more than six months, and her difficulty in being able to concentrate on schoolwork.

As the younger sister of an unpredictable, rebellious, angry girl, Tracy felt obligated to be a "problem-free" child for her parents. She had witnessed countless fights between her parents and sister and listened endlessly to her parents complaining about her sister. Tracy was praised by her parents for being a good student, responsible, and considerate. Tracy had become entirely oriented toward pleasing others. She learned to hide her negative feelings, conceal different opinions, and become exceptionally intuitive about other people's wishes and needs.

Whenever possible, Tracy kept her problems to herself. She carried her silence even to the point of telling no one when she was attacked and raped on the way home from school when she was 14.

As high school graduation grew closer, Tracy began to restrict her food intake. She counted calories constantly, began to eliminate whole food groups from her diet, and spent hours inspecting her body for fat. She knew that she was afraid to go away to college. She feared that her mother would become depressed without her. She felt guilty about starting a life of her own and confused about what her parents really wanted her to do about going to college. Tracy did not realize that her overwhelming terror of making a mistake played a major part in her anorexia nervosa.

Family and friends expressed concern about Tracy's weight loss, but she held them off with excuses and with promises to gain. She decided on her own to pursue psychotherapy because of worries about her physical health. After Tracy and I discussed her diagnosis of anorexia nervosa, we agreed to the following treatment plan: a complete medical evaluation by a physician familiar with eating disorders; weight gain at the rate of one to two pounds a week; a target weight of 122 pounds; weekly weigh-ins at the doctor's office (in a hospital gown, after voiding, and supervised by the doctor or nurse); and psychotherapy once or twice weekly, depending on her progress.

Tracy took more than one and a half years to reach her target weight. She would gain and lose. For a long time, she described her food intake as "huge," when in fact she was eating under 2,000 calories per day (on which she could not gain). Her fatigue and poor concentration, which she correctly understood as the effects of malnutrition, helped motivate her to stop restricting her food.

Psychotherapy centered on three broad topics: her "addiction" to food restriction and how to recover from it, her feelings about her family and about herself as a part of her family, and her body-image problems.

Tracy was able to grasp the concept of "addiction to restriction" very easily. She also saw that she would have to learn new coping skills in place of her "addiction." She remained, however, very guarded on the topic of her family. She was able to express some resentment toward her sister, but she just couldn't acknowledge any negative feelings toward her parents. Her body-image problems had a lot to do with the rape at age 14. Tracy did come to feel and express her reactions to that trauma, her self-blame, her shame, and last of all, her anger.

Tracy achieved her goal weight and maintained it for more than six months before ending her psychotherapy. She would return to anorexic ways of thinking when pressured or stressed, but she could resist the temptation to restrict her food. She had also expanded her social network at school, was able to participate in "fun things," share intimate stories with friends, and be silly when she felt like it.

ANOREXIA, BULIMIA, AND DRUG ABUSE

When I first met Allie she was 22, and her eating disorder had put her in the hospital four times: three for medical emergencies and once, for an entire year, for psychiatric treatment. Her problems with food had begun at about age 12. Allie had also abused cocaine for more than two years. Although she drank alcohol frequently, when she did, she drank to get drunk.

Over the years, Allie had seen a number of qualified outpatient therapists, only to become frustrated with them and drop out of treatment. She had, however, been trying to stick it out with her most recent therapist, who had then moved to another state. She told me that she had benefited a lot from her year in the hospital and that she was serious about getting well. Her perseverance with her previous therapist seemed to be a positive sign against a not very hopeful picture.

At 5'7" tall, Allie's weight had ranged from 87 to 128 pounds. She would make herself vomit after eating almost anything: An apple was as good an excuse as a huge binge on cake, ice cream, and candy. At times she used laxatives (up to 20 times the recommended dose), medicines to bring on vomiting, and appetite suppressants (over-the-counter or street drugs). She had often vomited blood and had blood in her stool. On occasion, Allie had intentionally cut or burned herself and once had made a suicide attempt.

Allie's background was brutally traumatic. Her parents separated when she was six, after years of vicious fighting. Her older brother was often left in charge, and he regularly beat her. During and after their separation, the parents made Allie and her brother deliver messages from one parent to the other. Sometimes those messages included threats or insults that provoked a rageful response from the recipient. The parental combat continued unabated throughout the time that Allie came to see me; it seemed to heat up whenever they could get the children or their friends to watch.

When Allie was eight, two older neighborhood boys picked on her for what became years of sexual abuse. At first, they approached her nicely, which she found flattering and confusing. As they attempted to coax her into sexual acts, she became more reluctant and afraid. Their tactics changed from gentleness to force and threats of more force. They warned her never to "tell" or they would hurt her mother. She was raped, sodomized, made to perform fellatio, called names, and forced to call herself names, such as "slut" and "pig." Allie was pretty sure the abuse began to taper off during her 10th year, and she recalled no further abuse after the age of 11.

Allie was a good student in grammar school and well liked because of her intelligence, wit, and beauty. By junior high school she was skipping classes, cutting school altogether, and sampling many drugs. She also began to binge, to induce vomiting, and to lose weight. It was at this point that school authorities insisted that her parents take her for psychiatric treatment.

Allie was helped very little by outpatient therapy, inpatient hospital treatment, medication therapy, or me. She and I worked together intensively (two to three sessions per week). She attended eating disorders group once a week. However, her symptoms lessened only temporarily. After nearly a year, she had yet another medical crisis (dehydration, with an electrolyte imbalance), and I referred her for another inpatient eating disorders treatment. Further information about her progress is not available.

People like Allie sometimes die of their illnesses, but some do get better. Many factors contribute to their ability to recover. Parents who continue to abuse the patient or blame the patient are hard to fight. Friends who support recovery can help a lot; sticking with friends who abuse food or drugs can undermine treatment. People give up addictions when they "hit bottom"; this point seems to be harder to reach for those who have been the most severely abused.

LONG-TERM TREATMENT OF BULIMIA NERVOSA

This case represents a successful treatment. It took three and a half years, half of which the patient spent in twice-weekly therapy, and a year during which the patient was also treated with antidepressant medication for her binge urges.

Jamie was 23 when she came to me for psychotherapy. She had a five-year history of bingeing and inducing vomiting while maintaining a normal weight. She was a graduate student, continuing a college romance which was now "long distance," had a number of good friends, and a dog she adored. When Jamie started therapy she was bingeing and purging about four times per week. She felt "fat" all of the time and devalued her looks overall. Her only previous treatment occurred at age 15 when she saw a psychiatrist three times after she had made a suicide attempt.

An only child, Jamie believed that family was especially important to her. She was close to her mother and stepfather (her parents divorced when she was seven), father, and maternal grandmother. Her friends and boyfriend saw her with her parents frequently and thought they were all "great."

It was not surprising to find that Jamie was better at recalling events in her history that made her happy rather than those that hurt her. She was accepted at a special grammar school for gifted children and enjoyed herself there very much. After her parents split up she saw her father most weekends and had a wonderful time with him. Although her mother would occasionally make insulting remarks about her father, neither her mother nor father was especially indiscreet in this area.

Jamie was popular throughout her schooling and was always free to invite other children to her home. When her mother remarried and moved, Jamie made friends easily and adjusted to the new school well.

In spite of her high intelligence, Jamie had practically no insight into her illness. She thought she had an eating disorder because she "liked to eat too much." As therapy progressed she reported that her mother frequently criticized her appearance, always begging Jamie to lose weight and be beautiful like her. (Her mother was quite beautiful and probably also had an eating disorder.) Jamie wanted to retract any bad reports she gave me about her mother, blaming herself for being so "one-sided" and feeling guilty about being so "unappreciative" of all that her mother had done for her. Although she was much more comfortable poking fun at her father for being a rigid, compulsive person, she was unable to give examples of him rejecting or mistreating her.

The first six months of treatment helped Jamie reduce her bingeing and vomiting to once a week or every other week. We worked on regulating her eating habits, identifying signals that she was getting "bingey," and establishing alternative stress release behaviors. As we also worked on identifying "triggers" of binge urges, we found multiple examples that pointed to contact with her mother as a primary trigger. This made it easier for Jamie to give an honest account of her life with her mother.

Jamie had very few memories prior to her parents' divorce. Once her parents separated she remembered very well that her mother would scream at her for no apparent reason, cry uncontrollably, and tell Jamie that she was a bad girl and a bad daughter. Sometimes her grandmother was there and intervened on Jamie's behalf. Most of the time her grandmother would explain that Jamie had to understand that her mother was going through a hard time. When Jamie was nine her mother remarried and became somewhat calmer. Even so, Jamie recalled that her mother would initiate fights with Jamie, Jamie would eventually become hysterical, and her stepfather would come home to a scene in which Jamie was out of control and her mother was cool, calm, and feigning ignorance about Jamie's upset. The other source of tremendous frustration came from her mother's teasing of her in front of a friend, persisting until Jamie would burst into tears. Both of these patterns were continuing in Jamie's adult life.

During the next six to 12 months, Jamie and I tried to develop strategies for Jamie to protect herself from such hurts by her mother. She tried very hard but never seemed to successfully preserve her self-respect in these encounters. The aftereffects of her contacts with her mother were still usually eating-disordered behavior. We agreed to have Jamie evaluated for treatment with medication for her binge urges. She began to take antidepressants, and within a month, all bingeing and purging had stopped. However, she found she could not handle her visits with her mother without feeling a loss of self-esteem and self-respect. At this point Jamie decided to cut off all contact with her mother, explaining to her that she needed time to get well and sort out her problems.

Into the third year of Jamie's treatment, she received a number of angry communications from her stepfather and grandmother berating her for her "cruel" treatment of her mother. She was able to tell them that she intended no harm to her mother but needed time for herself. They did not understand.

Now free of the continued pressure to be a "good daughter," Jamie worked hard on coming to terms with her past and present relationship with her mother. Feelings of hatred, fear, and hurt surfaced with intensity. In the final phases of our work together Jamie came to grips with the fact that her mother was emotionally impaired, which was probably caused by or worsened by her abuse of alcohol. She realized that the "closeness" she had felt with her mother was actually based on a one-sided relationship, and that her yearning to have a truly "motherly" mother would not be fulfilled.

Jamie was free of bulimic behavior, her body image was good, and she was maintaining her progress without medication. She stayed in touch with me for several years to tell me of her marriage and the birth of her first child. She had chosen to include her mother in these events but did not find herself reacting to her in the old ways.

Using Individual Psychotherapy to Treat Anorexia Nervosa and Bulimia Nervosa
by Linda P. Bock, M.D.

Individual psychotherapy is always a part of the recovery in anorexia or bulimia nervosa. Sometimes, for someone who is severely compromised or very thin, the initial phases of treatment revolve around nutritional stabilization. It is impossible to do adequate individual psychotherapy when the patient is starving or metabolically in danger. Just as one does not try to reason with an intoxicated alcoholic but waits instead for a sober and lucid period before attempting talking therapy, the eating-disordered person must be medically stable before talking therapy can be helpful. Furthermore, food work needs to keep pace with the talking work. Thus, a severely emaciated anorexic who seems to be "making excellent strides in the cognitive or emotional understanding in her therapy" is actually receiving unbalanced and inadequate therapy. If she were to risk gaining weight, the depth of her psychotherapy would be enhanced. Often with increased body weight (for the anorexic) or with eating and retaining high-risk foods (for the bulimic), the increase in intensity of affect can actively fuel psychological change and growth.

THE STRUCTURE OF INDIVIDUAL PSYCHOTHERAPY

Individual psychotherapy refers to the treatment of psychological disorders by a method that in-

volves interaction between a professionally trained therapist and a patient in a one-on-one, individual structure rather than in a group or a family structure.

A wide range of individual psychotherapies exist, including cognitive-behavioral psychotherapy, Gestalt therapy, rational-emotive therapy, supportive therapy, insight-oriented psychotherapy, psychodynamic psychotherapy, and psychoanalytic therapy (Garner, Vitouser, & Pike, 1997; Herzog, 1995). These types of treatment differ in the amount of activity of the therapist, the use of information and teaching, and the manner and depth of emotional expressivity.

Therapists who specialize in the treatment of eating disorders often work with other colleagues interested in eating disorders, are affiliated with a specialized treatment program, or attend national conferences on eating disorders. Several national information clearinghouses can provide referrals to a specialized therapist.

After an evaluation wherein individual psychotherapy is prescribed, the patient and the therapist must develop a working alliance, reaching agreement on appointment times, fees, and goals of treatment. The frequency of appointments can vary from a rare appointment to regular appointments once, twice, or more times per week. The frequency chosen depends on many factors. If the interest and insight of the patient are high, frequent sessions may be helpful. The patient who is overwhelmed and fearful may need frequent or infrequent sessions. In active psychotherapy, it is common for sessions to be held at least once or twice a week. The sessions must be frequent enough so that the process stays alive and fresh for the patient and the therapist and yet not so frequent that the patient cannot manage to conduct his or her own life of work and play.

ROLES IN PSYCHOTHERAPY

In cognitive-behavioral therapy, the underlying belief systems that support the illness are elucidated. The therapist offers cognitive corrections, education, and information. The patient agrees to observe and document various behaviors and to observe for the ideas that make those behaviors seem appealing or appropriate. Relapse prevention planning, exercises, and rehearsal tasks are assigned, and journaling is often helpful.

In insight-oriented psychotherapy (also called psychodynamic psychotherapy), the therapist agrees to be open to anything that the patient wishes to discuss. The patient is to speak freely without censoring ideas and thoughts. In this way, the patient can come to know his or her own feelings, memories, hopes, and dreams.

In interpersonal psychotherapy the main focus is the here and now, in actions taken outside therapy as well as inside therapy. (Wilson, Fairburn, & Agras, 1997). Past conflicts are not revisited. Therapy become a time to practice new interpersonal attitudes and techniques. Often the therapist directs the patient through various tasks and assignments.

In supportive therapies, the therapist serves as a coach or trainer (Johnson, 1995). Often the therapist will eat meals with the patient or be available for multiple phone contacts. Usually this level of therapy is reserved for severely impaired patients.

Behaviors such as maintaining low body weight, severely uncontrolled eating, lawbreaking, drug abuse, or self-mutilation can prompt hospitalization for the patient's own protection. A contract is helpful to delineate those behaviors that will exceed the limits of outpatient therapy as well as the consequences of such behaviors.

COURSE OF THERAPY

Therapy, especially insight-oriented psychotherapy, can be thought of as having a beginning, a middle, and an end. Ideally, a patient completes all three parts, but many people leave therapy before true completion.

The Beginning Stage of Therapy

The main tasks in the initial phase of treatment are to establish trust in the therapist and to develop a language for emotions. So often with eating disorders, food becomes the means to express all variety of human experience. This task of labeling affect (i.e., emotions) is often very difficult because most people with eating disorders are poorly skilled at using words to express emotions (Goleman, 1995). The word *alexithymia* describes this no-words-for-feeling state.

Trust is a major problem for patients with anorexia nervosa and bulimia. Often people with eating disorders experience closeness in a human relationship as dangerous, with a high potential for rejection, rather than as a source of comfort, warmth or nurturance. Trust, therefore, is often difficult to establish. Another impediment to trust is shame. Most individuals with eating disorders are dominated by feelings of self-loathing and guilt. The drive for thinness and outer beauty is a reflection of the inward sense of worthlessness. Because of the expectation that others will see the person's "badness," the person expects to be rejected and abhorred. One defense to protect themselves from rejection is compliancy, or "people-pleasing." With the "sham" self as armor, any rejection is muffled or dampened. The consequence, however, is that the individual's true self is clouded from view, and genuineness and trust do not develop easily.

As trust and word skill become stronger, overt symptoms in the person's life decrease. This marks the beginning of the middle phase of psychotherapy.

The Middle Stage of Therapy

During the middle phase, whatever tension that caused major problems in the patient's life becomes less problematic in the patient's "real" life and more operationally active in the therapy "life," that is, in the relationship between the patient and the therapist. For example, a patient who is overly dependent on her parents may become more assertive with her parents and feel safer about growing up, but become more dependent on the therapist instead. As another example, a patient who was so involved in people-pleasing that she had no identity of her own may try in the session to please the therapist even as she becomes better able to stand up for her own likes and dislikes outside of therapy.

Once the sources of tension are compartmentalized within the therapeutic relationship, they are studied in three contexts: (1) the patient-therapist relationship, (2) the relationships of the past, and (3) the relationships of the present. As an example, a patient with conflict over dishonesty may find herself caught in a deceit by her boyfriend or husband. During treatment the patient and therapist would look for tensions or feeling states about deceits in her current life (e.g., with her boyfriend or husband) as well as in her past (perhaps with her parents or teachers) and now in treatment (with her therapist).

By using these three areas of focus, the conflicts unravel and a clear meaning emerges. As the protective functions of the symptoms are more clearly seen, the person can develop new skills and defenses to protect oneself—better defenses than those the illness had offered. With the replacement of symptoms with new skills the end phase of therapy is at hand. Resolution occurs, and the patient no longer needs old symptoms to manage previously misunderstood or unconscious conflicts.

The End Stage of Therapy

As termination begins, it is common for some symptoms to return. In part these reappearing symptoms reflect the terror of leaving. The exacerbation of symptoms also allows a reworking of conflicts in a synoptic or review manner. Just as learning to trust the therapist was the challenge in the initial phase, learning to trust oneself is the accomplishment at the termination of treatment.

CONFLICTS ADDRESSED IN THERAPY

Some commonly encountered conflicts that can underlie an eating disorder are listed below as side-by-side polarities or tensions:

• Abandonment/Engulfment
• Dependence/Independence
• False Identity/Compliance

These extremes are often the feeling states occupied during illness. The optimum or healthy, normal position involves a mid-zone stance between the poles—comfort in human relationships, interdependence, and a genuine sense of self. Often problems arise with the developmental task of separation and individuation. This normal developmental process usually peaks from six months to three years of age. During normal adolescence, the separation-individuation struggles reawaken. The task within both age groups is to manage as a separate person and yet relate safely and competently with the surrounding world of people.

Commonly, though not universally, individuals with anorexia and bulimia have had problematic childhood or adolescent years. Often the families are dysfunctional, with one emotionally overwhelming parent and one emotionally unavailable parent. Parent alcoholism or workaholism, parent anxieties, child neglect, physical abuse, sexual abuse, date rape, abortion, or other major traumas are very common.

These burdens make the usual tasks of separation and individuation impossible for children to accomplish. An eating disorder, with all its defensive protections, serves to delay separation and individuation, provide safety from trauma, and draw forth caretaking from the very people the child needs developmentally to leave. If trauma is a significant component of the illness, safety becomes an essential aspect of therapy. Relapse into starving or purging as a method of emotional numbing substitutes if real safety is not present.

AFTER THERAPY

If the termination phase allows adequate time, the patient leaves treatment with self-reliance and the ability to continue the self-modulating, self-observing process without the therapist's presence.

The beginning, middle, and end phases of therapy can take equal amounts of time. For instance, in a three-year course of therapy, roughly 12 months may be spent in each phase. Other times, one phase can be protracted. For example, the death of a significant person (in the current or past) can make the termination phase richer and more time-consuming. If a patient is highly word-skilled or trusting, the initial phase may be quite brisk.

Although many patients can and do successfully complete treatment, not all patients who stop therapy have "finished" their therapy. Some patients start with one therapist, work for a while, then leave and later begin anew with another therapist. Often in the course of the second treatment, using the new skills acquired in the first therapy can enable treatment to progress more rapidly. Other people return to treatment, even after a full and successful therapy, when life's problems provoke distress and dysfunction. These new life stressors can reawaken old, dormant defenses and dysfunctional patterns.

THERAPY COMBINATION

Individual insight-oriented psychotherapy is typically augmented by nutritional counseling, cognitive-behavioral therapy, family therapy, and group therapy. Some patients benefit greatly from one therapy in the initial stages of recovery and from another therapy at a later time. Thus at first, fam-

ily therapy may, for one patient, be helpful to conquer denial; however, family therapy may be minimally significant as the patient approaches the close of therapy (Johnson, 1995; Wilson, Fairburn, & Agras, 1997).

The overall goal of therapy is to maximize discovery, to minimize symptoms and acting out, and to maintain fullness of life.

REFERENCES

Garner, David M., Vitousek, Kelly M., & Pike, Kathleen M. (1997). Cognitive-behavioral therapy for anorexia nervosa. In *Handbook of Treatment for Eating Disorders* (pp. 94–144). New York: Guilford.

Goleman, Daniel. (1995). *Emotional Intelligence.* New York: Bantam.

Herzog, David. (1995). Psychodynamic psychotherapy for anorexia nervosa. *Eating Disorders and Obesity: A Comprehensive Handbook.* New York: Guilford.

Johnson, Craig. (1995). Psychodynamic treatment of bulimia nervosa. *Eating Disorders and Obesity: A Comprehensive Handbook.* New York: Guilford.

Wilson, G. Terence, Fairburn, Christopher G., & Agras, W. Stewart. (1997). Cognitive-behavioral therapy for bulimia nervosa. *Handbook of Treatment for Eating Disorders.* New York: Guilford.

Group Therapy for Bulimia Nervosa

by Lillie Weiss, Ph.D., Melanie Katzman, Ph.D., and Sharlene Wolchik, Ph.D.

Has your eating gotten out of control? Do you eat too much and then throw up? Do you get depressed and disgusted with yourself afterwards? Do you feel that you would simply die if anyone discovered your "secret"?

YOU ARE NOT ALONE!

Many other people in your situation experience the same problems you do. They binge regularly, then vomit, take laxatives or water pills, or starve themselves. They feel guilty, embarrassed, and ashamed and think that they are alone with their suffering. Actually, the binge-purge cycle, or bu-

limia, as it is called, is fairly common. It is estimated that 8.3 percent of high school girls fulfill diagnostic criteria for bulimia (Johnson, Lewis, Love, Lewis, & Stuckey, 1984) and that one in five regularly engages in binge eating (Levine, 1987).

Group therapy can be very helpful for bulimics, who often feel isolated, alone, and misunderstood. In a group setting, you can learn, change, and share your experiences with others who have similar problems.

WHAT IS GROUP THERAPY?

Group therapy involves a variety of people with similar problems who meet in a warm, supportive, and confidential setting to discuss their common concerns and learn to deal with their problems through mutual sharing, support, and feedback. Most groups meet on a weekly basis, usually for one and a half to two hours, and are led by one or more therapists.

WHY IS GROUP THERAPY HELPFUL?

Group therapy affirms, first of all, that you are not alone. No longer do you have to feel isolated or believe that "nobody can understand." When you see others in your situation, you begin to make more personal connections that start you on the path of coping with problems by relying on people, not food. Many bulimics think that they are the only ones who binge and purge or have an extreme dislike for themselves and their bodies. They are often relieved to find that others have similar fears, preoccupations, and feelings. For teenagers in particular, it is such a relief to be able to finally express feelings of shame and hurt and be understood! The experience of sharing negative feelings and still being accepted by the group can help free them from these emotions.

Groups provide a "safe" place where you can express your concerns and not feel that you are going to be judged. You can learn to accept yourself and no longer feel ashamed or abnormal, or that you would "die" if anyone found out. Instead, through your experience and the experiences of others, you can learn to understand the reasons behind your preoccupation with food and weight.

Group therapy also provides the support you need to make changes. It is much easier to work on getting better when you have a whole team rooting for you and encouraging you along the way. Group members can help you through the rough times. In some groups, members talk with each other at times other than in the group sessions. These relationships can provide support for the changes group members make.

Group therapy also gives you a chance to learn. By seeing how others solve their problems, you can learn new ways of looking at and dealing with yours. You can learn much just by listening and vicariously sharing in the experiences of others. For example, listening to another group member's distorted view of her body may help you to recognize similar distortions in your perceptions of your body. Group members can also provide you with valuable feedback on your behavior, which you can use to make meaningful changes.

A group can also educate you about your eating problems and provide you with new tools to break out of old patterns. Group leaders can provide information about bulimia and dispel common myths and misconceptions. They can also teach you new coping skills to deal with your stresses.

Groups give you a chance to practice what you have learned. Jamie, for example, learned that she ate uncontrollably whenever she disagreed with someone but didn't speak up. In the group, she was encouraged to express herself whenever she had an opinion. Being able to practice her assertiveness skills in a group helped her to do so outside the therapy setting. She came to learn that she didn't need to "eat" her feelings, but that she could express them to others.

Probably one of the most important functions of a group is to offer hope. When you see someone with a similar problem making progress, it lets you know that you can change, too. As many have told us, "If she (or he) can do it, I can do it!"

TYPES OF GROUP SUPPORT

Several types of groups serve persons with eating disorders. Some groups are *closed* groups. In closed groups the same group members meet every session with no new members allowed. Closed groups are generally, but not always, short-term, meeting for a certain number of sessions with a beginning and ending date. *Open* or ongoing groups are open to new members. These tend to be longer-term and may go on indefinitely, with new members coming in and old ones leaving. Sometimes a beginning group member may start out in a closed group of limited duration, then join an open, long-term group for follow-up and maintenance.

Groups can also be *structured* or *unstructured*. Some groups have certain themes or topics for each week and follow a specified format. Generally, short-term, closed groups have a definite format or structure. Psychoeducational groups, or groups that combine psychotherapy and education, tend to be fairly structured and have planned teaching materials for each session. Group members can share their experiences and feelings within the context of that structure. Many long-term, open-ended groups tend to be unstructured, with no specific topic or agenda planned. In these groups, members discuss problems that have arisen since the last meeting and learn about how they deal with relationships by discussing the interactions that occur among the group members.

Homogenous groups and *heterogenous* groups also serve people with eating disorders. Homogenous groups are only for persons with bulimia, whereas heterogenous groups include individuals with all types of eating disorders. Although an argument can be made for mixing patients, it has been our experience that it is generally not useful for persons with different eating problems to be in the same group. In particular, we believe that individuals with anorexia should not be in the same group as those with bulimia because their dynamics differ (Weiss & Katzman, 1984).

When we speak of group therapy, we are generally referring to groups led by trained therapists. Peer support groups, or *self-help* groups, are organized and run by persons who have had eating disorders in the past. One function of these groups is to provide ongoing support.

In addition to groups for the person with the eating problem, there are support groups for family members. These groups can provide information, give support, and help your family give you the encouragement you need. Many families want to be helpful but may not know how. In addition, they may be misinformed about bulimia; groups can help correct these misconceptions and provide accurate information.

WHAT KINDS OF GROUPS ARE AVAILABLE?

Group treatments for eating disorders vary across a number of theoretical orientations and take place in inpatient, day hospital, or outpatient environments (Harper-Giuffre & MacKenzie, 1992; Polivy & Federoff, 1997). In addition, intensive "marathon" workshops for group participants are conducted in resort settings or other neutral environments. Here, we will briefly describe some typical group therapies for eating disorders.

Behavioral and Cognitive-Behavioral Group Therapy

As the name implies, behavioral approaches focus on the eating behavior. Group members keep track of the conditions that lead to disturbed eating and learn to substitute other behaviors for the bingeing and purging. Behavioral approaches use such techniques as relaxation, stress management, nutritional management, and strategies to change "triggers" for bingeing. For example, if skipping breakfast and lunch triggers bingeing behavior in the evening, group members learn to eat three meals a day to prevent nighttime binges.

Whereas most behavioral groups concentrate on the bingeing behavior, some focus on preventing vomiting by exposing the bulimic participants to food and not letting them vomit afterwards (Gray & Hoage, 1990). Some groups use a group meal as an opportunity for bulimics to reduce anxiety without vomiting afterwards (Franko, 1993). Most groups, however, do not involve therapists exposing group members to food and staying with them for several hours to prevent them from vomiting. In addition to its questionable effectiveness, it is time-consuming and unpleasant to many clients (Fairburn, 1988).

More common than pure behavioral approaches to group treatment are cognitive-behavioral approaches. Here the emphasis is not only on changing behaviors but on changing cognitions (thoughts and beliefs). Many bulimics, particularly women, have faulty beliefs and values about eating, weight, and body image—such as "I've found an easy way to diet" or "I need to vomit this gross bulge in my stomach"—that lead to their bingeing or purging. In cognitive-behavioral therapy, group members learn to recognize and change the way they think about weight, food, and eating. Cognitive-behavioral group therapy has been found to be a very effective treatment approach for bulimia (Dedman, Numa, & Wakeling, 1988).

Psychoeducational Group Therapy

Psychoeducational groups combine psychotherapy and education. Many cognitive-behavioral and other groups use a psychoeducational framework where information about bulimia is presented in an educational format with an opportunity for group participants to discuss and relate the information learned to their own particular situation. Most meetings in a psychoeducational group are fairly structured with specific, preassigned topics. Therapists frequently use intensive and detailed manuals to conduct the sessions, and group members complete structured exercises within the group as well as homework assignments. A psychoeducational group is in many ways like a class, with opportunities for learning and applying knowledge to one's own situation. Psychoeducational groups, like classes, usually have a syllabus and a limited number of sessions. They are frequently short-term, ranging from several weeks to several months.

Psychodynamic/Interpersonal Group Therapy

Unlike the above-mentioned approaches, which are heavily structured and intent on teaching specific content, psychodynamic group therapy is relatively unstructured, focusing on the "here and now." It attempts to provide an emotional experience where group members can learn about themselves and how they relate to others through their interaction with other members in the group. The group can be seen as a laboratory where group members can make self-discoveries and explore their relationships with others. Through these interactions, they can reexperience and reexamine problems related to interpersonal relationships. Psychodynamic groups focus more on the psychological and interpersonal issues behind the eating disorder, rather than on managing the eating behavior. The emphasis is on what happens within the group—the group process— rather than on providing specific informational content. Psychodynamic groups are usually long-term, six months or more, up to several years (Harper-Giuffre, MacKenzie, & Sivitilli, 1992).

Psychodynamic approaches have been used with behavioral, cognitive, and educational components. Many group therapies are eclectic, that is, they combine features of different treatment approaches. Most focus in varying degrees on both content (what members talk about) and process (what happens within the group).

A form of group therapy to help group members develop insight into their personal and eating problems is psychodrama. As the name suggests, it involves the use of drama to bring about psychological change. Group members act out their conflicts and emotions, with the therapist serving as director. As they role-play their situations, they release pent-up emotions, see their problems in a new light, and work through them within a supportive group atmosphere. Psychodrama uses some powerful techniques to bring about change. In "doubling," for example, the

therapist or another group member physically joins the protagonist or central character within the psychodrama and speaks his or her unexpressed thoughts and feelings aloud. Hearing and seeing one's "drama" on stage can be quite illuminating. "Role reversal," where one participant reverses roles with another and "becomes" that person, helps a group member see the world through that person's eyes and also how he or she is seen from the other's point of view.

Little research has examined the use of psychodrama specifically with bulimics. Psychodrama used specifically for bulimia focuses on eating behavior, body image, intimacy issues, and feelings about oneself (Callahan, 1989). An example of an exercise related to food and eating is the Clock exercise where group members walk silently in a circle, mentally passing through the hours of the clock, and then stop at a time when food becomes a problem for them. They then role-play and discuss their feelings. In the Mirror exercise for body image, group members face an imaginary mirror and describe what they "see." In these and other exercises, group members can play the parts of different foods, different body parts, or different people in their lives. Although psychodrama may at times have a playful quality, such as, for example, when people "become" ice cream, it can also quickly bring about very intense emotional experiences. It is important that psychodrama be conducted in a "safe" setting with a skilled and trained therapist, and only with group members who can separate fantasy from reality and withstand the emotional intensity of some very powerful psychodramatic techniques.

The Addiction Model

Some therapists view binge eating as an addiction like alcohol or substance abuse and use treatment approaches similar to Alcoholics Anonymous (AA). Overeaters Anonymous (OA) is an example of a group approach that views eating disorders as addictive and teaches abstinence from binge eating. In this approach, the person's relationship with food is viewed as an addiction, and within the group he or she is given support for abstaining from problem foods. Whereas some treatments for bulimia have used an addiction-oriented treatment model (Mitchell, Hatsukami, Goff, Pyle, Eckert, & Davis, 1985), it is one that has been much criticized (Wilson, 1991). Viewing their binge eating as an addiction rather than a learned habit or a coping mechanism leaves many with bulimia feeling out of control and not in charge of their behavior. In addition, teaching "abstinence" from food may encourage dieting, which is a known trigger for bingeing. Finally, the addiction model assumes that all women with eating disorders are the same and may ignore differences between bulimics and compulsive overeaters.

Intensive Short-Term Therapies

Whereas most groups meet on a weekly basis, some groups are more intensive, ranging from marathon weekend retreats to treatment retreats lasting several weeks. One benefit of intensive retreats is that group members can focus exclusively on their behavior without the distractions of "real life." Also, the relaxed setting and intensive group experience help participants develop a level of intimacy and sharing with others.

A rather innovative group experience is the two-day intensive group process-retreat or "bulimia workshop," which has been effective in changing women's eating habits and their feelings about themselves (Bohanske & Lemberg, 1987; Gendron, Lemberg, Allender, & Bohanske, 1992). The purpose of the retreat experience is to help women redirect the "problem" away from food and weight issues and toward developing more satisfying relationships with others and more meaningful personal goals. In addition to learning to change eating habits and receiving nutritional information, group members are taught ways of building self-esteem, being assertive, and communicating effectively. In these groups, they learn to view their bulimia as a personal problem requiring choice and responsibility rather than as an "identity" or a "disease." Some group members view the intensive experience as a "turning point," and many find the "togetherness" they experience with others as the most useful aspect of the retreat model. Although brief group retreats are not meant to supplant other long-term treatments, they can help in breaking through personal blocks and strengthening the commitment to change for those already in treatment.

Other intensive treatments include the Breaking Free workshops developed by Geneen Roth (1984) to help women break free from compulsive eating. In these eight-week workshops, participants learn to incorporate a philosophy of trusting yourself, nourishing yourself, and accepting yourself into daily actions and beliefs. Roth was a compulsive eater herself who decided that she could eat anything she wanted without guilt and would never diet again. She teaches women strategies that have worked for her to break free from compulsive eating such as learning to eat what you want and trusting yourself to make healthy choices. Roth's workshops are for all compulsive eaters.

A day hospital program provides another type of intensive treatment in a group setting. Patients attend the program in the hospital for about eight hours a day, going home for evenings and weekends. Some programs are limited to 12 patients at a time, but aside from the initial evaluations, typically all treatment occurs in groups (Kaplan, Kerr, & Maddocks, 1992). Patients are expected to attend all of the groups in the program, which can roughly be divided into two categories: eating and noneating groups. The eating groups consist of groups that eat meals together, menu groups, nutrition groups, and eating-attitude groups. Noneating groups include assertion, leisure and time management, creative arts, and body image. Most of the groups have an educational component. Day hospital programs have been developed particularly for women with serious anorexic and bulimic symptoms, particularly for those whose eating disorders have become medically dangerous. An advantage of a day hospital program is that patients can use many of the resources that a hospital setting provides without the financial burden of overnight hospitalization.

Inpatient group treatment is another short-term intensive treatment for individuals with eating disorders. When the eating disorder becomes physically harmful or life-threatening, hospitalization may become necessary. Inpatients tend to have longer and more severe eating-disorder histories, and the goals of the inpatient treatment program for bulimics are to break the binge-purge cycle and promote normal eating (Duncan & Kennedy, 1992). Because inpatient treatment is frequently limited to a few weeks, many patients may see this as an impetus to engage in the group and not waste time. Inpatient groups, like day hospital groups, are usually not restricted to bulimics, but include patients with other eating disorders as well. Like the other intensive, short-term treatments, inpatient groups can provide the momentum and serve as a good starting point for further outpatient therapy to maintain the progress made during this brief time.

Self-Help Group Therapy

Self-help groups differ from therapy groups in that they are not led by a professional therapist. They can be a good source of education and information and can also offer support and acceptance. Such groups are not meant to replace therapy and are frequently used in addition to professional treatment. They differ from regular therapy groups in that there is generally no charge to group members, and attendance is optional. Their biggest benefit is that they offer ongoing support; their biggest drawback is that there is usually very little control over who attends these groups.

WHAT CAN I EXPECT TO HAPPEN IN GROUP THERAPY?

In a typical group therapy session, a small number of people, usually between five and 12, discuss their eating habits and their feelings about themselves. They receive feedback from other group members and learn other ways of dealing with their feelings besides bingeing and purging.

In our groups (Weiss, Katzman, & Wolchik, 1985, 1986), we offer a combination of education and a chance to share feelings and experiences. Topics include information about bulimia, its medical and psychological complications, and myths and misconceptions about it. In addition to discussing proper nutrition and eating in a healthy manner, we discuss how eating is often used as a coping strategy and provide group members alternative ways of dealing with their stresses. Some of our sessions are devoted to such topics as perfectionism and anger management, as many bulimics set unrealistically high standards for themselves and have difficulty asserting themselves. We also talk about our feelings for our bodies and societal pressure for women to be thin. Reading materials, exercises, and homework in each session address these topics, and group members practice what they learn outside the therapy session.

IS GROUP THERAPY ENOUGH, OR DO I NEED SOME OTHER TYPE OF HELP AS WELL?

Group therapy is not the only treatment for bulimia and does not preclude individual treatment. Group therapy is frequently most effective in conjunction with individual therapy. It can also be used for follow-up and maintenance after a person has been in individual therapy for some time and wants to continue to have ongoing support when therapy is completed.

ARE ALL GROUPS BENEFICIAL?

The answer to that question is, unfortunately, no. Although group therapy, conducted by properly trained professionals, is, for the most part, very helpful, there are "bad" groups that may have some negative consequences. These groups are frequently led by persons who are knowledgeable about neither eating disorders nor group therapy. Make certain to check out the therapist's training and credentials before you join a group. It is important that the therapist be sufficiently familiar with eating disorders so that you can receive accurate information and help.

Although it is natural to feel uncomfortable at first when joining a new group, if you feel very ill at ease, belittled, or attacked, trust your instincts and find a group where you feel more comfortable. Although sometimes in a group you may hear feedback from the therapist that is uncomfortable, it should not feel disrespectful or humiliating. If you believe it to be so, discuss it with the therapist after the session.

One unfortunate consequence of some groups is that the members may want to talk about new ways of purging rather than to learn other ways to cope with their feelings and problems. If you find that the main topic in the group is a comparison of the most effective vomiting techniques, this is clearly the wrong group for you. A good group will encourage you to *decrease* your bingeing and purging, not teach you new ways to promote it. A good group will focus on feelings and the meaning of food, not just on what you ate.

Another feature of a "bad" group is pessimism. If you come out of a group feeling as though there is no hope, then you are probably being misinformed. In a good group, you will be given encouragement, hope, and healthy tools to help you break your habit. However, be aware that it may take several meetings to judge whether the group is right for you.

WHEN IS GROUP THERAPY MOST AND LEAST HELPFUL?

A common misconception about group psychotherapy is that it is a cheaper, second-rate treatment inferior to individual psychotherapy. The research literature concludes that groups are effective forms of treatment and that there appears to be no significant advantage to individual treatment where such comparisons are made (Polivy & Federoff, 1997). Also, no particular type of therapeutic approach produces consistently better or worse outcomes than others. It seems safe to conclude that groups are not inferior to individual therapy and are by themselves a useful and cost-effective means of treatment for bulimia. Some people may do better in a group setting than in individual therapy (and vice versa).

If you are motivated to change and commit yourself to attending all of the sessions, actively participating in them, and following through on homework assignments, you will likely do well in either individual or group therapy. If you have problems in addition to the bingeing and purging, such as alcohol or substance abuse, suicidal behavior, other medical risk, or have been diagnosed as having a personality disorder, you may need treatment for those conditions first. If you have a history of sexual or physical abuse, you may find that some highly structured group formats do not allow you to explore important connections between eating and abuse unless these topics are specifically addressed as part of the curriculum. If you are in a severe crisis that demands immediate attention, that may take precedence over anything else. Not only will your problems keep you from participating fully in the group program, but they may also be disruptive for the other group members. Most therapists will see you for an initial interview and do some screening and preparation before assigning you to a group. With a screening interview, the chances of being placed in an unsuitable group decrease. The initial interview not only allows you to see if the group is a good fit for you but also prepares you for the group experience. Screening patients and preparing them for group therapy helps reduce the dropout rate and improve the overall quality of the group.

Although the support and understanding received from other group members enhance the group's effectiveness, some group members may become too dependent on others. For this reason, and also to prevent some members from feeling excluded, socializing by members outside of the sessions is discouraged in some therapy groups. However, other groups, particularly support groups, may encourage friendships outside the sessions. Each group has its own rules, and you will have to decide whether a particular friendship is helping you or sapping your strength.

As the typical bulimic is a young, white woman, most group members will fall into that category. If you are a male, a minority, an adolescent, or an older woman, you may feel awkward about attending such a group session. Make certain to discuss these issues with the group leader beforehand. Look into category-specific groups, such as those for high school students, which may be more relevant for you if you are an adolescent. However, keep in mind that many eating issues relate to most group members, regardless of age, sex, or ethnic group.

Who conducts the group is as important as who attends it. Group therapy is often conducted by co-therapists, either female pairs or male-female pairs. Some therapists see a male-female pair as important in re-creating the parent figures in the group and allowing group members to see how they interact with both males and females (Bohanske & Lemberg, 1987). Others feel that a male therapist may inhibit female group members from talking about body image or sexuality (Hall, 1985). Who is most appropriate to work with the largely female eating-disordered population? The issue is a complicated one, yet a practical one as well. Who the best therapist is for you should be guided by your needs (Katzman & Waller, in press). In our experience, we have had success with groups led by both male-female pairs as well as female pairs. It appears that the other qualities of the therapist, such as warmth, caring, and competence, are more important than gender. It is crucial that you have a therapist you trust and can relate to, whether that person is male or female.

What type of group to join is another consideration. We have already reviewed the different types of groups, most of which are eclectic, combining aspects of different theoretical approaches. Reviews of the studies find no clear advantages to any given therapy, and group treatment seems to be as effective as individual methods (Garner, Fairburn, & Davis, 1987). There is a general consensus, however, that both group leaders and group members must play an *active* role in the therapy. Leaders teach, guide, and give information; group members observe their behavior, set their own goals, and communicate and participate in the group (Oesterheld, McKenna, & Gould, 1987).

Where to have group therapy—in an outpatient or inpatient setting—is another decision. As we said before, one advantage of both day hospital and inpatient treatment is that it takes you away from the demands of "real life" so that you can focus exclusively on the eating problems. Inpatient hospitalization may be necessary if there is a strong medical or suicidal risk. Anorexic patients are frequently hospitalized because of medical complications. In our experience, bulimics often can be very successfully treated in an outpatient setting. Although it is advantageous at times to get away from the pressures of everyday life, we feel that it is important for individuals to learn new eating habits and practice them in their day-to-day lives. We view bulimia as a learned habit and not as an illness. Thus, if there are no medical or psychiatric problems that warrant hospitalization, outpatient therapy is frequently sufficient to change disordered eating habits.

HOW CAN I FIND THE RIGHT GROUP FOR ME?

Contact your family physician, a school nurse or counselor, or the nearest university to get the names of some groups in your area. Remember, eating problems can be medically serious and psychologically draining, but you *can* change your eating habits and gain control over them. Remember, *you are not alone!*

REFERENCES

Bohanske, J., & Lemberg, R. (1987). An intensive group process-retreat model for the treatment of bulimia. *Group 11,* 228–37.

Callahan, M. (1989). Psychodrama and the treatment of bulimia. In L. M. Hornyak & E. K. Baker (Eds.), *Experiential therapies for eating disorders* (pp.101–20). New York: Guilford Press.

Dedman, P. A., Numa, S. F., & Wakeling, A. (1988). A cognitive-behavioral group approach for the treatment of bulimia nervosa: A preliminary study. *Journal of Psychosomatic Research 32,* 285–90.

Duncan, J., & Kennedy, S. H. (1992). Inpatient group treatment. In H. Harper-Giuffre & K. R. MacKenzie (Eds.), *Group psychotherapy for eating disorders* (pp. 149–60). Washington, DC: American Psychiatric Press.

Fairburn, C. G. (1988). The current status for the psychological treatments for bulimia nervosa. *Journal of Psychosomatic Research 32,* 635–45.

Franko, D. L. (1993). The use of a group meal in the brief therapy of bulimia nervosa. *International Journal of Group Psychotherapy 43,* 237–42.

Garner, D. M., Fairburn, C. G., & Davis, R. (1987). Cognitive-behavioral treatment of bulimia nervosa: A critical appraisal. *Behavior Modification 11,* 398–431.

Gendron, M., Lemberg, R., Allender, J., & Bohanske, J. (1992). Effectiveness of the intensive group process-retreat model in the treatment of bulimia. *Group 16,* 69-78.

Gray, J. J., & Hoage, C. M. (1990). Bulimia nervosa: Group behavior therapy with exposure plus response prevention. *Psychological Reports 66,* 667–74.

Hall, A. (1985). Group psychotherapy for anorexia nervosa and bulimia. In D. M. Garner & P. E. Garfinkel (Eds.), *Handbook of psychotherapy for anorexia nervosa and bulimia* (pp. 213–39). New York: Guilford Press.

Harper-Giuffre, H., & MacKenzie, K. R., (Eds.). (1992). *Group psychotherapy for eating disorders.* Washington, DC: American Psychiatric Press.

Harper-Giuffre, H., MacKenzie, K. R., & Sivitilli, D. (1992). Interpersonal group psycho-therapy. In H. Harper-Giuffre & K. R. MacKenzie (Eds.), *Group psychotherapy for eating disorders* (pp. 105–45). Washington, DC: American Psychiatric Press.

Johnson, C. L., Lewis, C., Love, S., Lewis, L., & Stuckey, M. (1984). *Incidence and correlates of bulimic behavior in a female high school population.* Journal of Youth and Adolescence 13, 15–26.

Kaplan, A. S., Kerr, A., & Maddocks, S. E. (1992). Day hospital group treatment. In H. Harper-Giuffre & K. R. MacKenzie (Eds.), *Group psychotherapy for eating disorders* (pp. 161–79). Washington, DC: American Psychiatric Press.

Katzman, M. A., & Waller, G. (in press). Gender of the therapist: Daring to ask the questions. In W. Vandereycken (Ed.), *The brain of the therapist.* London: Athlone Press.

Levine, M. P. (1987). *How schools can help combat student eating disorders.* Washington, DC: National Education Association.

Mitchell, J. E., Hatsukami, D., Goff, G., Pyle, R. L., Eckert, E. D., & Davis, L. E. (1985). Intensive outpatient group treatment for bulimia. In D. M. Garner & P. E. Garfinkel (Eds.), *Handbook of psychotherapy for anorexia nervosa and bulimia* (pp. 240–53). New York: Guilford Press.

Oesterheld, J. R., McKenna, M. S., & Gould, N. B. (1987). Group psychotherapy of bulimia: A critical review. *International Journal of Group Psychotherapy 37,* 163–84.

Polivy, J., & Federoff, I. (1997). Group psychotherapy. In D. M. Garner & P. E. Garfinkel (Eds.), *Handbook of psychotherapy for anorexia nervosa and bulimia* (2nd ed.) (pp. 462–75). New York: Guilford Press.

Roth, G. (1984). *Breaking free from compulsive eating.* New York: Signet.

Weiss, L., & Katzman, M. A. (1984). Group treatment for bulimic women. *Arizona Medicine 41*(2), 100–04.

Weiss, L., Katzman, M. A., & Wolchik, S. A. (1985). *Treating bulimia: A psycho-educational approach.* New York: Pergamon Press.

Weiss, L., Katzman, M. A., & Wolchik, S. A. (1986). *You can't have your cake and eat it too: A program for controlling bulimia.* Saratoga, CA: R. & E. Publishers.

Wilson, G. T. (1991). The addiction model of eating disorders: A critical analysis. *Advances in Behavior Research and Therapy 13,* 27–72.

Eating-Disordered Families: Issues Between the Generations

by Bonnie L. Pelch, A.C.S.W.

HAND ME DOWN HURT[1]

Hand me down hurt,
It's nothing new
As was done unto me now
I do unto you.

Like his daddy's daddy,
and his father's son,
over and over the same course is run.

You're so damn stupid,
That's what you are
Thru generations those words
travel far.

Please break the cycle,
Help stop the pain
Don't keep repeating this
Sad, sad refrain.

This poem wasn't written by a family member of an eating-disordered victim but by a fiancé. He realized that unresolved issues in past relationships are revisited in new relationships and in new generations. Therapists and writers in the fields of psychiatry, social psychology, family therapy, and self-help talk about issues among generations in families in a variety of ways. Virginia Satir (1972) refers to "scripting"; Judith Viorst (1987) points out the need to grieve the loss of dreams as well as the loss of loved ones; Charles Whitfield (1987) addresses the dynamics of shame and low self-esteem; Harriet Goldhor Lerner (1989) explains that overfunctioners need as much understanding and attention as do chronic underfunctioners. I would venture to say that you can't give what you didn't get.

To better understand multigenerational issues in eating-disordered families, we will first take a look at healthy families to see that, in family therapy, the patient is the family, not the individual. Comments regarding the healthy family will provide specific signs and symptoms that distinguish healthier from less healthy families.

Common traits of eating-disordered families, which may be similar to those of other dysfunctional family systems, will be discussed. Finally, the role of the family in the recovery of the eating-disordered victim and the healing of the family as a whole will be explored through the eyes of a family therapist.

HEALTHY FAMILIES

Family systems share at least eight characteristics that provide a natural pulse to the progress of a family unit in its life cycle. Those characteristics are:

- Quality of parental relationships
- Allocation of power
- Problem-solving ability
- Ability to discuss feelings
- Commonality of values
- Communication
- Intimacy and autonomy
- Tolerance to change

If the primary goal of the family is to support the development of all of its members, then these eight characteristics must be monitored regularly.

For example, allocation of power in healthy families is democratically distributed; no one person dictates decisions and plans for the family or its individual members. Functional systems avoid dominant-submissive interactions. A healthy family has open communication, with members able to discuss negative and positive feelings. Autonomy and intimacy are not privileges reserved for the adults only. Harriet Lerner (1989) clarifies intimacy as requiring "authenticity in the context of connectedness. Authenticity means we can be who we are in a relationship . . . it requires that we allow the other person to do the same."

---

[1] Copyright 1991 by Steve Finazzo. Used by permission.

Problem solving is a shared task, negotiated by two or more family members. The success of that task is not measured by a unanimous decision. Instead, asserting one's ideas and understanding other family members' points of view are the most important goals.

The ability to discuss one's feelings is critical to healthy individual and family development. The acceptance of emotions as valid, without labeling them as negative or positive, is a priority for the growth-conscious family. (See Sater, 1972.)

Because of space constraints, all eight family characteristics are not examined here. Instead, the chapter focuses on characteristics as they relate to the psychosomatic or eating-disordered family.

FAMILIES: SECONDHAND VICTIMS OF EATING DISORDERS

All families pass through their own unique life cycles. If one views the system as traveling horizontally through time, the phases are as predictable as those of the individual. The phases are leaving home, marriage, birth of children, parenting, children exiting the nuclear family, and retirement. What complicates this picture is that the family experiences a vertical, intergenerational dimension at the same time. Members of the family are pushed to change or recognize change at each phase (their horizontal task), while coping with whatever legacy has been passed down from previous generations (their vertical task). Attitudes about illness, money, sex, divorce, and death are a part of that legacy, which may be more or less functional. The difference between healthy and less healthy families is in the management of these vertical and horizontal phases. The less functional family gets derailed or stuck in either the normal or the unexpected life crises.

Superimposed on the family system and burdening the family further are purported risk factors for eating-disorder development, including the pressure on women to please others at their expense; the idealization of thinness; and the myth of the superwoman who can "do it all." If the family tends to magnify the aforementioned cultural attributes, an eating disorder has fertile ground in which to grow. (See Zerbe, 1995: pp. 101.)

Eating disorders do not thrive in a healthy cultural or familial environment. Be clear, however, that no parent sets out to have a child with an eating disorder. Although each family is different, eating-disordered families share common problems. The family often mirrors the difficulties experienced by the eating-disordered individual. In such a case, common family themes are preoccupation with food, weight, and/or appearance; perfectionism; a preoccupation with success (particularly financial); hypersensitivity toward one another (not distinguishing where one member's problem ends and the other member's begins); poor conflict resolution skills; and an absence of flexibility regarding family rules or expectations.

The eating-disordered family has at least four vulnerable areas of family functioning that deserve mention:

- Perfectionism
- Life in the extremes
- Suppression of one or more inherent human emotions (sadness, anger, gladness, fear, or confusion)
- Conflict related to one's sexuality

Perfectionism is a thread that may run from appearance to eating only healthy foods to being number one at school or work. Just being "good enough" is rarely acceptable to the success-driven individual or family. Even one's choice of sport or recreation ultimately depends on having the perfect or best score/performance.

Life in the extremes (all-or-nothing thinking) can be a trap that fuels the eating disorder. Moderation is seen as boring, mediocre, or insignificant. Obsessions and compulsions are some extreme forms in action. Alcoholism is by far the best-known compulsion/addiction, but the list of "-holic" states grows yearly. Some commonly recognized states seen in families are "workaholics," "rageholics," "sadaholics," and "hypochondriaholics."

A third area of vulnerability is suppression of one's emotions. The very response (fight or flight) that has preserved generations of humans as well as other life forms is discouraged in obvious and not so obvious ways within the dysfunctional family. A person's emotions instruct the individual how to react and behave. Being cut off from one's emotional self is a sure way to repeat the dysfunctional behavioral patterns of generations past.

How does the fourth area, conflicted sexuality, fit into this dysfunctional family picture? If

If the family environment is one in which communication related to sexual relations is considered shameful or inappropriate, one's body and sexual urges are perceived as bad or negative. Therapists of eating-disordered families have long noticed that the family and the individual with an eating disorder have a harder time than most in accepting adult sexuality.

FAMILY THERAPY OF THE EATING-DISORDERED FAMILY

The above paragraphs may paint a rather fatalistic picture for chances of recovery, but individuals and families need not be prisoners of their past. For the most part families do the best they can, and they truly want greater health and happiness than experienced with their families of origin. A primary goal of the family therapist is to assist families in becoming healthier and happier. Although the process of examining unacknowledged, unsettled issues from the past is painful, doing so frees the parent, spouse, or child to live life in a more positive way. A family member may want to have a different kind of family system than the one from which he or she came. However, without competent therapy, support, and education, the member may end up repeating old family patterns. (See Garfield & Garner, 1997: pp. 316.)

Often the overprotectiveness of a family member contributes to maintenance of the eating disorder. Such overprotectiveness may be motivated by love, but the end result is to stunt the separation process that occurs in adolescence (the usual time when eating-disorder symptoms surface in the patient of the eating-disordered family).

A dynamic in eating-disordered families that requires immediate attention is preoccupation with weight and appearance. If family members or significant others who reside with the victim of the eating disorder continue to focus on food, and obsessive weighing of oneself, any individual movement toward recovery is likely to be sabotaged; throwing out the family scale is always a good first step.

The selection of a family therapist should be tailored to the needs of the family. If the parents relate to the therapist and yet one or more children don't feel comfortable, the family should find a different therapist (and vice versa). If one family member consistently finds fault with the therapist, the family may need to move on without that individual being in treatment. Start family therapy with the idea that the family has reasons for being in this place at this time. Let the family therapist accompany you into the new and scary places you will need to go to become healthy.

CONCLUSION

Family therapy plays a crucial role in the recovery of the eating-disordered family. When used in connection with individual treatment, chances for a full recovery are greatly improved. Rarely can eating-disordered family systems survive the collision of the dysfunctional vertical and horizontal intergenerational dimensions of family members without professional therapy intervention. Goals of family therapy include accepting family as good enough, moving away from perfectionistic thinking, seeing guilt and self-doubt as dead end, and recognizing that healthy traits as well as unhealthy ones pass from generation to generation. With multitherapy intervention, full recovery is possible.

REFERENCES

Garfield, Paul E., & Garner, David M. (Eds.). (1997). *Handbook of treatment for eating disorders* (2nd ed.). New York: Guilford Press.

Lerner, H. G. (1989). *The dance of intimacy*. New York: Harper & Row.

Satir, V. (1972). *Peoplemaking*. Palo Alto, CA: Science and Behavior Books, Inc.

Viorst, J. (1987). *Necessary losses*. New York: Ballantine Books.

Whitfield, C. (1987). *Healing the child within*. Deerfield Beach, FL: Health Communications, Inc.

Zerbe, Kathryn J. (1995). *The body betrayed: A deeper understanding of women, eating disorders, and treatment*. Carlsb CA: Gurze Books.

The Intervention Process: Working with Eating-Disordered Clients, Their Families, Significant Others, and Friends

by Kathy Jo Dennison, R.N.

On any given day, a professional Interventionist may receive calls such as these:

"I'm Frightened She's Going to Die!" … "Amy's been anorexic for about 15 years and it's getting worse. She's only eating about 300 calories a day now and she won't quit exercising. I stay home from work so that I can fix food for her hoping that she might eat a little bit. I know she must feel weak but promises to see the doctor keep getting broken.

"Amy is so bright! She graduated from college with a business degree, but she's so weak, she hasn't been able to work for the past three years. Every time I mention getting some help, she starts yelling and screaming. She told me that if I 'went behind her back' and spoke to anyone, she'd leave and I'd never be able to find her. I'm frightened … I was told that you specialize in working with eating disorders. Can you help her? You're our last hope."

"She's Out of Control and She's Ruining Our Lives!" … "I'm not even sure why I'm calling you—I know Sara isn't going to change! She's been bulimic since before we were married 14 years ago. She told me about it, but I never thought it was that bad. Now it's all the time! Sara used to be so attractive—everyone liked her. Now, no one even wants to be around her. And about three years ago, she started drinking. Between the money she spends on food and in the bars, we're in deep financial trouble. I'm about ready to throw in the towel. Last week I think I saw Susan, our 11-year-old daughter, throw up after dinner, and that really scared me. I guess that's why I'm calling you. Can you fix Sara?"

"I Know Alan's Not Happy … All He Does Is Eat" … "He tells me that he isn't eating that much, but I know that he's gained at least 50 or 60 pounds just in the last six months! When I

try to talk to him, he gets really mad at me and tells me I'm fat, too. I guess I am overweight, but I try to eat the right foods and take care of myself. I think he needs to see a doctor—he's always coughing and out of breath; he complains about pounding headaches and sore knees. I think it's related to his weight. He tells me that he'll see a doctor, but he never does. We used to have so much fun together but now he's just moody. When I get home from work, I never know what I'm going to find. Half the time he's angry and hateful and this frightens me. I want to leave him, but I'm afraid to. Can you put us back together?"

The preceding case-history vignettes were taken from actual intervention calls received and are typical of how the intervention process is initiated. Some of the details have been altered to protect the identities of the clients and their family members.

INTRODUCTION TO THE INTERVENTION PROCESS

In the late 1970s when the intervention process was developed, it was not uncommon to hear stories about shaming, disrespectful, and heavy-handed interventions. The initial "confrontive" model worked toward the goal of "breaking down" the client to the point of acquiescence and coercion into prescribed treatment recommendations. This early process had high potential for leaving both the client and intervention team participants with deep emotional scars. Who among us hasn't seen a television portrayal of an intervention that both shamed and frightened all the participants? In many instances, those early interventions left negative memory images imprinted in the minds of all who were exposed to them about the intervention process. In addition to the creation of a shaming, negative environment, many times the facilitator or interventionist would also misrepresent specific terms of treatment recommendations. An example of this tactic would be to mislead the client about the length of treatment stay, freedoms and privileges associated with treatment, and expectations about the client's role in the treatment process. God help the poor admissions staff member who had to deal with this dishonesty and anger from the client on the day of admission!

FROM SHAME-BASED MEMORIES TO A FAMILY-SYSTEMS APPROACH IN INTERVENTIONS

Thankfully, the hard-core, shame-based, confrontational model has become a thing of the past for most interventionists. As we've evolved our clinical expertise, a more respectful intervention model has emerged. With the presentation of this newer model, it has become possible for the interventionists to work with the complete family system and to admit their clients into treatment in far better psychological condition, thus preparing the client for the treatment process without having to "lose" treatment time while the client heals from the intervention.

This newer model, the Invitational Model, incorporates the complete family system into the intervention process and replaces shaming, disrespectful tactics with care, concern, support and an invitation to the client to join his or her family and support system in recovery. The basic premise is that the behavior, and not the person, has negatively impacted all members of the family. As the family system is integrated in the intervention, it frequently becomes clear that there is more than one "patient" in the system, and the need for clinical assessment becomes essential. The family is no longer an "adjunct" to the identified patient's treatment, but rather a "part" of the treatment and recovery process. An added value of the "Family Centered" approach is recognition of the dynamics of the entire family system from which the identified patient emerges prior to entering the treatment process. An integral component of the "Family Centered" process includes working closely with each family member and helping each individual to set goals for his or her own recovery process as well as a plan for the family reintegration.

COMPONENTS OF THE INVITATIONAL INTERVENTION

Assessment and Evaluative Process

After being contacted by a family member, friend, or referring professional, the interventionist begins to gather information, initiates the assessment process, makes a clinical judgment as to the appropriateness for an intervention, and selects the "intervention team." During this stage, it is extremely important that back-up plans for psychiatric crisis episodes and/or medical emergencies are developed with all members of the team. The identified "patient" is brought into the process and invited to join the group by the interventionist. She or he is encouraged to be part of the process and to actively participate in all family meetings. Dates, times, and locations for the intervention are decided and agreed upon.

Didactic Sessions and Processing Segments

As the group comes together and begins to work as a "team," therapeutic components include allowing each member of the team to discuss and process how the eating-disordered dysfunctional behaviors have impacted them. It is essential that the interventionist carefully facilitate this group, allowing recognition for each individual while maintaining the direction of the intervention process.

It is extremely important that all members of the intervention team are included in the psychoeducational segments and that the information disseminated is clear and understandable. Some recommended didactic segments may include those listed below. Educational segments should be added that are specific to family dynamics and presenting issues—i.e., chemical dependency, sexual or physical abuse, self-injurious behaviors, gambling, grief management, and trauma.

- The Eating Disorder Disease Process
- The Addiction Cycle
- Addressing Guilt & Shame Issues
- Family Systems & Family Building
- Characteristics of the "Alive" Family
- Effective Communication Skills
- Intervention Goals

- Treatment Options, Expectations, & Plans
- The Recovery Process
- The Reintegration of the Family Unit

GROUP PROCESSING AND THE DEVELOPMENT OF SUPPORT LETTERS

Throughout the intervention process, the need for team members to actively claim their feelings and concerns is critical. Many clinicians specializing in the treatment of eating disorders have found that both their eating-disordered clients and the clients' families share misconceptions about the disease/addiction processes and that, through exposure to clear, factual information, questions and feelings are resolved.

Letters of support, concern, and encouragement for the identified patient are at the very core of the intervention process. The interventionist assists each team member in targeting and expressing their support in written form which will be read at the final intervention process meeting. The importance of having each team member prepare a written letter cannot be underestimated. As emotions run high and the potential for engagement in disputes is viable, the letter serves as both a "point of focus" and a means of assisting each team member to honestly express their support and concern, regardless of the emotional climate.

DRESS REHEARSAL—INTERVENTION REVIEW

The "Dress Rehearsal" provides all team members the opportunity to read their letters of support, process their feelings, and receive support from both other team members and the professional interventionist. It is during this segment that team members are able to offer encouragement to one another and correct, remind, and bond with each other as emotional hurts and painful memories are revealed.

It is important during this phase that the interventionist maintains group structure while therapeutically providing for the processing of feelings by each member of the group. Needless to say, clinical experience and expertise is necessary for this group process. At the conclusion of the dress rehearsal meeting, participants will be prepared for the final intervention meeting.

THE INVITATIONAL INTERVENTION

It is at this juncture, the Invitational Intervention, that the intervention process is culminated. Whether the "identified client" has been an active team participant from the beginning and now feels a strong part of the team, or if the client decides to join the group at this last meeting only, the emphasis is on care, concern, support, and encouragement for recommended treatment.

During the Invitational Intervention, each team member has the opportunity to read their letter of support and to discuss with the group their own personal goals for recovery. Although emotions may run high and anger may be expressed as truths are revealed, the client is always treated with respect and dignity.

It is extremely helpful if the interventionist is trained and experienced in expressive therapy modalities as these can be of tremendous benefit to the client and team members. Of particular value is a psychodramatic family sculpting through which the client and other team participants can visualize the impact that the eating-disordered behaviors have had on the entire family system. Indeed, "a picture can be worth a thousand words."

At the conclusion, the client is invited to join the family in recovery. His or her role in the treatment/recovery process is discussed and options for treatment are presented from which the client can choose, thus assuming an active part in the course of their own recovery.

Plans for treatment are implemented at this time and a program for team members' involvement in the treatment process is presented. The commitment of each team member to the treatment/recovery process can be very helpful in preparing for treatment successes.

A program for future family meetings is introduced and the "mechanics" for family meetings—i.e., chairman assignments, agenda items, conflict resolution techniques, etc., are presented by the interventionist for discussion by team members. This intervention process closure assists the team in becoming goal-oriented and provides a platform for family/team reintegration.

THE PROFESSIONAL INTERVENTIONIST: QUALIFICATIONS, TRAINING, AND SUPERVISION

Throughout the past decade, the percentage of higher acuity patients and complex cases has risen dramatically. These higher ratios of clients presenting with multiple addictions plus depression, physical and sexual abuse trauma, personality disorders, mood disorders, anxiety disorders, and resulting medical problems have increased the demand for well-trained, experienced interventionists to meet these clinical challenges. It is of the utmost importance that the professional interventionist has a solid clinical background with experience specific to eating disorders as well as a clear understanding of the psychodynamics of the pathology relating to associated behaviors. Ongoing training for the interventionist is vital to professional proficiency and credibility.

In addition, it is extremely important that the professional interventionist find a confidential source, or sources, for clinical supervision and the processing of their work. The profession of intervention is often one of isolation and aloneness in which the only "system" the clinician spends time in is the dysfunctional system of his or her client's. It is therefore essential that the interventionist builds a strong support network of caring colleagues.

In conclusion, for interventionist clinicians who "go straight into the eye of the tornado" and who do not have the opportunity to observe the "success" of those we introduce into treatment, it is important that we always hold onto those "rainbow rewards" that come our way. What follows is one of my treasured "rainbows"…

Dear Kathy Jo,

Words seem totally inadequate to express my gratitude to you. I owe you a debt I will never be able to repay whether my daughter lives or dies. For so long, I have struggled with getting her into some form of treatment, but was unable to find anyone who seemed to have an understanding of the illness enough to be able to advise me as to how to put all of the pieces together to find the help she so desperately needs. There are no words in the English language to express to you what it has been like watching my daughter die and not know how to intervene to prevent her death! Your phone call to me as we began the intervention process was one I shall never forget! Thank you, Thank you. Thank you. I am forever grateful to you.

(Excerpt from letter reprinted with permission)

Cognitive-Behavioral Therapy and Eating Disorders

by Carol B. Peterson, Ph.D., and James E. Mitchell, M.D.

INTRODUCTION

Of the various psychological and pharmacological approaches that have been used for the treatment of eating disorders, cognitive-behavioral therapy (CBT) has been studied most extensively. Cognitive-behavioral approaches for the treatment of eating disorders were adapted from techniques used to treat depression and anxiety (Beck & Emery, 1985; Beck, Rush, Shaw, & Emery, 1979). In general, CBT aims to change behavioral and cognitive patterns that contribute to and maintain eating-disorder symptoms. In contrast to many other types of psychotherapy, CBT is a short-term, highly structured approach in which the clinician takes an active role in providing information and in working with the client for symptomatic change.

A large number of investigations have found that CBT is effective for the treatment of bulimia nervosa. Preliminary studies have in-

AUTHORS' NOTE: The preparation of this chapter was supported in part by the Center Grant for Eating Disorders Research from the McKnight Foundation and the Minnesota Obesity Center Grant #P30 DK50456 from the National Institutes of Health.

dicated that CBT is also effective for the treatment of binge eating disorder, a type of eating disorder in which the individual, who is usually overweight, engages in recurrent binge eating episodes but does not use regular compensatory behaviors such as self-induced vomiting, laxative or diuretic abuse, fasting, or excessive exercise. Although a considerable amount has been written about the use of CBT with anorexia nervosa, only a few studies have evaluated its effectiveness, with mixed results.

RESEARCH INVESTIGATING CBT AND BULIMIA NERVOSA

At least 20 controlled studies to date have evaluated the efficacy of CBT for the treatment of bulimia nervosa. The majority of them found that CBT led to a greater reduction in binge eating and purging compared with wait-list control groups not receiving treatment and with minimal intervention treatment conditions, and that both group and individually administered CBT are effective in reducing symptoms (for reviews, see Mitchell & Peterson, 1997; Peterson & Mitchell, 1995). CBT was found to be more effective than psychodynamic psychotherapy in one study (Garner et al., 1993), and another study found that although CBT was superior to interpersonal therapy (IPT) and behavioral therapy (BT) at the end of treatment (Fairburn et al., 1991), CBT and IPT were comparable and superior to BT at longer-term follow-up (Fairburn, Jones, Peveler, Hope, & O'Connor, 1993; Fairburn et al., 1995).

Studies comparing CBT with antidepressant medication have generally found that CBT is more efficacious in reducing binge eating and purging (Wilson, Fairburn, & Agras, 1997). Investigations that evaluated the combination of CBT with antidepressant medication have yielded inconsistent results, with only one finding a higher remission rate from bulimic symptoms compared with CBT alone (Walsh et al., 1997), one finding that the addition of medication to CBT was beneficial only for mood and anxiety symptoms (Mitchell et al., 1990), and one finding that the combination was superior to CBT alone on measures of some psychological variables (Agras et al., 1992).

In summary, CBT has been found to be a useful treatment for bulimia nervosa in a number of studies. Although the results with IPT may be comparable at long-term follow-up

based on preliminary evidence, the vast amount of research substantiating the use of CBT with bulimia nervosa makes it the current treatment of choice.

RESEARCH INVESTIGATING CBT AND BINGE EATING DISORDER

Techniques that have been used successfully for the treatment of bulimia nervosa have been adapted for the treatment of binge eating disorder, a type of eating disorder that has gained increasing attention. A number of studies have demonstrated that CBT is effective in reducing the frequency of binge eating episodes among individuals with binge eating disorder (Smith, Marcus, & Kaye, 1992; Telch et al., 1990; Wilfley et al., 1993). One study found that CBT was comparable to IPT (Wilfley et al., 1993), although another found that those who did not respond to CBT did not show further improvement with subsequent IPT treatment (Agras et al., 1995).

Although CBT appears to be helpful in reducing binge eating, most research participants with binge eating disorder did not lose weight as a result of treatment, a significant finding because the majority of such individuals are overweight or obese, and many seek treatment for the explicit purpose of losing weight. However, one study using CBT did observe that individuals who remained in remission from binge eating were most likely to have lost weight at one-year follow-up (Agras et al., 1997). One study using behavioral approaches that targeted weight loss found that both weight and binge eating were significantly reduced, and that weight loss and the dietary restriction involved were not associated with increased binge eating (Marcus, Wing, & Fairburn, 1995).

RESEARCH INVESTIGATING CBT AND ANOREXIA NERVOSA

Although a fair amount has been written on the use of CBT in treating anorexia nervosa (Garner & Bemis, 1985; Garner, Vitousek, & Pike, 1997; Pike, Loeb, & Vitousek, 1996), few studies have evaluated its efficacy. One study found that CBT was equally as effective as BT (Channon, De Silva, Hemsley, & Perkins, 1989). A more recent investigation observed that CBT was useful in preventing relapse among individuals who were recovered to a normal weight range following hospitalization (Pike, 1996).

USING CBT WITH EATING DISORDERS

A number of manual-based CBT programs have been developed to treat eating disorders. The one used most widely was written by Fairburn (1985; Fairburn, Marcus, & Wilson, 1993) for the treatment of bulimia nervosa. Most CBT programs focus initially on nutritional rehabilitation and behavioral techniques, with a later emphasis on cognitive restructuring and relapse prevention.

After introducing the treatment program, providing a rationale for treatment, and emphasizing the importance of self-monitoring, the clinician uses the initial sessions to focus on normalizing eating patterns, which requires the client to consume regular, well-balanced meals and snacks. For individuals who are significantly underweight, a focus on weight restoration is necessary. Early phases of CBT implement behavioral techniques to interrupt problematic patterns, including stimulus control (e.g., avoiding high-risk situations, substituting alternative behaviors for eating-disorder symptoms) and contingency management, in which consequences of symptoms are modified. Cognitive restructuring, in which thought patterns are modified, is a crucial aspect of CBT. Although cognitive restructuring may focus initially on eating patterns and concerns about weight and shape, addressing underlying beliefs about self-esteem and interpersonal relationships may be valuable later in treatment. Because relapse rates are high (Olmsted, Kaplan, & Rockert, 1994), the final phase of CBT usually consists of relapse prevention. Psychoeducation is used throughout treatment to illustrate aspects of eating-disorder symptoms and recovery procedures.

CBT can be conducted in individual therapy or in groups. Unlike other types of psychotherapy, it is usually short-term and focuses on the present, rather than attempting to identify developmental precursors of eating problems. In CBT, the therapist takes an active role in providing information and assigning homework.

CASE EXAMPLE

Jane[1] was a 21-year-old, 5'6" unmarried female who was completing her senior year in college at the time of her initial evaluation. She had decided to seek treatment at the urging of her roommate, who had noticed that food was missing from their dormitory room and confronted Jane about obtaining help for her eating disorder.

The clinician began by conducting a full history of Jane's eating-disorder symptoms. Jane admitted that she had been binge eating and vomiting since the beginning of her sophomore year in college. At that time, she was concerned about having gained weight during her freshman year and thought she was unattractive. She was also experiencing increased academic demands since deciding to major in pre-business. She started to diet by restricting her caloric intake to 1,000 kcal/day and increasing her exercise to one hour of aerobics six days per week. After one month, her weight had dropped from 140 to 130 pounds. Over time, however, she found it increasingly difficult to maintain her strict diet. During midterms, she experienced her first binge eating episode, in which she consumed a box of cookies in 30 minutes, and felt a sense of loss of control. Terrified about the possibility of gaining weight, she self-induced vomiting, which she had heard about on television shows and from other women with eating disorders.

At first, Jane engaged in binge eating and vomiting episodes only once or twice a month. However, during final exams, she began to binge eat and vomit more frequently, as often as twice a day. At the time of her initial evaluation, Jane was binge eating and vomiting five days a week. Her binge eating episodes typically consisted of a pint of ice cream, 20 cookies, and a medium-sized bag of potato chips. Outside of the binge eating episodes, Jane restricted her calorie and fat intake. She exercised for 90 minutes a day, six days a week, using a combination of aerobics and weight training. Although she experimented with laxatives and diuretics as weight-control techniques on a few occasions during her junior year, she did not use them regularly. She denied any history of chewing and spitting food, ruminating, or using syrup of ipecac.

At the time of her evaluation, Jane weighed 135 pounds. She believed that she was extremely unattractive at this weight, and thought that her ideal weight was 115 pounds. Jane's shape and weight strongly influenced how she felt about herself as a person. For example, if the scale indicated a one-pound weight gain, she believed that she was a shameful person with no self-control. She would feel better about

---

[1] The name has been changed to protect the individual's identity.

herself on days when she lost weight. She was also extremely embarrassed about the fact that she engaged in binge eating and vomiting episodes, and she believed that the only way she could stop was by using more self-discipline and restricting her food intake.

In addition to obtaining a detailed history of Jane's eating disorder, the clinician evaluated her for symptoms of depression, anxiety, and alcohol and drug abuse, all of which Jane denied. The clinician also referred Jane for a medical evaluation, in particular to determine if she had abnormal serum electrolytes, the most common medical complication of bulimia nervosa.

To begin the treatment, the clinician described the rationale for using CBT. She explained that CBT is a short-term treatment, one that is very focused on changing symptoms using behavioral and cognitive strategies. She emphasized that in a number of research studies CBT has been found to be the most effective approach for treating binge eating and vomiting. The clinician also introduced self-monitoring, in which Jane would write down everything she ate while she was in treatment, along with thoughts and feelings that accompanied food consumption. The clinician emphasized that self-monitoring is one of the most important components of CBT because it provides useful data during the sessions and facilitates awareness of patterns between sessions.

After introducing CBT, the clinician explained the nature of bulimia nervosa to Jane. She emphasized that for many women, extreme concerns about shape and weight lead to restrictive dieting. The clinician then explained the risks of excessive dieting and described research that had been conducted in the 1950s in which healthy men were placed on extremely restrictive diets (Keys et al., 1950). As a result of caloric restriction, the men experienced mood swings, concentration impairment, social withdrawal, and preoccupation with food. After being allowed to resume eating, the men experienced binge eating episodes, in which they consumed large amounts of food. This research suggests that binge eating may be an outcome of extreme food restriction, perhaps a behavior that served an important evolutionary function at times when the food supply was scarce. Although bulimia nervosa is characterized by overeating, the extreme dieting may be an important causal factor for many individuals.

After explaining the risks of dieting, the clinician emphasized the importance of eating regular meals and snacks and worked with Jane to develop a plan to improve her nutritional intake. For example, Jane would typically skip breakfast, eat a salad for lunch, and end up binge eating in the afternoon. The plan specified eating larger amounts of food for breakfast and lunch, with scheduled snacks in the morning and afternoon.

Jane expressed great interest in what the clinician explained to her. However, she was frightened that eating regular meals and snacks would lead to weight gain. The clinician emphasized that most normal-weight individuals do not gain weight as a result of eating regular meals and snacks. In fact, eating regular meals and snacks might serve to increase Jane's metabolism, which would help stabilize her at a healthy weight. Furthermore, the clinician explained to Jane that the vomiting associated with bulimia nervosa is ineffective in ridding the body of the food ingested during a binge. Although Jane was convinced that she "got all the food out" while purging, the clinician explained that the body absorbs a portion of the food eaten during a binge eating episode.

Nonetheless, Jane remained skeptical. The clinician suggested a technique called hypothesis testing, in which she and Jane would devise an experiment to "test" her belief. They considered possible ways of experimenting to see whether Jane's belief that she would definitely gain weight eating regular meals was true. They agreed to a one-week trial period, in which Jane would eat according to the meal plan and weigh herself just once at the end of the week (to avoid confusion from normal weight fluctuations that she might observe during more frequent weighings).

When Jane weighed herself one week later, she noted that her weight had not increased. In addition, she was struck by how much less she was binge eating and vomiting. Jane discovered that eating regular meals and snacks and increasing the amount of food she was consuming made her much less hungry and less likely to binge eat in the afternoon. She realized that she had only had two binge eating episodes in the past week, which was a significant reduction in frequency.

As the sessions progressed, the clinician and Jane continued to review her self-monitoring sheets and noted patterns of precursors or cues associated with binge eating and vomiting. The clinician introduced techniques to interrupt behavioral patterns associated with bulimic symptoms. Working together, Jane and her clinician developed a list of situations that appeared to trigger her bulimic symptoms and identified specific strategies for each one. For example, Jane discovered that she was much more likely to binge eat in the afternoon and evening when she was alone in the apartment. Because these conditions served as a powerful stimulus to binge eat and vomit, Jane developed strategies to modify them. She began to study in the library at night. In the afternoon, she would invite a friend to visit, or she would go to the common area instead of back to her room. Jane also evaluated situations in which she was less likely to binge eat and attempted to increase their frequency, for instance, sleeping at least eight hours per night and attending movies with friends.

The clinician also explained the importance of examining contingencies of bulimic symptoms that may maintain them. Jane determined that as much as she disliked binge eating and vomiting, it was positively reinforcing because it allowed her a break from homework. She and the clinician selected other forms of relaxation while studying so that she would not rely on binge eating for this purpose. In addition, they identified ways of rewarding Jane for not binge eating and vomiting. Jane decided to put a dollar in a jar for every 24-hour period she was free of bulimic symptoms. She agreed that after one month, she would use the money to purchase compact discs for herself. The clinician also emphasized the importance of Jane providing herself with "mental" rewards, for example, praising herself each time she was able to refrain from binge eating.

The nutritional and behavioral changes were effective in reducing the frequency of Jane's symptoms to once a week. When Jane and the clinician examined the precursors of the remaining symptoms, they determined that Jane was still self-inducing vomiting because she believed that she was overweight and she was concerned about gaining weight. The clinician introduced the idea of changing cognitions, or the thoughts that an individual experiences privately. The clinician explained that cognitions strongly affect feelings and behaviors. For example, two individuals receive a score of 95% on an exam. One of these individuals says to herself, "This is great. I studied hard, and I hoped to do well. A 95% is a good score." She feels happy and goes out with her friends to celebrate. The other individual thinks, "I wanted 100%. It's not a perfect score, so I guess I didn't do very well." She feels sad, disappointed, and frustrated, and stays alone in her room.

The clinician explained that changing an individual's thoughts can influence associated feelings and behaviors. She first gave Jane a list of examples of maladaptive thought patterns common to women with eating disorders (Garner & Bemis, 1985; Peterson & Mitchell, 1996). Examples included minimizing, in which success is discounted (e.g., "I might have gone the whole day without binge eating, but anyone could do that"); catastrophizing, in which the worst outcome is assumed (e.g., "I just ate a cookie, and I'm certain to gain five pounds"); and dichotomizing, in which only the extremes of a situation are considered (e.g., "There are good foods, like carrots, and bad foods, like ice cream; if I eat a bad food, I've blown it and I might as well binge") (Beck et al., 1979). Jane recognized a number of these patterns and determined that they were likely to contribute to her bulimic symptoms.

The clinician then explained cognitive restructuring, in which a thought is examined systematically and revised to be more realistic. She explained that the first step is to identify the thought, then to evaluate alternative explanations and evidence for and against its validity, and, finally, to modify the thought to make it more realistic. As an example, they selected Jane's cognition that often precipitated vomiting episodes in which she thought to herself, "I have to get rid of this ice cream by vomiting, or otherwise I'll gain weight." Jane and the clinician evaluated the evidence supporting this belief. Jane admitted that although she would feel less anxious if she vomited, she knew that, realistically, a dish of ice cream was not likely to lead to weight gain. Other evidence that refuted the cognition was that vomiting was not effective in ridding the body of food. For the final step, Jane revised the thought and stated, "Even though I may be anxious about gaining weight, I won't gain weight from eating a dish of ice cream, and vomiting is ineffective for weight control anyway."

Jane was quite pleased with her success in reducing her binge eating and vomiting but continued to believe that she was overweight. She and the clinician conducted cognitive restructuring that focused on her thoughts about body image (Cash, 1996; Rosen, 1997). The clinician also explained the difficulty in feeling comfortable with what was probably a biologically healthy weight for Jane when current societal expectations of thinness are so unrealistic, and recognizing the cultural context of eating disorders (Striegel-Moore, Silberstein, & Rodin, 1986). They also worked together using cognitive restructuring to help Jane separate her sense of self-worth from her weight and shape. By the third month of treatment, Jane found that although she was still dissatisfied with her appearance at times, she was more accepting of herself as a person and recognized that her body weight was healthy for her, even if it did not meet the societal ideal.

By the beginning of the fourth month of treatment, Jane was free of binge eating and vomiting. She had reduced her exercise to 45 minutes, four days a week, and noted that she exercised for health and a sense of well-being rather than to "get rid of calories." For the final four weeks, she and the clinician focused on relapse prevention. The clinician emphasized that there is a risk of relapse among individuals with eating disorders. She suggested that Jane may struggle at times in the future, and that it would be important to view such struggles as challenges rather than as indications that she has failed, which could lead to a worsening of symptoms. They devised specific plans of what she would do after treatment ended to get back on track if she experienced difficulties, for example, resuming self-monitoring, reviewing her written homework exercises from therapy, or reading a self-help book (e.g., Fairburn, 1995). They also agreed that if she had more than one episode of binge eating and vomiting in a month, she would contact the clinician. Finally, they reviewed her progress in therapy and identified the techniques that had been most helpful that Jane could continue to use in the future.

LIMITATIONS AND CONCLUSIONS

Cognitive-behavioral therapy for the treatment of eating disorders has been widely used and studied. The research literature suggests that CBT is the first treatment of choice for bulimia nervosa, and probably for binge eating disorder as well. CBT's role in the treatment of anorexia nervosa is less clear, although it appears promising for the treatment of this condition as well. However, CBT is ineffective for a minority of individuals with eating disorders, and many of those who improve initially show a relapse of symptoms. Further research is required to understand why CBT is ineffective in some cases and to identify treatments that can be used alternatively. An additional limitation of CBT is that although many eating-disordered individuals show improvement, many remain symptomatic to a lesser degree (Mitchell et al., 1996). Studies need to determine ways of promoting complete remission and preventing relapse using CBT or additional interventions. Finally, although CBT has been used extensively in research settings, more attention must be paid to how these techniques are used by clinicians in the community and ways that CBT can be used in community settings to promote maximum recovery among individuals with eating disorders.

REFERENCES

Agras, W. S., Rossiter, E. M., Arnow, B., Schneider, J. A., Telch, C. F., Raeburn, S. D., Bruce, B., Perl, M., & Koran, L. M. (1992). Pharmacologic and cognitive-behavioral treatment for bulimia nervosa: A controlled comparison. *American Journal of Psychiatry 149*, 82–87.

Agras, W. S., Telch, C. F., Arnow, B., Eldredge, K., Henderson, J., & Marnell, M. (1995). Does interpersonal therapy help patients with binge eating disorder who fail to respond to cognitive-behavioral therapy? *Journal of Consulting and Clinical Psychology 63*, 356–60.

Agras, W. S., Telch, C. F., Arnow, B., Eldredge, K., & Marnell, M. (1997). One-year follow-up of cognitive-behavioral therapy for obese individuals with binge eating disorder. *Journal of Consulting and Clinical Psychology 65*, 343–347.

Beck, A. T., & Emery, G. (1985). *Anxiety disorders and phobias*. New York: Basic Books.

Beck, A. T., Rush, A. J., Shaw, B. F., & Emery, G. (1979). *Cognitive therapy of depression*. New York: Guilford Press.

Cash, T. F. (1996). The treatment of body image disturbance. In J. K. Thompson (Ed.), *Body image, eating disorders, and obesity: An integrative guide for assessment and treatment* (pp. 83–108). Washington, DC: American Psychological Association.

Channon, S., De Silva, P., Hemsley, D., & Perkins, R. (1989). A controlled trial of cognitive-behavioural and behavioural treatment of anorexia nervosa. *Behaviour Res Therapy 27*, 529–535.

Fairburn, C. G. (1985). Cognitive-behavioral treatment for bulimia. In D. M. Garner & P. E. Garfinkel (Eds.), *Handbook of psychotherapy for anorexia nervosa and bulimia* (pp. 160–92). New York: Guilford Press.

Fairburn, C. G. (1995). *Overcoming binge eating*. New York: Guilford Press.

Fairburn, C. G., Jones, R., Peveler, R. C., Carr, S. J., Solomon, R. A., O'Connor, M. E., Burton, J., & Hope, R. A. (1991). Three psychological treatments for bulimia nervosa. *Archives of General Psychiatry 48*, 463–69.

Fairburn, C. G., Jones, R., Peveler, R. C., Hope, R. A., & O'Connor, M. (1993). Psychotherapy and bulimia nervosa: The longer-term effects of interpersonal psychotherapy, behavior therapy, and cognitive behavior therapy. *Archives of General Psychiatry 50*, 419–28.

Fairburn, C. G., Marcus, M. D., & Wilson, G. T. (1993). Cognitive-behavioral therapy for binge eating and bulimia nervosa: A comprehensive treatment manual. In C. G. Fairburn and G. T. Wilson (Eds.), *Binge eating: Nature, assessment, and treatment* (pp. 361–404). New York: Guilford Press.

Fairburn, C. G., Norman, P. A., Welch, S. L., O'Connor, M. E., Doll, H. A., & Peveler, R. C. (1995). A prospective study of outcome in bulimia nervosa and the long-term effects of three psychological treatments. *Archives of General Psychiatry 52,* 304-312.

Garner, D. M., & Bemis, K. M. (1985). Cognitive therapy for anorexia nervosa. In D. M. Garner & P. E. Garfinkel (Eds.), *Handbook of psychotherapy for anorexia nervosa and bulimia* (pp. 107–46). New York: Guilford Press.

Garner, D. M., Rockert, W., Davis, R., Garner, M. V., Olmsted, M. P., & Eagle, M. (1993). Comparison of cognitive-behavioral and supportive-expressive therapy for bulimia nervosa. *American Journal of Psychiatry 150,* 37–46.

Garner, D. M., Vitousek, K. M., & Pike, K. M. (1997). Cognitive-behavioral therapy for anorexia nervosa. In D. M. Garner & P. E. Garfinkel (Eds.), *Handbook of treatment for eating disorders* (2nd ed.) (pp. 94–144). New York: Guilford Press.

Keys, A., Brozek, J., Henschel, A., Mickelsen, O., & Taylor, H. L. (1950). *The biology of human starvation* (2 vols.). Minneapolis: University of Minnesota Press.

Marcus, M. D., Wing, R. R., & Fairburn, C. G. (1995). Cognitive treatment of binge eating versus behavioral weight control in the treatment of binge eating disorder. *Annals of Behavioral Medicine 17,* S090.

Mitchell, J. E., Hoberman, H. M., Peterson, C. B., Mussell, M., & Pyle, R. (1996). Research on the psychotherapy of bulimia nervosa: Half empty or half full? *International Journal of Eating Disorders 20,* 219–29.

Mitchell, J. E., & Peterson, C. B. (1997). Cognitive-behavioral treatment of eating disorders. In L. J. Dickstein, M. B. Riba, & J. M. Oldham (Eds.), *Review of psychiatry* (Vol. 16) (pp. I-107-I-134). Washington, DC: American Psychiatric Press, Inc.

Mitchell, J. E., Pyle, R. L., Eckert, E. D., Hatsukami, D., Pomeroy, C., & Zimmerman, R. (1990). A comparison study of antidepressants and structured intensive group psychotherapy in the treatment of bulimia nervosa. *Archives of General Psychiatry 47,* 149-157.

Olmsted, M. P., Kaplan, A. S., & Rockert, W. (1994). Rate and prediction of relapse in bulimia nervosa. *American Journal of Psychiatry 151,* 738–43.

Peterson, C. B., & Mitchell, J. E. (1995). Cognitive-behavior therapy. In G. O. Gabbard (Ed.), *Treatments of psychiatric disorders, volume 2* (2nd ed.) (pp. 2103–28). Washington, DC: American Psychiatric Press.

Peterson, C. B., & Mitchell, J. E. (1996). Treatment of binge-eating disorder in group cognitive-behavioral therapy. In J. Werne (Ed.), *Treating eating disorders* (pp. 143–86). San Francisco: Jossey-Bass.

Pike, K. M. (1996, April). *Relapse prevention for anorexia nervosa.* Paper presented at the Seventh New York International Conference on Eating Disorders, New York, NY.

Pike, K. M., Loeb, K., & Vitousek, K. (1996). Cognitive-behavioral therapy for anorexia nervosa and bulimia nervosa. In J. K. Thompson (Ed.), *Body image, eating disorders, and obesity: An integrative guide for assessment and treatment* (pp. 253–302). Washington, DC: American Psychological Association.

Rosen, J. C. (1997). Cognitive-behavioral body image therapy. In D. M. Garner & P. E. Garfinkel (Eds.), *Handbook of treatment for eating disorders* (2nd ed.) (pp. 188–204). New York: Guilford Press.

Smith, D. E., Marcus, M. D., & Kaye, W. (1992). Cognitive-behavioral treatment of obese binge eaters. *International Journal of Eating Disorders 12,* 257–62.

Striegel-Moore, R. H., Silberstein, L. R., & Rodin, J. (1986). Toward an understanding of risk factors for bulimia. *American Psychologist 41,* 246-263.

Telch, C. F., Agras, W. S., Rossiter, E. M., Wilfley, D., & Kenardy, J. (1990). Group cognitive-behavioral therapy for the nonpurging bulimic: An initial evaluation. *Journal of Consulting and Clinical Psychology 58,* 629–35.

Walsh, B. T., Wilson, G. T., Loeb, K. L., Devlin, M. J., Pike, K. M., Roose, S. P., Fleiss, J., & Waternaux, C. (1997). Medication and psychotherapy in the treatment of bulimia nervosa. *American Journal of Psychiatry 154,* 523–31.

Wilfley, D. E., Agras, W. S., Telch, C. F., Rossiter, E. M., Schneider, J. A., Cole, A. G., Sifford, L., & Raeburn, S. D. (1993). Group cognitive-behavioral therapy and group interpersonal therapy for the nonpurging bulimic: A controlled comparison. *Journal of Consulting and Clinical Psychology 61,* 296–305.

Wilson, G. T., Fairburn, C. G., & Agras, W. S. (1997). Cognitive-behavioral therapy for bulimia nervosa. In D. M. Garner & P. E. Garfinkel (Eds.), *Handbook of treatment for eating disorders* (2nd ed.) (pp. 67–93). New York: Guilford Press.

Pharmacological Management of Eating Disorders

by Sheldon P. Wagman, D.O.

In considering the treatment of eating disorders one has to conceptualize them in biopsychosocial dimensions. The etiology of eating disorders is not well understood. Thus treatment must be considered in a multidimensional manner. Medications play a role, but they should be just one part of a holistic approach that includes individual and group psychotherapy, nutritional education and counseling, examination of social-cultural issues, and behavior modification.

Prior to initiating treatment for an eating disorder, the health care professional should perform the following: a complete medical history; a complete physical examination; complete psychiatric assessment, and baseline laboratory tests, including: a complete blood count, serum electrolytes, liver function test, kidney function (including blood urea nitrogen and creatinine), thyroid profile, electrocardiogram, and fasting blood glucose.

The blood tests are usually ordered as either SMA-22 or biochem profile #2. These may indicate the need for more specific tests, such as an endocrinological workup, a neurological workup, and a bone density study.

What follows is a summary of the known pharmacological treatments for anorexia nervosa, bulimia nervosa, and binge eating disorder.

ANOREXIA NERVOSA

No one medication is effective in treating anorexia nervosa. What is known is that medications can treat the psychological symptoms often associated with anorexia nervosa (e.g., depression, anxiety, obsessions, and compulsions).

Antipsychotic Medications

The use of antipsychotic medications is based on the concept that anorexics have so distorted their body image and their perception of themselves in their emaciated state that they are considered to be delusional. Chlorpromazine[1] was thought to be effective in promoting weight gain, but the side effects of seizures, hypotension, constipation, liver impairment, and a variety of gastrointestinal symptoms led to its disuse. Other neuroleptic agents such as Pimozide[2] and Sulpiride[3] have not been shown to offer any advantages to a placebo, and their side effects of potential seizures and tardive dyskinesia place the patient, whose health is already compromised, in an even more vulnerable state.

Antidepressant Medications

Depression is commonly found in conjunction with anorexia nervosa. It has been reported that patients with anorexia have a high lifetime risk for major depressive episodes. Studies have shown little efficacy for using Clomipramine or Amitriptyline[4] in the treatment of anorexia nervosa. They did not seem to help the depression or effect weight gain. The side effects—sedation, tachycardia, constipation, and dry mouth—made them intolerable.

Studies of Fluoxetine seem to demonstrate some positive results: weight gain and diminished depressive symptoms.[5,6] A preliminary report of a placebo-controlled study of Fluoxetine in patients with anorexia nervosa indicates that it helped maintain the weight gain that had occurred during treatment.[7] The idea that an antidepressant may increase weight and reduce obsessions, thus preventing relapse, has been shown to have value clinically. What has been found in patients who are anorexic and clinically depressed is that sometimes when their nutritional state improves, the depression also diminishes. One must take care in prescribing antidepressant medications for anorexic patients because of their weight loss and the emaciated state. Changes in body protein and fat consumption can significantly affect how the medication works. The person with a low protein level due to inadequate nutrition tends to experience many problems with antidepressant medication because that medication often binds to protein. If there is insufficient protein for the medication to bind to, the result may be a higher percentage of the unbound drug in the system. This could lead to increased side effects and less tolerance for the medication.

Anxiolytics

No specific controlled studies have reported on the use of anxiolytic medications (i.e., those that reduce anxiety) in the treatment of anorexia nervosa. Some reports describe the use of a short-acting benzodiazepine (i.e., Lorazepam: 0.25–0.5 mg 20—60 minutes before mealtime), which may reduce the level of anxiety that surrounds food intake.[8] It should only be used briefly due to its addictive quality. I have used Clonazepam in a like manner with good results (i.e., the reduction of pre-meal anxiety, which then enables the person to eat).

Appetite-Enhancing/Stimulating Agents

Studies have found modest weight gain with the use of Cyproheptadine, an antihistaminic, antiserotonergic drug. The sedating side effect tended to negate any positive results, however, and the results reported are not impressive.[9,10] Clonidine, an antihypertensive drug, was found ineffective in promoting weight gain despite early research suggesting it might induce eating behavior.[11] Tetrahydrocannabinol, the active component of marijuana, was also thought to enhance appetite. Further studies indicated that it was no better than a placebo.[12]

Trace Metal Replacement

Zinc deficiency has been studied as it relates to anorexia nervosa. No studies have demonstrated that a zinc supplement is superior to a healthy diet.[13]

Prokinetic Drugs

Delayed gastric emptying of the stomach, with associated bloating, abdominal distention, and early satiety, has been noted with anorexic patients. Medications such as Metaclopramide, Domperidone, and Cisapride have been administered to enhance the gastric emptying, thus leading to better overall compliance with nutritional programs.[14,15,16] These medications may be indicated when there is significant abdominal distention associated with meals. It should be kept in mind that refeeding in of itself also accelerates the rate of gastric emptying.[17]

Electroconvulsive Therapy

Electroconvulsive therapy has been used to treat patients with intractable anorexia nervosa—where all treatments have failed and the patient's life is at stake. No evaluated controlled studies have been reported to date; most of the information provided has been anecdotal.[18]

Lithium

Lithium has been studied in a double-blind placebo-controlled study. Some weight gain resulted, but no other behavioral changes were evidenced. The medical concern is being able to stabilize lithium levels with people who have erratic food and fluid intake.[19]

BULIMIA NERVOSA

In considering pharmacotherapy for patients with bulimia nervosa it is important to consider that the symptoms may reflect the presence of psychiatric disorders. Often the bulimic patient has a depressive disorder, anxiety disorder, substance abuse disorder, or personality disorder. They tend to self-mutilate and may have a greater disturbance of perceptions of their body, their shape, and their personality. In considering pharmacotherapy for patients with bulimia, it is important to keep in mind the possible presence of a co-existing disorder. On occasion the co-existing disorder may begin to improve once the nutritional state improves.

Antidepressant Medications

Tricyclics (TCAs)

Imipramine was the first TCA to demonstrate a marked positive response, compared with the placebo, in reducing the bingeing and purging behaviors of bulimia nervosa.[20] The problem with imipramine and other TCAs relates to their side effects which include sedation, dry mouth, blurry vision, constipation, hypotension, and weight gain. Desipramine has been widely studied in patients with bulimia nervosa, and reports indicate the bulimic behavior diminishes as long as the person continues to take the medication.[21,22] When the medication was solely used to treat bulimia nervosa and was discontinued after improvement, significant rates of relapse resulted.[23]

Monoamine oxidase inhibitors (MAOs)

The problem with MAOs lies in the need for dietary restrictions and the potential for serious medical problems and drug interactions, which can be fatal. This is especially so with patients who are also substance abusers and have personality disorders. Because of this, these drugs are rarely used.

Selective serotonin reuptake inhibitors (SSRIs)

Four SSRIs are on the market: Fluoxetine, Sertraline, Paroxetine, and Fluvoxamine. Fluoxetine has been the most studied. A breakthrough study demonstrated that the dose of 60 mg per day was highly effective in reducing the frequency of binge eating episodes.[24] A second study confirmed the advantages of the Fluoxetine at the 60-mg-per-day level versus a placebo over a 16-week period.[25] More recently, evaluating the effectiveness of Fluoxetine with a number of psychological variables demonstrated significant improvement in the short term.[26] No placebo-controlled studies of the use of Paroxetine and Sertraline have been published, although one recent study of Fluvoxamine showed no advantage when used only to prevent relapses after clinical improvement was achieved.[27]

Trazodone

Trazodone has been demonstrated to be superior to a placebo for treating bulimic behaviors in a short-term trial study.[28]

Bupropion

Bupropion has been studied and found to increase the risk of seizures. It is therefore contraindicated at this time for the treatment of bulimia nervosa.[29]

Mood Stabilizers

Lithium carbonate and carbamazepine have been studied under controlled conditions and have not been found to be effective in the treatment of bulimia nervosa.[30,31]

Anxiolytics

No reported double-blind studies have demonstrated the efficacy of an anti-anxiety medication. Furthermore, because the anti-anxiety medications tend to be addictive, and people with bulimia nervosa are prone to develop substance abuse or dependence, they should be used with great caution, if at all.

Opiate Antagonist

Naltrexone was studied to determine if it might be effective in changing the appetite. No evidence of benefit for the treatment of bulimia nervosa was found.[32]

Appetite Suppressants

Trials of Fenfluramine have been conducted in the hopes of promoting satiety so the bulimic patients will consume fewer calories.[33] Subsequent trials using Dl-Fenfluramine and desipramine plus cognitive behavior therapy failed to support the effectiveness of Fenfluramine, possibly because the cognitive behavior therapy may have obscured the benefits of the medication.[34,35] Dl-Fenfluramine and Fenfluramine have since been removed from the market due to life-threatening complications.

A Final Note on Bulimia Nervosa

It has been shown that the most effective treatment for bulimia nervosa is cognitive behavior therapy. Medications may serve an adjunct function, but when used to treat bulimia nervosa solely, the relapse rate is significant once the medications are discontinued. Evidence supports the use of cognitive behavior therapy and medication in tandem.

BINGE EATING DISORDER

Binge eating disorder is currently under study to determine whether it should be included in the *DSM-IV* as a separate entity under eating disorders. (It is now listed under the general heading of the DSM-IV Eating Disorders Not Otherwise Specified.) Only a few studies have looked at the effects of antidepressant medications,[36] appetite suppressants, and the opiate antagonist Naltrexone on this disorder. Desipramine, in a placebo-controlled study, was shown to diminish the binge eating behavior.[37,38] Fluvoxamine, in an unpublished placebo-controlled study, was also shown to be more effective than the placebo in diminishing binge eating behaviors.

Dl-Fenfluramine has also been shown to be more effective than a placebo in reducing the number of episodes of binge eating in obese women. However, no weight loss resulted despite the fact that binge eating had been reduced.[39] Fluoxetine has also been studied for the treatment of binge eating disorders in obese women. The study suggests that it may be a useful adjunctive treatment in this group of patients.[40,41] The opiate antagonist Naltrexone has also been studied in conjunctive with psychotherapy and found to be more effective than psychotherapy alone in treating binge eating disorders.[42]

When prescribing medications for eating disorders, it is important to do so as part of a team effort. The psychiatrist should discuss with, and get feedback from, the team regarding the use of medication as it fits into the total treatment picture for the person with an eating disorder. The psychiatrist should also sit down with the patient and his or her family and discuss the medication in detail including the choices of medication, the reason for the choice, possible side effects, and the length of time the person would be on the medication. If the psychiatrist does not take the time to do this, the effectiveness of the medication may not be nearly as great as one would hope.

MEDICATIONS BY CATEGORIES

Antipsychotic Medications
Chlorpromazine (Thorazine)
Pimoziede (Orap)
Sulpiride (Dogmatil—not available in U.S.)

Antidepressant Medications
Tricyclic Agents
Amitriptyline (Elavil)
Clomipramine (Anafranil)
Desipramine (Norpramin)
Imipramine (Tofranil)

Monoamine Oxidase Inhibitors (MAOIs)
Phenelzine (Nardil)
Isocarboxazie (Marplan)

Selective Serotonin Reuptake Inhibitors
Fluoxetine (Prozac)
Fluvoxamine (Luvox)
Paroxetine (Paxil)
Sertraline (Zoloft)

Atypical Agents
Bupropion (Wellbutrin)
Trazodone (Desyrel)

Anxiolytic Medications
Clonazepam (Klonopin)
Lorazepam (Ativan)

Appetite Stimulants
Cyproheptadine (Periactin)
Clonidine (Catapres)

Appetite Suppressants
Fenfluramine

Prokinetic Agents
Cisapride (Propulsid)
Domperidone (Metilium)
Metaclopramide (Reglan)

Mood Stabilizers
Carbamezepine (Tegretol)
Lithium Carbonate (Escolith-Lithobid)

Opiate Antagonist
Revia (Naltrexone)

ENDNOTES

1. Dally, P., & Sargent, W. (1966). Treatment and outcome of anorexic nervosa. *British Medical Journal 2*, 793–95.
2. Vandereycken, W., & Pierloot, R. (1982). Pimozide combined with behavior therapy in the short-term treatment of anorexia nervosa: A double-blind placebo-controlled crossover study. *Acta Psychiatric Scand 66*, 445–50.
3. Vandereycken, W. Neuroleptics in the short-term treatment of anorexia nervosa: A double-blind placebo-controlled trial with Salpiride. *Br. J. Psychiatry 184*(144), 288–92.
4. Biederman, J., Herzog, D. B., Rivinus, T. N., et al. (1985). Amitriptyline in the treatment of anorexia nervosa. *J. of Clin. Psychopharmacol 5*, 10–16.
5. Gwirtsman, H. E., Guze, B. H., Yager, J., & Gainsley, B. (1990). Fluoxetine treatment of anorexia nervosa: An open clinical trial. *Journal of Clinical Psychiatry 51*, 378–82.
6. Kaye, W. H., Weltzin, T. E., Hsu, L. K. G., & Bulikem, C. M. (1991). An open trial of Fluoxetine in patients with anorexia nervosa. *Journal of Clinical Psychiatry 52*, 464–71.
7. McConaha, C., Kaye, W. H., Sohol, M. S., et al. (1996, April). Double-blind Fluoxetine study in anorexia nervosa. Presented at the 7th International Conference on Eating Disorders, New York.
8. Anderson, A. E. (1987). Uses and potential misuses of anti-anxiety agents in the treatment of anorexia nervosa and bulimia nervosa. In P. E. Gurfinle & D. M. Garner (Eds.), *The role of drug treatments for eating disorders* (pp. 59–72). New York: Brunner/Mazel.
9. Halmi, K. A., Eckert, E., La Du, T. J., et al. (1986). Anorexia nervosa: Treatment efficacy of cyproheptadine and amitriptyline. *Arch. Gen. Psychiatry 43*, 177–81.
10. Vigersky, R. A., & Loriaux, D. L. (1977). The effect of cyproheptadine in anorexia nervosa: A double-blind trial. In R. A. Vigersky (Ed.), *Anorexia nervosa*. New York: Raven Press.
11. Casper, R. C., Schemmer, R. F., & Javaid, J. I. (1987). A placebo-controlled crossover study of oral clonidine in acute anorexia nervosa. *Psychiatry Res 20*, 249-260.
12. Gross, H. A., Ebert, M. H., Faden, V. B., et al. (1983). A double-blind trial of delta-9-tetrahydrocannabinol in primary anorexia nervosa. *J. Clin. Psychopharmacol 20*, 165–67.
13. Lash, B., Fosson, A., Rolfe, V., et al. (1993). Zinc deficiency and childhood onset of anorexia nervosa. *J. Clin. Psychiatry 54*, 63–66.
14. McCallum, R. W., Groll, B. B., Lange, R., et al. (1985). Definition of a gastric emptying abnormality in patients with anorexia nervosa. *Digestive Diseases and Science 30*, 713–22.
15. Domstad, P. A., Shih, W. J., Humphries, L., Deland, F. H., & Digenis, G. A. (1987). Radionuclide gastric emptying studies in patients with anorexia nervosa. *Journal of Nuclear Medicine 28*(5), 816–19.
16. Kamal, N., Chamit, T., Anderson, A., et al. (1991). Delayed gastrointestinal transit times in anorexia nervosa and bulimia nervosa. *Gastroenterology 101*, 1320–24.
17. Rigaud, D., Bedig, G., Merrouch, M., et al. (1998). Delayed gastric emptying in anorexia nervosa is improved by completion of a re-nutrition program. *Dig. Disorder. Sci. 33*, 919–25.
18. Ferguson, J. M. (1993). The use of electroconvulsive therapy in patients with intractable anorexia nervosa. *Int. J. Eat. Disord 13*, 195–201.
19. Gross, H. A., Ebert, M. H., Faden, V. B., et al. (1981). A double-blind controlled trial of Lithium Carbonate in primary anorexia nervosa. *J. Clin. Psychopharmacol 1*, 376–81.
20. Pope, H. G., Hudson, J. I., Jonas, J. M., et al. (1983). Bulimia treated with imipramine: A placebo-controlled, double-blind study. *Am. J. Psychiatry 140*, 554–58.
21. Hughes, P. L., Wells, L. A., Cunningham, D. J., et al. (1986). Treatment of bulimia with desipramine. *Arch. Gen. Psychiatry 43*, 182–86.
22. Barlour, J., Blouin, J., Blouin, A., et al. (1988). Treatment of bulimia with desipramine: A double-blind crossover study. *Can. J. Psychiatry 33*, 129–33.
23. Walsh, B. T., Hadigan, C. M., Devlin, M. J., et al. (1991). Long-term outcome of antidepressant treatment for bulimia nervosa. *Am. J. Psychiatry 148*, 1206–12.

24. Fluoxetine Bulimia Nervosa Collaborative Study Groups. (1992). Fluoxetine in the treatment of bulimia nervosa. *Arch. Gen. Psychiatry,* 139–147.

25. Goldstein, D. J., Wilson, M. G., Thompson, V. L., et al. (1995). Long-term Fluoxetine treatment of bulimia nervosa. *Br. J. Psychiatry* 166, 660–66.

26. Goldbloom, D. S., Olmsted, M. P. (1993). Pharmacotherapy of bulimia with fluoxetine: Assessment of clinically significant change. *Am. J. Psychiatry* 150, 770–74.

27. Fichter, M. M., Kruger, R., Rief, W., et al. (1996). Fluvoxamine in prevention of relapse in bulimia nervosa: Effects on eating—specific psychopathology. *J. Clin. Psychopharmacol 16,* 9–18.

28. Pope, H. G., Kech, P. E., & McElvoy, S. L. (1989). A placebo-controlled study of Trazodone in bulimia nervosa. *J. Clin. Psychopharmacol 9,* 254–59.

29. Horne, R. L., Ferguson, J. M., Pope, H. G., et al. (1988). Treatment of bulimia with bupropion: A multicenter controlled trial. *J. Clin. Psychiatry 49,* 169–76.

30. Hsu, L. K. G., Clement, L., Stanthouse, R., et al. (1991). Treatment of bulimia nervosa with Lithium: A controlled study. *J. Nerv. Ment. Disorder 179,* 351–55.

31. Kaplan, A. S., Garfinkel, P. E., Darby, P. L., & Garner, D. M. (1983). Carbamazepine in the treatment of bulimia. *Am. J. Psychiatry 140,* 1225–26.

32. Mitchell, J. E., Christensen. G., Jennings, J., Huber, M., Thomas, B., Pomeroy, C., & Morley, J. (1989). A placebo-controlled, double-blind crossover study of naltrexone hydrochloride in outpatients with normal weight bulimia. *J. of Clin. Psychopharmacol 9,* 94–97.

33. Blouin, A. G., Blouin, J.H., Perez, E. L., et al. (1988). Treatment of bulimia with fenfluramine and desipramine. *J. of Clin. Psychopharmacol 8,* 261–269.

34. Russell, G. F. M., Chechley, S. A., Feldman, J., & Eisler, I. (1988). A controlled trial of dl-fenfluramine in bulimia nervosa. *Clin. Neuropharmacol 22*(suppl), S146–S149.

35. Fahy, T. A., Eisler, I., & Russell, G. F. M. (1993). A placebo-controlled trial of d-fenfluramine in bulimia nervosa. *Br. J. of Psychiat 162,* 597–603.

36. Hudson, J. I., Carter, W. P., Pope, H. G. (1996). Antidepressant treatment of binge eating disorders: Research findings and clinical guidelines. *J. of Clin. Psychiatr 57*(suppl 8), 73–79.

37. Walsh, T. & Devlin, J. (1995, November-December. Pharmacotherapy of bulimia nervosa and binge-eating disorders. *Addictive Behaviors 20*(6), 757–64.

38. McCann, U. D., & Agras, W. S. (1990). Successful treatment of non-purging bulimia nervosa with desipramine: A double-blind, placebo-controlled study. *Am. J. Psychiatr 147,* 1509–13.

39. Stanford, A., Berkowitz, R., Taurikut, C., Reiss, E., & Young, L. (1996, November). D-fenfluramine treatment of binge-eating disorders. *Am. J. Psychiatry 153*(11), 155–59.

40. Marcus, M. D., Wing, R. R., Ewing, L., Kern, E., Gooding, W., & McDermott, M. (1990). A double-blind placebo-controlled trial of fluoxetine plus behavior modification in the treatment of obese binge eaters and non-binge eaters. *Am. J. Psychiatry 147,* 876–81.

41. Green, C., & Wing, R. R. (1996). A double-blind, placebo-controlled trial of the effect of fluoxetine on dietary intake in overweight women with and without binge eating disorders. *Am. J. Clin. Nutr 64,* 267–73.

42. Marrazzi, M. A., Markham, K. M., Kinzie, J., & Luby, E. D. (1995, February). Binge-eating disorder: Response to naltrexone. *Inter. J. of Obesity & Related Metab. Disorders 19*(2), 143–45.

Undermining Anorexia through Narrative Therapy

by Stephen P. Madigan, Ph.D. and
Elliot M. Goldner, M.D.

Despite numerous theoretical and therapeutic approaches to the problem of anorexia, it remains slippery and difficult to locate. Anorexia has a way of desecrating prized theories and beliefs, and an inflexible approach to it would be foolhardy. Over the years, we have had to shift away from certain practiced assumptions and adopt others. Without flexibility, anorexia will certainly gain the upper hand.

We do not wish to add to the already long list of theories and practices that claim to offer the "correct" approach and correct understanding of the "underlying issues" in anorexia nervosa. It is our view that our therapeutic professions have too often produced additional suffering for clients and families by insisting to focus on controlling mothers, abusive fathers, enmeshed family boundaries, chemical imbalances, etc.

We believe it is best for us to acknowledge that the particularities of the problem are complex, and that reductionistic assumptions will not adequately apply to each of the individuals who come to receive help from us. What we hope to relate in this chapter is not a catch-all theory, but rather a set of ideas and approaches that appear to be helpful to most of the people we have worked with who are struggling against anorexia.

A narrative approach to anorexia nervosa (Madigan & Goldner, 1997) assists in the reauthoring of lives and relationships, and views persons as separate from the totalizing and problematic anorexic identity (Madigan, 1992, 1995, 1996). The person and problem are viewed as mutually influenced within a given cultural context, and the problem is not solely located within the body of the person. Persons struggling with anorexia are imagined to be coping alongside, and being shaped by, powerful sets of dominant beliefs.

LOCATING THE PROBLEM

The Western myth of the individual is best placed in context by anthropologist Clifford Geertz (1973, p. 229) when he writes: "The Western conception of the person as a bounded, unique, more or less integrated motivational and cognitive universe, a dynamic centre of awareness, emotion, judgment and action, organised into a distinctive whole and set contrastively against a social and natural background is, however incorrigible it may seem to us, a rather peculiar idea within the context of the world's cultures."

Therapists from every discipline have developed the compelling habit of describing persons as "things." The "thingifying" of persons is supported and given a "truth status" through the technologies of science, government, and the popular press. The conventional culture of psychotherapy participates in the manufacturing of these solitary personhoods through totalizing techniques which place the problem inside the person's body, thereby decontextualizing the subject and the problem.

Our therapeutic approach abandons the idea of the self-as-object-of-knowledge, and the self as the identified problem in therapeutic practice. We suggest, in contradistinction, that a narrative description for the identity of persons rejects:

- notions of the self as an inner wealth of deep resources in combat with primitive impulses.

- ideas of a self alienated from a universe, an environment that it seeks to rejoin through rational comprehension of mysteries (scientific discovery) and through intense emotional attachments (romantic love).

- a sense of self as a consistent, knowable, enduring identity (humanism) which is nurtured or limited and can be known, measured, and directed.

- therapies for the self which focus on discovering historical (psychoanalysis, family of origin) or environmental (behaviourism, cybernetics, systems) truths about the self and which relegate to themselves the power to set the self in new directions.

What is important in a narrative approach to problems is also the golden rule of real estate buying: Location, Location, Location! If therapists can take the step to no longer locate problems entirely inside person's bodies, then persons and problems begin to look very different. This is by no means a trivial step, as it paradigmatically shifts the therapist and client outside and beyond 100 years of psychological science.

EXTERNALIZING INTERNALIZED ANOREXIC CONVERSATIONS

From our experience of working on an eating-disorder ward, in the community, and in independent practice, the way the problem of anorexia seems to work is to trap people into a set of intense fears and beliefs. It is tenacious and insidious.

It is critical for a person to be freed from anorexia's relentless discursive grip in order to rediscover his or her life. If the trap is still active, it is far too likely that anorexia will take hold again. This might be why treatments that focus primarily on weight gain rarely lead to prolonged recovery. It might also explain why "forcing" weight gain is so often ineffective in the long term. As long as the dominant fears and beliefs that comprise anorexia entrap the individual, it is highly likely to regain its ground.

Recognition of the importance of deconstructing debilitating beliefs and meanings is not unique to narrative approaches. Cognitive, motivational interviewing and other frameworks have stressed the centrality of core beliefs in providing an opportunity for change. In helping someone put anorexia behind them, there are other activities that may also be very important, including medical, nutritional, and emotional components (see Goldner & Birmingham, 1994). However, in almost all situations, a key area involves attention to the dominant narratives that emanate from the problem, and the institutional structures that support them. As these dominant narratives are deconstructed, the steel jaws of anorexia's trap can be released.

Madigan (1991, 1995) has described the therapeutic practice of externalizing internalized problem discourse as an elaboration of ideas advanced by White and Epston (1990). This aspect of our work aims to discursively separate the person from the problem as a way to deconstruct taken-for-granted notions of anorexia and reconsider ideas of who constitutes the "self" who struggles against anorexia (Madigan & Epston, 1995).

In the case of anorexia, the discursive scaffolding is complex. Pro-anorexic systems that support anorexia have many discursive forms, and are manufactured through archives of dominant knowledge and carried out through powerful disciplinary practices (Law & Madigan, 1997). They may include specific cultural trainings around perfection, safety, and control; gender trainings of body surveillance, and less than worthy identities; religious beliefs regarding body purity, self-sacrifice, guilt; and the cultures of self-help who promote the politics of condemnation; and many more.

By externalizing anorexia's internalized problem conversation, we create a linguistic separation of the problem and open space to consider the influences which promote the life of anorexia. Hence, anorexia is not viewed as "living inside" the person, nor is it seen as a manifestation of an act of control on the part of the person or a means of "getting attention." When anorexia is situated within a community's textual discourse there is no need to pathologize the person's family. Anorexia is considered within a domain of language and viewed in terms of discursive body politics (Bordo, 1990).

By affording ourselves the opportunity to reconsider what constitutes persons and problems from a post-structural position, a different set of therapeutic practices is instigated and the therapeutic relationship shifts. Where we decide to discursively situate the problem and person locates the therapist's ideological practice beliefs.

The discourses of fear, perfection training, patriarchy, and guilt appear to be very common

externalizations. Locating these internalized beliefs and the meanings within specific sets of dominant institutional, familial, cultural, and religious norms is extremely important.

We do not practice externalizing the problem as a therapeutic technique, nor do we propose it as a strategy or trick. Externalizing internalized problem discourse is stationed within a landscape of specified political and philosophical thought. In brief, externalizing internalized problem discourse

- establishes a context where persons taken by anorexia experience their identity as separate to the problem;

- proposes that the person's body/mind/relationships to others are not the problem; the problem is the problem (counters the effect of labeling, pathologizing, and totalizing descriptions);

- enables people to work together to defeat the effects of the problem;

- uses cultural practices of objectification to objectify anorexia, instead of objectifying the person as being anorexic;

- challenges the individualizing techniques of scientific classification and looks at the broader context for a more complete problem description;

- introduces questions that encourage the persons taken by anorexia to outline the devastating effects of the problem and locate the discourse of the problem within the trainings of a pro-anorexic community;

- deconstructs the pathologizing 'thing-ification' and objectification of individuals through challenging taken-for-granted social norms;

- allows for the possibility of multiple re-remembered descriptions of themselves, by bringing forth alternative versions of a person's past, present, and future; and

- counters the dis-membering effects of anorexia by encouraging persons towards re-membering themselves back towards membership groups, activities and community (see Madigan, 1997).

REFLEXIVITY AND EARLY-ON STRUGGLES

Working in close quarters with anorexia demands an enormous amount of internal reflection and questioning by everyone involved. We find that a regular practice of reflexivity (Lax, 1990)— the practice of asking ourselves questions about our questions and therapeutic beliefs—enhances accountability to the client and allows the therapy to remain flexible. In considering how we might be helpful to a client, there are a number of reflexive questions we would consider asking ourselves and each other:

- In what ways might I get trapped into reproducing the most common misconceptions of anorexia in the session?

- In what ways can I avoid getting caught up in anorexia's trap of pitting the person against all those that wish to help?

- What are the untried and unique ways that I can show how much disrespect anorexia has for this person's life?

- How can I show a sincerity to help this person without scaring her/him off?

- What questions can I ask to allow this person to consider taking up their own personal protest against anorexia?

- In what ways can I be aware of my professional position to acknowledge and not misuse my power as a therapist?

When we meet clients early on in their struggle with anorexia we considered inquiry into the following areas:

- Why have you come to see someone like me at this time?

- Do other people's descriptions of anorexia fit your description of yourself?

- Why might this be a fitting description?

- What name might we come up with to describe the current situation?

- Has anorexia in any way taken things from your life that you value?

- In what ways has anorexia affected your relationship with yourself, friends, family, etc.?

- Are there ways in which anorexia has tricked your mind into thinking that an anorexic life is the best life possible?

- Do you think it tricks other young people's minds?

- If you could make a prediction, what kind of a future does anorexia hold for you?

From our first meeting with clients and their families we try to unpack the discourses supporting anorexia, those that support the view of a privatized anorexia within the client, and anorexia's tactics which act to create a discursive wedge that disconnects the person from any hope of support and recovery. When a narrative approach is introduced into a person's relationship with the problem of anorexia, much of the symmetrical escalation between persons is diffused for the first time. Our intent is to break the either/or, black/white position of anorexia and by so doing open discursive space for alternative possibilities.

CONSIDERING FAMILY

Many families we work with often describe their "early on" experience with anorexia in terms of fear, shame, anger, frustration, and paralysis. They will have often encountered blame for the pain their child was experiencing from the professional and non-professional community, and explain that the blame has had a debilitating effect on their family's ability to cope. Their experience is often constituted through a dominant discourse about anorexia, backed up by an archive of popular psychological, philosophical, and biological theories that hold the family, and specifically the mother, responsible for their "anorexic child." Despite the stories of incompetence told about families, they will often report that they were able to take up multiple "anti-anorexic" strategies in an attempt to find a solution, and assist the client in becoming free of the problem. They include both a tactic of "tough love" and, a more passive position they described as a "walking on eggshells" approach.

When we meet up with families early on in the struggle with anorexia, these are some of the questions we would consider asking:

- What have you been led to believe about the causes of anorexia?

- Why is it that professionals seem to blame parents as the cause of anorexia?

- What sorts of worry and worst-case scenarios do you picture when you consider your child's/sibling's struggle?

- What have you noticed that you do that helps your child's/sibling's health and undermines anorexia's grip?

- Can you think of any reasons why anorexia would not want this family to work together on this problem?

- Do you have any reason to believe that your child/sibling can someday be free of anorexia?
- What is it about this family that anorexia could never destroy?

A narrative approach to therapy helps to unpack dominant stories acting in support of the problem. The intent of our questions in the initial session is to bring forward hope through re-remembering experiences of courage, competence, appreciation, and change. Answers to our conversational inquiries often contradict how the family had been feeling "under the influence" of the professional community and their local culture.

Our questions act to open space for new descriptions, exceptions, and information previously restrained by the problem. The intent of the questioning is to include news of information and difference that weakens anorexia's version of the client and their family. Questions are grammatically designed to predict possible futures, moments of freedom, and victories over anorexia across the temporal plain. Throughout the session, therapist questions provide an alternate historical explanation for the onset of anorexia.

We often send families an anti-anorexia survey prior to the first session and ask each member of the family to fill it out.

ANTI-ANOREXIA SURVEY

Thank you for participating in our anti-anorexia survey. We are currently surveying people who were at one time or another taken with anorexia, as well as a number of family members, partners, friends, and therapists. We will be using your replies to assist us in better serving your needs. Please take no more than 30 minutes to answer the following questions. Feel free to expand your reply beyond the space provided. Remember, there are no right or perfect answers.

1. How do you understand the problem of anorexia?

2. What are the ideas that you have come across about anorexia that have been helpful or not helpful to you in your life? Please explain by giving examples.

3. From your experience, in what ways have you found therapy helpful/not helpful?

4. Are there specific techniques through which anorexia recruits its victims?

5. Are there certain structures/beliefs of our society which may be viewed as supporting anorexia? If so, please describe these pro-anorexic structures.

6. In your experience what is anorexia's most effective weapon/strategy? Please explain.

7. In your experience are there any therapeutic practices that you have experienced that you would consider to be pro-anorexic? Please explain.

8. In your opinion, why does anorexia recruit so many more women than men?

9. What effect does anorexia have on relationships, e.g., family, couples, friends?

10. What effect does anorexia have on relationships to professionals?

11. In what ways have you witnessed other people standing against anorexia? Please explain.

12. Please name the three main pro-anorexic activities that you have experienced?

13. Please name the three main anti-anorexic activities that you have experienced?

14. What advice would you give to a person presently being recruited by anorexia?

15. What advice would you give to a professional presently working with people who are suffering the effects of anorexia/bulimia?

16. What advice would you give to a family member presently living with a person who is suffering the effects of anorexia/bulimia?

17. Where are the sites of anti-anorexic education most needed?

18. What are the most effective ways that anorexia finds to manipulate a person?

19. How many people do you think anorexia recruited in 1997?

20. How many people do you think anorexia will recruit during the year 2000?

21. Are there any anti-anorexic activities that might be viewed as responsibilities of our community?

22. Do you think anorexia is genetic? Please explain.

23. Do you think anorexia will soon be exported to other countries? If yes, please specify how?

24. If you could have a few minutes "face to face" with anorexia, what do you think you would say?

25. How would it feel to utter these words to anorexia/bulimia?

26. Final comments.

During the first session we discuss the family's answers to the survey. Often we sit quietly in witness to the family's intimate knowledge of anorexia, and appreciate their hard-won ability to say "no" to the possibility of surrender. In ensuing sessions, we might pursue these questions with the family:

- How has anorexia made attempts to divide and conquer this entire family?

- As a parent, how has anorexia turned you against yourself? Has it tried to convince you that perfect parenting is possible?

- Are there times when you are able to see and/ or remember your child/sibling free from the grip of anorexia?

- What is it that you notice about your child/sibling during these times of freedom?

- What is it that you notice about yourself as a parent during these times of freedom?

- What are your feelings now that we know that your child/sibling is not to blame for anorexia's hold?

- Who is it that sits behind the rules of anorexia? Have they ever tried to discipline you?

ONGOING CLIENT WORK

We consider a position of reflexivity to be crucial to our ongoing client work, since anorexia, in our experience, can be very defeating of therapists. We consider the following reflexive questions:

- How can I bring out this client's hard-won knowledge about anorexia in a way that is client supporting and anorexia defeating?

- In what ways can we draw out the marginalizing effects of anorexia in the client's life without them feeling ashamed and less than worthy?

- How can my enthusiasm for them not scare them away from help?

- How best can I take a position to "cheerlead" from behind?

- What can I do to respect the client's story of struggle without supporting an increase in anorexia?

- How might I ask this client about the horrendous effects of anorexia without humiliating and silencing them and causing them to despair?

- What is the best way to ask the client about their starved physical and emotional life?

- What is going to help me remain most hopeful about this client's life?

In the first few meetings with clients, we put forth the following questions that are intended to contradict anorexia's story of who the client is as a person and to debilitate anorexia's relationship with her/him. We have categorized the questions to assist readers in following our intent.

DECONSTRUCTION OF ANOREXIC RECRUITMENT TACTICS

- In what ways has anorexia affected your relationship with yourself by telling you that you are unworthy? That you are its special protégé? That you are only an anorexic person?

- In snatching your concentration away from you, does anorexia push you further into its concentration camp?

- How did anorexia manage to wedge you away from your own thoughts and version of the world?

- Do you believe that you are only the person anorexia tells you you are?

- By what means did anorexia entice you into isolation and despair? Would a good friend do this to you?

- How did anorexia trick you into thinking that hospitals and death were a better alternative to life in the free world?

- Do you think that the rule book of anorexia self-specialization specializes in torture and assassination?

- How does anorexia get away with making people remember to forget their best qualities?

- How does anorexia trick people with promises of safety while it silently takes them towards its ultimate aim—death?

SITUATING ANOREXIA IN ALTERNATIVE HISTORY

As therapists, we would also be concerned with taking a historical account of the client's relationship with anorexia. Throughout the interview, the questions would be a mix of general and specific inquiry. Questions that generalize assist clients in connecting with others (breaking down the practices of isolation) and help them to reconsider and recollect alternative theories about anorexia (breaking down the practices of self-specialization). In researching the client's past relationship with anorexia, we might ask:

• What effect does being a slave to the idea of perfection have on anorexia overtaking a person?

• Were there factors in your life beyond your control that made anorexia look like an attractive option?

• What do you remember in your life that most helped anorexia along?

• When you think back upon your introduction to anorexia, were there promises made to you?

• Do you think anorexia makes these same promises to everyone, or has it made you think that you are its special student?

• Did the abuse you suffered at the hands of _____ help along this feeling of being less than a person?

• Did the abuse you suffered at the hands of _____ somehow assist in anorexia's recruitment of you?

• Does the culture of 'thinner is better' sway people's thoughts away from other unnoticed qualities in themselves?

RE-REMEMBERING COUNTER IDENTITIES (SEE MADIGAN, 1997)

That professionals are sometimes pejorative and blaming when working with persons taken by anorexia is well-documented (Tinker & Ramer, 1983; Garner, 1985). The problem of anorexia engenders strong feelings of anger, hopelessness, frustration, etc., in some caregivers. Often, when working with someone who has experienced blame and guilt and was labeled "controlling" and "narcissistic" by professionals, we have had to work carefully at asking questions that contradict these other professional discourses.

• Can you remember qualities of yourself prior to anorexia's onset that you would like to re-remember?

• Have there been stories told about you that help you to forget your finer qualities?

• Has there ever been a time during treatment that you disagreed with the popular and professional version of you?

• How were you able to keep your own positive thoughts of yourself alive, despite what others were saying?

• Can you name the quality in you that has kept you alive all these years despite anorexia's attempts to kill you?

• Can you remember qualities of yourself prior to anorexia taking you that you would like your therapists/family/friends to re-remember?

• What do you think has caused some professionals to forget your best qualities?

EXPERIENCING AND APPRECIATING FREEDOM

We highlight and support any and all anti-anorexic efforts clients make (Goldner & Madigan, 1997). Recognition of a person's counter-struggle while under anorexia's pressured regime is a magnificent experience for therapists and clients alike, and one truly worth appreciating. The following questions help outline, underline, and color in the picture of increasing freedom:

• At which time of the day are you most anorexic-free?

• How are you able to find this freedom?

• In what ways have you "stepped outside anorexia" this week, and what has this stepping out stepped you toward?

• Who on the ward noticed these fantastic anorexic-free achievements?

• Was the time spent outside anorexia delicious?

• Do you ever catch yourself living outside anorexia's prison camp? What is it like? What color is your freedom?

• Do you ever find other people enjoying your own mind rather than experiencing the mind anorexia gives you?

• If you were to string together all of these victorious anti-anorexic moments, what effect would it have on anorexia?

- What rules of anorexia did you have to breach in order to attend this meeting today?
- Do you think that your anti-anorexic "noticing" of yourself has put anorexia on notice?
- Who in your life would be just barely amazed by your leaving anorexia behind?
- What advice do you have for my many colleagues who find themselves befuddled on how to best help people go free of anorexia?
- Have you ever plotted an escape from anorexia?
- What plans do you think your own anorexic-free person has for you?
- Which parts of your life will you retrieve and which good qualities will be re-remembered and come back to you once you are free of anorexia?
- How do you think it will feel when you are free to just have to "measure up" to yourself and not to the culture of anorexia's nagging torment?
- How do you think your comeback to your own life might be inspiring for other people?

DECONSTRUCTION OF CULTURE QUESTIONS

- Why do you think anorexia attempts to devour some of the best individuals of our generation?
- Can you think of ways that anorexia "pushes its way" onto people?
- Can you identify anything in popular culture that feeds into a "not measuring up to" lifestyle?
- If someone wanted to make a public protest over the destructive effects of anorexia, what would you suggest they do?
- Is the violence that anorexia perpetrates on your body similar to or different from other forms of violence?
- What does our society promote that leaves most people with a distorted sense of their own bodies?
- Can you figure out what and who most promotes perfection training?

ANTI-ANOREXIA ANTI-BULIMIA LEAGUES

The Vancouver Anti-anorexia League was born out of anti-anorexic group work at St. Paul's Hospital in Vancouver, Canada (see Grieves, 1997). The Vancouver league activities include international networking, community education programs, letter-writing campaigns, community organizing and protests against cultural misrepresentations of the body viewed to be pro-anorexic, teaching therapists' alternative approaches to therapy, working alongside hospital staff assessing community needs, counseling high school students and teachers, running groups, and publishing the league's magazine, *Revive*.

Our Vancouver Anti-anorexia/Anti-bulimia League is now five years in operation, and we are proud to be the oldest anti-anorexia league of this kind. We are indebted to our friend David Epston for introducing league ideas to us and to his ongoing creativity and support. The Vancouver group has assisted the formation of leagues and communities of concern in numerous cities across North America and the Western world. The anti-anorexia groups and subsequent research groups entertained discussions of the following questions:

- Why is anorexia so bent on reducing the women of this group into second-class citizens?
- Does anorexia betray your human rights?
- Do you think it is right that anorexia forces the members of this group into lives of isolation, perfection, subordination, and suffering?
- During the group talk, were there ever times that you felt inspired enough to consider leaving anorexia behind?
- What was it like for you to sit among a group of anti-anorexic freedom fighters?
- Are there sometimes anti-anorexic qualities that you notice in one another that you may one day notice in yourselves?

Other questions that involve the specific unraveling of anorexic fear tactics include the following:

- How were you able to push back the anorexic fear, when fear had you boxed into such a tight corner?
- What are some of the specific techniques you used to rid yourself of the panic that fear brought?
- What does it feel like to know that slowly but surely you are now controlling your fears?
- When you have those times that you are free of fear, how does your world look different?

- Do you think that there are times when you are free of fear and you don't recognize it? If so, could you be even more free of fear than you think?
- Do you think this fear is an imperfect fear?

RESEARCH ON NARRATIVE METHODS AND ANOREXIA

In an effort to look more closely at a narrative approach to anorexia, we put together a pilot research study. We hypothesized that a short-term narrative anti-anorexia group might be more effective than a control situation in facilitating recovery in women who were beginning treatment in a hospital program because of anorexia (Goldner & Madigan, 1997). Women were randomly assigned to the narrative group (N=10) or the control situation (N=10), which was a support group facilitated by an experienced counselor. Women in both groups received eight sessions of group intervention which included two sessions with family members. We found that women assigned to the narrative group were more likely to attend and remain connected to treatment. Furthermore, a few weeks after the end of the final session, women in the narrative group reported more hopefulness about recovery, defined themselves as more separate from the problem of anorexia, and reported less shame about the problem. Although this pilot study was too small to draw conclusions and has not yet followed the longer-term course of the participants, it suggests that a narrative approach holds some promise in providing an opening for people to move through in their escape from the hold of anorexia.

We hope that our narrative approach to anorexia may help to free some of those who could not otherwise find a way out.

REFERENCES

Bordo, S. (1994). Unbearable Weight: Feminism, Western Culture and the Body. Berkeley: University of California Press.

Garner, D.M. (1985). Iatrogenesis in anorexia nervosa and bulimia nervosa. *International Journal of Eating Disorders*, 4, 701–26.

Geertz, C. (1973). The interpretation of cultures. New York: Basic Books.

Goldner, E.M., & Birmingham, C.L. (1994). Anorexia nervosa: Methods of treatment. In L. Alexander-Mott & D.B. Lumsden (Eds.), Understanding Eating Disorders: Anorexia Nervosa, Bulimia Nervosa, and Obesity (pp. 135–57). Taylor & Francis.

Goldner, E.M., & Madigan, S.P. (1997, April). Narrative ideas in family therapy. Proceedings of the 2nd London International Conference on Eating Disorders. London, U.K.

Grieves, L. (1997). Beginning to Start: The Vancouver Anti-anorexia, Anti-bulimia League. In I. Law (Ed.), *GECKO: a journal of deconstruction and narrative therapy.* Vol. 2, (pp. 78–88), Adelaide, Australia: Dulwich Centre Publications.

Law, I., & Madigan, S. (1997). Discourse, Power and Identity: a discursive approach. Unpublished manuscript.

Lax, W. (1991). The Reflecting Team and the Initial Consultation. In T. Andersen (Ed.) *The Reflecting Team in Action,* New York: Norton.

Madigan, S., & Goldner, E. (1998). A Narrative Approach to Anorexia: reflexivity, questions and discourse. In Michael Hoyt (Ed.), *Constructive Therapies,* Jossey-Bass, New York.

Madigan, S. (1997). Re-considering memory: re-remembering lost identities back towards re-membered selves. In D. Nylund & C. Smith (Eds.) *Narrative Therapy with Children,* Chapter 13, pp. 127–42. New York: Guilford.

Madigan, S. (1996). The Politics of Identity: Considering community discourse in the externalizing of internalized discourse. *Journal of Systemic Therapy,* Vol 15, #1, pp. 47-63, New York: Guilford.

Madigan, S., & Epston, D. (1995). From Psychiatric Gaze to Communities of Concern: from professional monologue to dialogue. In Stephen Friedman (Ed.) *The Reflecting Team in Action.* New York: Guilford Publications.

Madigan, S. P. (1993). Questions about questions: situating the therapist's curiosity in front of the family. In S. Gilligan & R. Price (Eds.), *Therapeutic Conversations* (p. 219–36). New York: Norton.

Madigan, S. P. (1992). The application of Michele Foucault's philosophy in the problem externalizing of Michael White. *Journal of Family Therapy,* 14, 265-279. London, UK.

Tinker, D.E., & Ramer, J.C. (1983). Anorexia nervosa: Staff subversion of therapy. *Journal of Adolescent Health Care,* 4, 35–39.

White, M., & Epston, D. (1990). *Narrative means to therapeutic ends.* New York: Norton.

Narrative Therapy: Introduction to "Death of a Scalesman": In Her Own Voice

by Ray Lemberg, Ph.D.

Meredy is a 29-year-old woman, an individual, and a person who has touched more lives than she can ever know. I've been her psychologist and therapist for seven years. She has had many therapists in the past and has been in the hospital many times for the treatment of anorexia, obsessive-compulsive behavior, depression, despair, and self-loathing.

Meredy looks skeletal (she must be approximately 60-some pounds at 5 feet 6 inches tall), although I know her inner beauty and imagine her as a pretty redhead who takes after her mother: a strong and vital woman. I know Meredy as a most extraordinary person despite the chains of anorexia that bind her. She is brilliant, creatively gifted, compassionate to the downtrodden, inquisitive, witty, and most of all, my friend.

Meredy is a true Renaissance woman with a noose around her neck that chokes her at every turn. We have tried *almost* everything together as a team to rid her of the check and balance system that rules her life and makes her rigid, edgy, and always tired. She struggles—day in and day out, in fact, I imagine hour by hour—except for the reprieve of sleep and a few stolen moments of creative bursts that take her out of the clutches of anorexia. Life is often painful for Meredy; full of conflict, full of "shoulds" and full of thoughts of not being worthy enough to live a fulfilled life.

Anorexic voices rule her, dictate her rituals and create regrets, which are countless. She is steadfast in not giving up and often glimpses visions of a life past; carefree as a solid Kansas girl playing softball with family and friends and maintaining an intense curiosity about everything around her. At other times she sees a future as a writer, a chemist, an artist, an inventor, a lover, an aunt, and most of all a healed person who graces the life of her caring family and friends without feeling different or a burden.

I hope you can come to know Meredy as I have through her own narrative statement which follows and through the excerpts of the many letters that her loved ones have written her about the person they know without anorexia. You will find a letter from me requesting information from family and friends followed by their sincere responses, which has been used as part of her narrative therapy.

Meredy is an incredible human being who deserves much more.

Dear

I am writing on behalf of Meredy Humphreys to those individuals who have touched her life in a significant way. Meredy is my client of several years and has been working to unlock herself from the grips of anorexia.

The intent of this letter is to help Meredy reconstruct her past and to promote healthy aspects of her present self, leaving behind the anorexic identity that has come to encompass her.

Meredy and I have spent a great deal of time identifying those people in her life that have made a difference. You are one of them. Your help would be greatly appreciated.

I am asking that you write back with information about Meredy from your own personal point of view. Letters that we collect will be used to help Meredy do a "life review" and reconstruct her sense of self. Please address the following concerns:

1. In what ways do you think you have influenced Meredy's life and, in turn, how has she influenced yours?

2. What was she like before the anorexia took over? Or

3. If you did not know her then, what is she like now when you know her apart from the anorexia?

4. What is Meredy like as a person, what are her qualities, what are her blind spots, what makes her distinct?

5. If you are aware of any price that Meredy has paid to the anorexia, what might that be?

6. If the anorexia has stolen from your life, how has it affected you, your relationship with Meredy, or significant others in your circle?

7. Once Meredy fully escapes the hold of anorexia, what do you see her future like without it?

I want to thank you in advance for helping Meredy and helping me to be of assistance to her. We are taking this endeavor very seriously and would appreciate your frank and thoughtful comments.

Sincerely,

Ray Lemberg, Ph.D.
Clinical Psychologist

MEREDY BEFORE ANOREXIA TOOK OVER

"When she was small I teased her quite a little: called her a 'Minnie' because at about age two or three she couldn't pronounce Meredy clearly (short for Meredith, her maternal grandmother's namesake); Merd-Bird; Chebubbins (chubby cherub). I thought she generally liked the pet names, but wondered after the anorexia set in if 'Chebubbins' bothered her. I later asked her if she resented being called 'Chebubbins' and her answer, as it oftentimes was, pretty oblique—bottom line, she was sensitive about being chubby, even a chubby cherub."

—father

"Meredy has influenced my life with her wonderful sense of humor, her fine and always curious mind, her keen desire to be helpful to her siblings and to us. As a child and before the anorexia, Meredy appeared to be fun-loving, laughing lots and enjoying her relationships with her brothers."

—mother

"She was quite a quiet girl, pretty, with big twinkling eyes lighting her round, very freckled face. Her auburn hair, cut in bangs and to just below the tips of her ears, was straight, thick, and beautiful. She sat in the bow of the canoe, conversing only in response to my attempts at con-

versation, but paddling ably in response to my commands. We negotiated swift high water that day and made it under the low water bridge without incident, to our destination where we waited for the others."

—aunt

"She was like a good book or a mini vacation—always interesting to listen to, and she always made me think twice about everything. She also liked art and had a great interest in good art. She couldn't threaten me or make me insecure because she was such a good friend, and I was aware and guarded against being manipulated. I could talk to her about almost anything; she even talked to me a little about her past, her childhood, her sister, playing football, eating ice cream and peanut butter, and a tiny bit about her parents..."

—Michelle H., friend

About an unpopular classmate in the fourth grade: "The boy's mother told us one time that he didn't want to go to school because 'no one liked him' but there was always Meredy, implying there was at least one person who would be nice to him. She was a very tender-hearted little creature, somewhat like her mother—she couldn't tell the mean kids from the well-behaved (or at least she drew no distinction between them)."

—father

MEREDY, THE PERSON APART FROM ANOREXIA

"We really didn't know each other before anorexia became part of your life. Even now, I feel like I only know you apart from the anorexia. To me, anorexia is only one aspect of your whole self. I don't remember discussing it with you very often, you usually seemed uncomfortable in sharing that part of yourself. I always wondered if I should have done more to encourage you to talk more openly. Sometimes it seems that a 'true friend' would have pushed you a little harder and maybe even confronted you about the way you are hurting yourself. Many times I wanted to do that, but I also did not want to upset you or lose your friendship. My own experience of wanting others to see me beyond my illness [her friend at this time had cancer] helped me to justify to myself that it was okay to just be your friend. I guess I felt that you probably already had enough people pushing you already and maybe I could show I care by just letting you be. Was that being a good friend? I'll never know, but I'll always wonder if I should have done more. I feel like there is much that I do not know about you. But I do know that you have many strengths. Your sarcastic wit and humor is the first thing that comes to mind. You are extremely intelligent, but also possess that rare ability to share your intelligence with others without seeming intimidating. From the way that we met to your ability to never forget a birthday or special occasion, your thoughtfulness and concern always touches me. As a friend, *you are a 'real cheerleader,'* encouraging and truly enthusiastic for others' success. Having tasted your baklava and read your newspaper editorials, I know that you have many achievements and talents for which you should feel great pride. I especially admire your courage to live on your own and pursue your goals, particularly in regard to your career."

—Michelle L., friend

"Meredy never says an unkind word about anyone. She is not the least bit vicious or gossipy."
—Kim, friend

" I know Meredy is generally thrifty with herself and overly generous with others. She loves to give gifts and no effort is too much to give the right one if she thinks it will please. She bought me a bracelet when she lived with me and ordered a watch with our company logo for me. Meredy is thoughtful, caring, bright, witty, and can have a great sense of humor when she is in a good mood. She remembers birthdays, takes time to illustrate her letters on the computer, likes helping people and enjoys people who enjoy her. Earning the Phi Beta Kappa key seemed to embarrass, but please her. It amazed me that she could perform to such high standards academically in view of the many days of school she missed because of her health. Also amazing was the number of voluntary activities she engaged in during college. She needs to be needed and, I think, likes to be acknowledged."

—aunt

"Despite her lack of physical energy, Meredy is one of the hardest workers I know. She often works herself into exhaustion. Some of her qualities include: sensitive, caring, persistent, analytical, perceptive, and fair. Meredy is distinct in her genuine concern for other people (a concern which, I believe, is greater than concern for herself), her intellect, her curiosity, her bargain-

hunting skills, and her ability to remember things (birthdays, anniversaries, etc.)."
—Hank, brother

"Meredy's most obvious blind spot—other than the anorexia and topic of food—is in not being able to see her genuine worth. She is not only very bright and capable, but she is also very lovable. She probably will have difficulty believing this statement, but I consider it a privilege to have known her, even during the first struggles of anorexia."
—Dr. Mike M., Professor, Bethany College

THE PRICE MEREDY HAS PAID TO ANOREXIA

"I have thought about Meredy's death a lot, more so than I have thought about the deaths of other siblings, since hers seems so always imminent; I think I do not want to be surprised when it happens. My *'death watch'* has—as best as I can tell—helped make me more unconcerned about my own death than I otherwise would be. It is not that I necessarily accept Meredy's death young as foregone, and, given a clear idea of what might assist her towards eating without fretting, it would make me 'feel good' to do 'my part'."

—Doug, brother

"She was home part of the summer after her ninth grade, one year after the onset of the anorexia, after having been in the hospital most of the year, but keeping her school work pretty current. She went back to 'playing' softball with her team. Her teammates from the previous year were very supportive, but she wasn't strong enough to swing the bat with any gusto, or throw from one base to another. She was trying to play first base for one inning and tried to field a little roller about ten to fifteen feet away but couldn't; she fell down and muffed an easy play. I was glad to be wearing sunglasses and a ball cap I could pull down, because I began to cry. The other girls were very understanding. The anorexia was robbing both of us of a lot of fun we had in earlier summers, would it ever end? Not yet!"

—father

" I worry that I will lose a good friend to this frustrating illness—*Meredy has paid a huge price to this disease.* It makes me so angry. I used to have dreams that she was well; she was happy and dating. Meredy's body was stunted. She was an incredible athlete. We played softball together. I'll never forget the summer after she'd gotten so thin, she still insisted on playing. She was so weak she struggled with every step. She fell once and we all thought she would just shatter. This disease has diminished the chance for her to find a man to love. Who wouldn't be afraid to date someone that could die any day?"

—Kim, friend

"Anorexia sometimes steals from my good feelings about our friendship and replaces those feelings with guilt and worry. At times, I feel that the anorexia prevents me from being myself in our relationship. For example, I want to let you know when I notice that you seem 'up' or that you are looking better. But I worry about how you might perceive those words prevents me from saying anything at all. I feel, too, that there is a lot you do not say to me. There is much that I don't know about you. Anorexia has stolen from both of our lives by keeping us apart in this way."

—Michelle L., friend

"One enduring image I have is of her attempting to reach first base in a softball game, falling, and ending up splayed by the effort all over the hard dirt of the infield.... She has forked over to some little inner fascist demagogue much of her freedom to decide (as many of us have—we're, however, less visible about it). She has, due to poor health, been unable to attend some family get-togethers—funerals and other holidays—though that could be looked on as a plus. She has squandered a small fortune in pursuit of a thing which should have been hers by luck of birth."

—Doug, brother

"In our family Meredy seems to be the focus of lots of anxiety, not because of who she really is but because of our impotent efforts to 'make her better.' Others in the family do much better than I in relating to her without the specter of anorexia—I suppose the main thing that anorexia has 'stolen' from my life is the naive, immature attitude that all our children were relatively 'happy.' Ironically, when I think about the anorexia, I mostly 'feel' a heaviness and sadness that is different from anything else I have known even when my father (whom I was close to) died suddenly..."

—mother

"Most of all, the anorexia filled me with sadness and fear. Meredy guarded her anorexia

and history, so I didn't feel I could bug her about it without upsetting her. I just left the anorexia out of the picture most of the time and enjoyed Meredy's witty humor, her poetry; abilities of analyzing and manipulating and synthesizing everything."

—Michelle H., friend

"Meredy has paid a huge price to anorexia and so have those who love her. My constant concern is that the price Meredy pays might be her life. I know she has suffered tremendously physically and emotionally. *Anorexia is like a demon that is trying to steal her soul.* I imagine that every day is a struggle for her. I also imagine that living with anorexia takes incredible physical and emotional energy. There are so many positive things that that energy could be going towards. The passion that is going into her illness could be directed in so many productive and positive channels rather than continuing to rob Meredy of a more normal life. (I know that the anorexia might 'feel or seem' normal, but if she is able to leave it behind, there is a whole different world out there for her.)"

—Alyson, sister

MEREDY AND HER FUTURE

"...It doesn't matter what I see her future as without the crutch of anorexia holding her back; it matters how she sees it, and whether she sees it as something worth unshackling herself for. With her intelligence, creativity, sincerity, and desire, she could accomplish a whole lot that she would, I believe, take satisfaction in. I don't know if she enjoys her life now."

—Doug, brother

"If Meredy beats this thing, I see her doing important things with her talents. Things that make her happy and satisfied with her life. I would love to travel somewhere with her—go hiking in the mountains, protect endangered wildlife somewhere. I could see us sitting in the sun, appreciating the beauty of nature, discussing the power of God, and figuring out ways to keep the world as wonderful as it is. And, of course, writing poetry and stories about our adventures."

—Kim, friend

"Meredy is a good person, with or without anorexia. However, I sincerely believe she will become a more productive and much happier person when she can overcome it. She might go on to get her Ph.D. which at one time she intended to do, she might marry, have a family. She loves children and is good with them. I know her chances for happiness and *my hopes for her will grow proportionately with her battle won over anorexia.*"

—aunt

"Meredy is a great person. She challenges others to think. She engages others in great conversations. She is willing to help others with math problems using several ways to solve the problems and she can relate math to real-life situations. Meredy is great in encouraging others to succeed. She likes to see people happy and enjoying themselves. Meredy is a word wonder. She can solve tons of puzzles, write poems, figure out solutions, configure tons. Meredy is a great cook. She is willing to try new recipes and share with others. Meredy is very distinct. Her journeys in life are extraordinary. *She walks with a grace and gangliness of a person who makes a difference. Meredy does what others say she cannot do.*

—Michelle H., friend

Note: Bold italics are added by the editor

Death of a Scalesman
by Meredy Humphreys, B.S.

"Hey, welcome, glad you could make it. Come in. Sit down."

"Yeah, well . . . I'm kinda in a hurry. . . ."

"Oh, do you have an appointment or something . . . ?"

"Uh, no . . . just got things to do, you know . . . ?"

My guest sits down, though nervously twitching.

"Relax," I say, "this isn't an interrogation. . . . I just want to discuss some things with you."

"Yeah, I know. I just have a lot of things on my mind."

"Would you like some coffee or something?"

"Yes, sure, coffee."

"Cream or sugar . . .?"

"Just black."

"Of course, how could I forget?"

As blank, boring, and bitter as you yourself, Bitch, I say under my breath.

"What . . . I couldn't hear you? Did I do something wrong . . . ?"

"No, not really," I say with a tinge of empathy. Sometimes I am lucky enough to forget the baggage of guilt and worry my guest lugs around constantly.

"So what is it you want from me? Let's get to the point and get done. I DO have other things I need to be doing," my guest impatiently blurts out.

Ah, I think, I am beginning to hear that rude, almost evil voice. I forget my empathy.

"Geez, what if I just invited you to have a cup of coffee and shoot the breeze."

"'Shoot the breeze'—like I have time or even want to do that—what the hell purpose is there to shooting the breeze??!! If that is what this little get-together is for, then I'm outta here."

"Oh, sit down. I don't think I'd want to shoot the breeze with you anyway, and I do have some important issues to discuss with you.

"We've been friends (acquaintances and enemies, I think, but don't say aloud) for about 15 years now—so what do you think we developed here—I mean, that is over half of my life. Frankly, I don't see it as a great investment. Sure, you've been a close friend at times, but I have come to realize that you are not a true friend—more like a friend of 'convenience'— and I'll be the first to admit you have been convenient and even comforting in the past. But you are becoming very tiring."

"Yeah, well, why do you continue to hang out with me—you think I need YOU???"

"As a matter of fact you do need me to survive. I am your cover. Most people never see you for what you really are. A lot of people see us as one entity. They think I AM you or you are me—whichever—I don't like it. At times you are so rude, disrespectful, and downright mean that you hurt people and scare them away. Then I have to go back and apologize or, worse yet, I just plain miss out on meeting someone."

"Yeah, sure, whatever, but you know you need me. You don't know how to function without my guidance. I mean when things are tough, I am always there. I help you cope with all those details that stress you out. I am there on the holidays, on the weekends, when you go to sleep at night, when you cry. . . ."

"But there are times that I can almost leave you behind. My mind is able to pursue other creative bents. I laugh, I make jokes, sometimes I even come up with an innovative idea, and to tell you the truth I don't think you have a whole lot to do with me then. In fact, most of my better friends and close family see this—they see you and they see me and we are NOT one."

"Well, believe as you will, but consider living without me. You would be like a fish in the middle of the Sahara. Flip flop, flip flop, no direction, no idea how to conduct yourself, and soon to shrivel under the hot sun. You would just be—not knowing which way to walk, how to spend the hours of your day, what comes next. Imagine yourself in the middle of a barren parking lot. No buildings, no cars—just you and blacktop for as far as the eye can see. That is you without me. And that is just your environment, on the inside you are so full of anxiety, your mind is aflutter with 'what now?'; and even with all that anxiety you are empty."

I am caught speechless. Is this true? I am beginning to doubt my beginning convictions about this individual—let me call this person Rex. Perhaps Rex is right. I mean I have had him around for 15 years—over half my life. I barely remember my life without him; and when I do, I am not sure that the person I remember is me!!?? Rex has helped me out in times past—I admit that. But the thought of Rex always being there is something I

have never been able to imagine. I have dreamed of leaving Rex behind and being a full individual of my own making. But I am not sure that I know what that "making" is. I am scared—if Rex is right. . . . Oh, I hope not—but I have long THOUGHT I wanted Rex to be gone and yet look where he still is—right there across the table from me. Sitting there smugly, confident in his hold on me. How strong is he? Doubts are flooding in. Rex smiles. Does he know how my head is swirling? I must assume he does—he probably knows me as well as himself. But does he know me as well as I know myself? Don't I have some secrets that he is not a party to? Of course I do. He only knows that part of me that he has invaded, and I said it myself—he and I are not ONE. So there is a whole other me that he doesn't know or understand. Perhaps that is the me that can lead me from the Sahara and out of that barren parking lot. But that part of me is so underdeveloped—I mean it really stopped serious development around age 13 when I met Rex. Sure it has had some spurts and creeps of growth and development along the way—but could this part of me take on all the facets of life if Rex left? God, I sound like a co-dependent woman speaking about her mate—but that is not far from the truth.

What would a "divorce" from Rex take? To begin with I need to develop my own new behaviors that are not dictated by Rex. Once that process is in gear and perhaps within that process I need to develop and define ME—not the Rex-Me duet—but the me solo. I am suddenly hit with an image of myself on a tight wire, teetering alone—struggling. Then, as I look around, I see a net—it is composed of the open arms of my therapist, my dietitian, my doctor—over there is my Mom and Dad—shoot, there's the whole family, and there is another part of the net that is interwoven with many of my friends. I feel big, questionable steps ahead and the net will be a vital tool—but I am also feeling a tug to scurry back to the platform at the beginning of the rope—I feel there is some sense of security there. I glance back over my shoulder.

I am brought back to reality and find myself staring at Rex. He is tapping his ugly, long, controlling fingers on the table.

"Have we finished here?" he chides. "I have better things to do with my time than to dwell on these issues—they are old and worn out. Listen, we've been friends for too long to part now. Besides, you've had these types of thoughts before, we always remain friends—just getting closer every day." He smiles with a sarcastic twinge. "Unless, you've got some real action plan, backed by some courage—let's just shake hands and call it a day—like any other in the past 15 years—doesn't that sound safe and comfy?" I feel a great ball of anxiety welling up inside. I feel trapped between hatred of Rex and a certain need for his companionship. It is often so easy to have him around. I admit he helps make a lot of decisions for me. In fact, the damage the two of us have inflicted on my body has ruled out a lot of the opportunities and activities from which I might otherwise have to choose. Also, due to my physical appearance, I tend to believe that many of those around me excuse me for some shortcomings that I might— as a physically healthy individual—have to take responsibility for.

"Face it," Rex continues his little speech of persuasion, "whether you want to admit it or not, we're as good as one. Sure, you have your individual fleeting fantasies of leaving me behind, but more often than not when action happens—it is us. We play the crazy games, and in these games no one is looking at us as two individuals. We are one in your body, or what's left of it," he snickers. Rex rises from his seat and paces a bit. "Granted, I am absolutely dependent on you for my existence. I am so much your creation. There are others out there that perform duties like I do—but I have my own particular characteristics—there is no other like me. And it is some of that very uniqueness that, I think, appeals to you. So let's just leave things status quo, as they say. You don't know anything different, you're surviving—you know me—I know you; we're always there for each other. Let's just call another truce and get on with our existence."

Fear, hatred, love, loss, anger, seasoned with lots of anxiety and confusion, are boiling within my inner cauldron. I fear the loss of Rex as if I love him, but at the same time I am so angry with him that I am driven as far as hate. But most of all I am tired of him. He is old. He is boring. He drags on me, often allowing the world to pass on by. He dominates so much of my time that I am unable to pursue the ideas that evolve in my head . . . the ideas of writing a book, drawing a picture, investigating an inventive idea.

Cloudy headed, I turn on the radio; hoping for some musical reprieve from all this tiring sparring. A light, melodic voice floats out. Karen Carpenter. Ever since one of Rex's cohorts killed her, I find myself listening to her a little closer, and I am sure I hear a certain longing in her words— something that I somehow relate to. As her words continue to flow from the speakers, I find the anger and fear welling up in me and I glare at Rex. He seems so aloof—doesn't he have any sorrow or remorse? I am now filled with a stinging rage that somebody like Karen Carpenter was taken at the hands of somebody like Rex, and I fear that Rex intends to do the same to me.

Adrenaline mixed with a great deal of courage propels me from my seat. I rush at Rex. Grasping his throat I begin choking him, then I grab a knife and plunge it into his heartless chest cavity. I watch him shrivel to death. A brief smile of satisfaction and relief brush across my face.

There is no blood on my hands; just a ton off my shoulders. No jury could ever find guilt with me—I just killed it. It was an act of self-defense— self-survival is perhaps a more accurate term. Ironic as it may seem, this is a murder which allows the admitted perpetrator to be freed from the imprisoning bars.

I shove his remains out the door. I feel a fresh breeze blow over me.

The Secret Wisdom Within: Solution-Based Brief Therapy and Eating Disorders

by Barbara McFarland, Ph.D.

You cannot teach a man anything. You can only help him to find it within himself.—Galileo

It is a misnomer to call medicine "the healing art." The healing art is the secret wisdom of the body. Medicine can do no more than facilitate it. (Weil, 1988, p. 76)

Effective treatment for an eating disorder requires that each person be treated as an individual and allowed to determine, in large part by his or her own reactions, what is the best approach and process for him or her. As Francis Bacon put it, "There is wisdom in this beyond the rules of medicine: A man's own observations, what he finds good of, and what he finds hurt of, is the best medicine to preserve health" (LeShan, 1989, p. 127).

Generally, when families seek treatment for an eating disorder, they feel guilty, overwhelmed, frustrated, and helpless. Depending on his or her level of readiness for treatment, the family member suffering from anorexia or bulimia is at best ambivalent regarding the need for clinical intervention.

Therapists have their own reactions to treating anorexic or bulimic families. Because these illnesses are, for the most part, viewed as perplexing, multifaceted, and complex clinical syndromes, these families, in turn, are generally viewed the same way. Selvini-Palazzoli (1978) believes that treating anorexics or bulimics often generates significant feelings of frustration, inadequacy, and aggression within the therapist. Cohler (1977) adds, "Psychotherapy with anorectic patients leads to intense emotional reactions in the therapist: perhaps the most intense encountered in a therapeutic relationship" (p. 353).

All of this, coupled with the limitations managed care has placed on mental-health benefits (a generous health plan may only allow 20 sessions per year), can make treating anorexia and bulimia a major challenge for both clinicians and families.

BRIEF THERAPY: SHIFTING PARADIGMS

Given the pressures of managed care, brief therapy has moved into the mainstream of clinical practice. Many clinicians who specialize in treating eating-disordered individuals as well as family members find it hard to believe that anorexia or bulimia can be treated "briefly." "Brief" doesn't necessarily mean short. I have treated clients within time spans ranging anywhere from six to 32 sessions, within one year or within two years, depending on the client's goals and needs. These sessions can be used intermittently or more intensely, again depending on the client's progress and needs.

Solution-based brief therapy has more to do with an "attitude" in that it operates within a paradigm of wellness, focusing on solutions and specific goal development, rather than the more traditional medical model paradigm, which explores underlying causes and tends to be nonspecific in its treatment focus. The major thrust of solution-based brief therapy deals with what is problematic for the client now and what needs to happen so that the situation can improve. Moreover, although essential for pathology-based paradigms, determining risk factors in solution-based brief therapy is of no consequence to the treatment process and, in fact, results in therapeutic detours that promote wastefulness in treatment and clutter the therapeutic relationship. Rather than reexamining and dwelling on the past, brief therapy focuses on the present and future. What difference does the client wish to see in his or her life today? What needs to happen so he or she can get on with life in a way that is meaningful to him or her?

Within this model, the therapeutic relationship shifts from a hierarchical one, in which the therapist is the expert, to a collaborative one, in which the client is the expert. With this shift in power, a cooperative and mutual relationship, in which the realities of the client are acknowledged and respected, precludes resistance and recalcitrance. Within a mutual, cooperative relationship, in which the therapist joins with the client, resistance is minimized.

Collaborating with eating-disordered clients also requires faith—faith in the self-healing and self-regulating capacity of the human organism. Following the homeopathic approach to medicine, which stresses the value of working with the body and its own natural healing powers, requires that faith be a part of self-healing. Friedman and Fanger (1991, p. 15) state, "We view the therapist as a guide who takes his cues from the client and relies on the client's natural momentum towards movement and change. The therapist needs to have faith in the healing power contained within the client's natural healing ecology."

SEVEN USEFUL PRINCIPLES

Having used solution-based brief therapy as a major focus of my work, I have found useful seven principles to guide my treatment with clients.

1. Focus on Client and Family Strengths

As brief therapy operates within a strength-based paradigm, clients are not viewed as "sick" or given diagnostic labels but rather are viewed as "stuck" but basically capable, competent, and able to surmount their own difficulties or to solve their own problems (deShazer, 1991). This paradigm shift is crucial in doing brief therapy. The therapist must help the client and family identify the strengths they possess and, when possible, use these in the treatment process.

Generally, when clients seek counseling, they are completely immersed in the problem, steeped in pervasive feelings of shame, inadequacy, and personal impotency. They have spent a vast amount of energy trying to figure out the "why" of their perplexing behavior. Brief therapy jars them out of the obsessive cycle.

Solution-based therapy maintains the premise that no experience occurs *all* the time; there are always exceptions or periods of nonproblematic behavior. The therapeutic task becomes one of assisting clients to discover these exceptions so that he or she can see that the solutions are already within the client's existing repertoire of behaviors and, thus, likely to be repeated.

Thus, exploring exceptions is a useful strategy that not only decreases patients' and families' sense of hopelessness but also helps them identify their strengths, helping them to increase their awareness of their mastery experiences. The therapist interviews the client when the purging or restricting behaviors are less rampant to determine what's different during those times. Exploring exceptions not only helps the client see that the eating disorder isn't always in control but also reinforces solution patterns that have been helpful in the past. An exploration of exceptions jars patients out of the obsessive cycle and into examining those times when their eating disorder is more manageable.

One client I worked with, who had just transferred to Cincinnati, Ohio, discovered that her bulimia was much less problematic on those weekends when she was socially active. By increasing her socialization and normalizing her feelings about moving to a new city, her bulimia decreased significantly.

As this case illustrates, solutions for certain clients may in fact be unrelated to their eating disorder. (Numerous case examples are presented in my book *Brief Therapy and Eating Disorders*, 1995). In other cases, especially with the more medically compromised client, treatment must focus on weight restoration and stabilization and/or binge and purge reduction.

2. Work with the Client to Build a Cooperative Relationship

Solution-based therapy makes no assumptions about the "real" nature of the problem, takes the client at his or her word, and focuses on finding a solution that is salient and unique to that particular individual. Working cooperatively with the client is a cornerstone of solution-based brief therapy. Thus, the therapeutic relationship is collaborative at its core. With eating-disordered clients this notion of collaboration and participation is especially critical as they generally feel "a paralyzing sense of ineffectiveness" (Bruch, 1973, p. 13) and suffer greatly impaired levels of self-esteem (Boskind-Lodahl, 1976; Johnson

& Maddi, 1986; Love, Ollendick, Johnson, & Schlesinger, 1985; Root, Fallon, & Friedrich, 1986; Slade, 1982; Striegel-Moore, Silberstein, & Rodin, 1986; Swift, Bushnell, Hanson, & Logemann, 1986). As partners and participants in the process, clients assume more of the responsibility for their own recovery, thus empowering themselves in the treatment experience. Instead of relinquishing control to the therapist, they take control of their own health and treatment.

However, before this is possible, the therapist and client must negotiate a goal that is salient to the client. Because many eating-disordered clients enter treatment under duress and generally don't believe they have a problem, negotiating such a goal is a major task in the very first few sessions of treatment.

Although each case is unique, the goals most identified by anorexic clients tend to center around two themes: (1) the avoidance of hospitalization and/or the discontinuance of outpatient therapy and (2) the desire to participate in some activity (e.g., athletics, dance, enrollment at college some distance from home, and driving) for which their physical condition will not allow. "What has to be different so that you don't have to come back here anymore?" or "What will you have to do so that you don't lose complete control and end up in the hospital?" With clients who are athletes, dancers, or exercise enthusiasts, we negotiate how they can continue these activities at their optimum performance level, which requires a certain number of calories or pounds to maintain.

3. Picture Life Without the Problem

One useful technique to help the client project himself or herself into a problem-free future is to ask the Miracle Question:

> Suppose you go home and go to bed tonight after today's session. While you are sleeping a miracle happens and the problem that brought you here is solved. Because you were sleeping, you didn't know that this miracle happened. What do you suppose will be the first small thing that will indicate to you tomorrow morning that there has been a miracle overnight and the problem that brought you here is solved? (Berg & Miller, 1992)

This question is a powerful frame around which clients can establish goals. Furthermore, as they describe what life will be like when the problem is solved, they come to believe that there is a solution to the problem and to actually behave in ways that will lead to fulfilling this expectation.

Another similar question is to ask the client and family, "How will this family be different without the eating disorder?" Exploring answers to this question generates a sense of hopefulness and leads to a discussion of goals.

Externalizing the eating disorder is another technique that is very helpful. The client is asked various questions such as, "How does the eating disorder affect or influence your self-esteem . . . friends . . . family . . . freedom?" "What can you do to stand up to the eating disorder?" "What must you do differently not to let the eating disorder get control of you?" "When are the times you have been able to stand up to the eating disorder?"

As therapy progresses, the therapist needs to remind the client and family that change *is* happening by highlighting, amplifying, and reinforcing the changes that have occurred. Given the tenacity of eating disorders, it is often very difficult to recognize that changes have occurred. The therapist must help to increase the client's awareness of these changes by focusing on them.

Client:	I'm so disgusted with myself. I've been bingeing and purging like crazy.
Therapist:	So, when have you been able to stand up to the bulimia since I've seen you?
Client:	(hesitating) Uh, well, I guess a few days last week. But, gosh, yesterday and today have been awful. Like it was before.
Therapist:	You mean to tell me that you had a few days last week when you didn't binge or purge at all?
Client:	Well, yeah. Actually, now that we're talking about it, I guess I did pretty good up until yesterday.

Focusing on change and what's different can help the client gain a new perspective on the manageability of the eating disorder.

4. Develop a Working Contract

If a client is medically compromised or the symptoms are beginning to spiral downward, we negotiate and develop a contract (reviewed at four- to six-week intervals) that typically includes

- a goal weight or a required number of calories needed to maintain athletic or dance performance;
- the degree of involvement with the nutritionist;
- a schedule of weigh-ins and blood tests;
- the frequency of therapy;
- and some specific task for the parent(s) such as "Mom can ask Mary Jo one time a day how she is doing with her eating."

5. Use a Team Approach

Once again, in the case of a more medically compromised client, the use of a team in the development and implementation of the contract is necessary. In addition to the therapist, the client, and the family, other members of the treatment team should include the client's primary care physician, an experienced nutritionist, and, in some cases, an exercise physiologist. The nutritionist helps determine ideal body weight range and what reasonable weight the client would have to achieve and maintain to accomplish his or her goals. We typically use the absolute lowest weight in the Ideal Body Weight (IBW) range and have sometimes negotiated one or two pounds less. The physician, along with the nutritionist, determines the weight at which hospitalization would be required.

I typically serve as the "case manager," making sure that everyone is kept informed of treatment progress or difficulties.

Case Example

Working together as a team and negotiating contracts is best illustrated by the following case. Leah, a 17-year-old anorexic, was coerced into treatment by her parents and in denial regarding her severely restrictive eating patterns. At 5' 9", her large frame carried 119 pounds. She had lost 30 pounds in the four months prior to entering treatment.

In our first session Leah was polite but reticent. She thought her parents were making too much of her weight loss. As far as she was concerned, there wasn't anything wrong with her. I tried my usual question I use to engage clients who are in therapy because someone else has sent them: "Now I know you don't want to be here, but your parents and your physician think otherwise. What do you suppose would have to happen so you and I don't have to meet anymore?" That question didn't result in any useful response as she was determined that she was not going to eat any more than she already was, which was about 500 calories per day.

I maintained my neutral posture but did share my serious concern regarding her weight loss. We negotiated that she did not have to come back to see me as long as she continued to be weighed in by her physician twice weekly, something she had negotiated with her mother and was already doing consistently.

I continued seeing her mother, who was more motivated to participate in treatment. Using the weigh-in as an indicator of Leah's willingness to cooperate and the "extremely close" relationship Leah and her mother perceived themselves as having, Leah's mother and I developed a contract, which she presented to Leah. (See next page.) Leah's mother further agreed to take responsibility for enforcing the contract with her daughter. The hospitalized weight of 116 pounds was identified by the physician while the corresponding restrictions and privileges were developed by Leah's mother and me. (Please note that her driving privileges were removed and her curfew was restricted only because of her physical symptoms, which included dizziness and passing out.)

Leah and her mother reviewed the contract and negotiated some of the details, and Leah agreed to adhere to it although, according to her mother, she was "not a happy camper." I established my role as that of "consultant" to Leah's mother, and we met once a month to review Leah's progress.

Leah gained three pounds within a month and became extremely anxious, at which time she requested a session with me. We talked about her anxiety and developed some strategies for coping with these "freaky" feelings. By the end of the session she agreed to attend a support group, and we further agreed that she would continue to see me when she felt it would be helpful. I continued to work with Leah and her mother on an "as needed" basis. By the end of the summer, Leah had gained 10 pounds, which was her goal weight to enter college. Although it may seem that much time and effort was put into Leah's treatment, my work with this mother and daughter lasted only six months, and we only used a total of nine sessions.

Contract Negotiated with Leah, a 17-Year-Old Eating-Disordered Patient

128 lbs. Can go away to college; however, must see a physician there for an initial weigh-in and continue having monthly weigh-ins and develop a relationship with a therapist or group on campus.

125 lbs. No weigh-ins.

123 lbs. Bimonthly weigh-ins; driving privileges reinstated; curfew extended and social activities increased.

120 lbs. Weekly weigh-ins.

119 lbs. Semiweekly weigh-ins; no driving privileges; restricted curfew and social activities as a result of lethargy and physical condition.

118 lbs. Weekly individual therapy; three times a week weigh-ins with physician.

117 lbs. Family therapy; intensive outpatient group therapy; three times a week weigh-ins with physician.

116 lbs. Hospitalization.

6. Negotiate the End of Therapy at the Beginning

For therapy to be brief, the client and therapist must be clear about where they are going and how they plan to get there. This future-focused orientation instills a degree of hopefulness within clients as they are no longer burdened by the possibility that they will be in therapy "forever," but rather can experience successes and use therapy intermittently.

This approach is not curative but rather intended to move clients in the right direction so that they can get on with the business of living their lives. The frequency and intensity of therapy are negotiated with the client and are dependent on his or her medical status. This may mean seeing one anorexic client for seven sessions over several months and another for 32 sessions, some of which may be weekly, depending on the client's medical status.

In solution-based therapy, the client is motivated to participate in treatment and to leave treatment with a mind-set that promotes a belief in his or her ability to manage the eating behavior and other challenges of life. Given the biophysical aspects of eating disorders, many of these clients are likely to use therapy intermittently throughout their early adult to mid-adult years as they continue to work to alter their relationship with food.

7. Assign Homework

Because the real therapy takes place between sessions, clients need to do homework between each

and every session. Therapy isn't about "talking" but about "doing." Because the relationship is collaborative, both the therapist and client have work to do.

Depending on the client and the flow of the session, I have found the following homework assignments to be helpful with eating-disordered clients:

• *Encourage the symptom.* Prescribing the symptom is useful for some clients and a very effective group task. I will frequently tell clients I want them to binge and purge every other day between sessions, with the other day being a normal food day. They are asked to note what's different on the normal days. Clients frequently report that being given permission to binge and purge makes the desire much less intense. We then explore what this really means for them.

• *Perform pattern intervention tasks.* Another assignment that is frequently useful is pattern intervention tasks, which attempt to alter any problematic eating rituals. For example, a client only purged at home, so we developed an intervention in which she was to go out two times and purge anywhere else but home. Although she agreed, she wasn't able to do the assignment, and thus came to realize that she had more control over her purging than she thought.

• *Monitor self-talk.* Having the client monitor self-talk, especially during an urge to binge and purge that is controllable, helps clients pay more attention to what is going on inside themselves. We work toward writing new self-talk scripts that are more supportive and encouraging.

- *Observe.* Observation tasks require the client to observe something specific like the times she feels more in control of her bingeing or least likely to restrict or times when she feels more self-confident. In addition to observing, the client is asked to notice what's different during those times.

- *Practice standing up to the eating disorder.* Self-talk, meditation, conversations with others, and moderate exercise are all strategies that the client uses to "stand up" to the eating disorder. This is a part of the externalizing technique used in therapy.

- *Keep a journal.* Daily journaling is very helpful in assisting clients to pay more attention to their feelings and to identify them.

- *Self-assign homework.* More often than not, I turn the responsibility over to the client and ask him or her what the homework should be.

Given the tenacity of compulsive eating, purging, or restricting behaviors, eating-disordered clients are prone to relapses. Therefore, therapists may ask themselves what they would like the client to leave treatment with. Should he or she leave with a mind-set that promotes ongoing attempts at insight into a never-ending problem and the belief that a cure will come with the magical key of understanding? Or should he or she depart with a mind-set that promotes a belief in his or her ability to manage the eating behavior and other challenges that life presents?

I have come to recognize that by shifting the underlying paradigm of therapy from disease to health, we clinicians make it possible for the eating-disordered clients we treat to achieve, more than anything else, an increased sense of self-efficacy, which empowers them to face other life challenges. As we continue to attend to what is *inside* the client that is good, worthwhile, capable, and competent, the client becomes more connected to these qualities within himself or herself. The client is empowered to believe in his or her own ability to manage life and she is much more likely then to see far beyond the looking glass.

REFERENCES

Berg, I., & Miller, S. (1992). *Working with the problem drinker.* New York: Norton.

Boskind-Lodahl, M. (1976). Cinderella's stepsisters: A feminist perspective on anorexia nervosa and bulimia. *Signs: Journal of Women in Culture and Society 2,* 342–356.

Bruch, H. (1973). *Eating disorders: Obesity and anorexia nervosa.* New York: Basic Books.

Cohler, B. (1977). The significance of the therapist's feelings in the treatment of anorexia nervosa. In S. Feinstein and P. Giovacchini (Eds.), *Adolescent psychiatry,* Volume 5, (pp. 352–384). New York: Jason Aronson.

de Shazer, S. (1991). *Putting difference to work.* New York: Norton.

Friedman, S., & Fanger, M. (1991). *Expanding therapeutic possibilities: Getting results in brief therapy.* Lexington, MA: Lexington Books.

Johnson, C., & Maddi, I. (1986). The etiology of bulimia: A biopsychosocial perspective. In S. Feinstein, J. Esman, A. Looney, A. Schwartzberg, A. Sorosky, and M. Sugar (Eds.), *Adolescent psychiatry,* Volume 13 (pp. 253–273). Chicago: University of Chicago Press.

LeShan, L. (1989). *Cancer as a turning point: A handbook for people with cancer, their families, and health professionals.* New York: Plume.

Love, S., Ollendick, T., Johnson, C., & Schlesinger, S. (1985). A preliminary report of the prediction of bulimic behaviors: A social learning analysis. *Bulletin of the Society of Psychologists in Addictive Behaviors 4,* 93–101.

McFarland, B. (1995). *Brief therapy and eating disorders: A practical guide to solution focused work with clients.* San Francisco: Jossey-Bass.

Root, M., Fallon, P., & Friedrich, W. (1986). *Bulimia: A systems approach to treatment.* New York: Norton.

Selvini-Palazzoli, M. (1978). *Self-starvation: From individual to family therapy in the treatment of anorexia nervosa.* New York: Aronson.

Slade, P. (1982). Towards a functional analysis of anorexia nervosa and bulimia nervosa. *British Journal of Clinical Psychology 21,* 167–179.

Striegel-Moore, R., Silberstein, L., & Rodin, J. (1986). Toward an understanding of risk factors in bulimia. *American Psychologist 41*(3), 246–263.

Swift, W., Bushnell, M., Hanson, P., & Logemann, T. (1986). Self-concept in adolescent anorexics. *Journal of the American Academy of Child Psychiatry 25,* 826–835.

Weil, A. (1988). *Health and healing.* Boston: Houghton Mifflin.

Nutritional Counseling for Anorexic and Bulimic Patients

by Annika Kahm, B.S.

Is there a need to educate eating-disordered patients about calories and nutritional balance? Don't most of them know it all?

There *is* a need even if the patients don't agree. Very often their parents, relatives, or friends ask: "Can't you just tell her to eat normally, like everybody else does?" We know, of course, it's not that easy. And patients know it, too. Actually, they often *know* all about good eating habits; they just cannot *follow* them. We see this in hospitalized patients who achieve weight gains in order to get privileges or be discharged. Though they may leave the hospital, they may never learn how to maintain their food intake at healthy levels or understand why this is so important. They will usually repeat the old pattern of restriction and weight loss because it's too scary to gain weight and feel out of control.

That's partly why nutritional counseling, with education and motivation, is an important part of the teamwork necessary to help these patients achieve full recovery. The counseling described here is done on an outpatient basis, and most visits are weekly. Treatment is individualized and can vary in length from a few weeks to over a year, depending on the patient's needs.

THE BASICS OF NUTRITIONAL COUNSELING

At the initial office visit a thorough nutritional history is taken. Its purpose is to learn about the patients' eating habits and certain psychological traits, as well as to gain relevant information about their families. It's important that patients understand the purpose of nutritional counseling. They should agree that the final goal is to be able to eat a meal when hungry, to stop when comfortably full, and to do so at least three to four times per day, without obsessing about food in between meals. It is also important that patients ultimately accept and like themselves at healthy body weights and trust that the scale won't go up after a meal (and they will know why if it does). In other words, they should feel in control over their food intake and weight.

Small, manageable steps should be presented to help the patient reach this long-term goal. A first step usually is a low-calorie meal plan designed jointly by the patient and the nutritionist. It is important to have the patient involved in these decisions. At this initial visit it's also crucial that a relationship be formed—a warm, trusting, nonthreatening relationship—so that the patient feels safe to express likes and dislikes.

THE MINIMUM CALORIC NEED

Nutritional education, then, is introduced as an integral part of the motivation to improve eating behavior. Only when patients can understand why and how the body responds to starvation, bingeing, and restriction can they dare to try to eat properly. Their metabolism, which has adapted to fasting by slowing down, will then speed up and function appropriately (Apfelbaum, 1975; Flatt, 1980). If they can accept that their metabolism has not been destroyed but has only been sluggish for as long as the eating disorder has been active, patients then have the greatest potential for normalizing their abnormal eating habits. Part of the education is to learn not only how many calories the body needs on a daily basis but also why it needs them:

1. The basic metabolic rate is approximately 1200 kcal (calories)/day (for breathing, blood circulation, etc.).

2. For growth and maintenance, the body needs approximately 150–300 kcal/day (renewal of blood cells, hair, skin, etc.).

3. Digesting and absorbing food requires approximately 150 kcal/day.

4. For maintaining body temperature, hydration, and chemical concentration in cells,

the body needs approximately 150 kcal/day.

This means that a human being who does not exercise needs about 1650 kcal/day. With physical activity we can add 300–500 kcal/day. An individual who eats less than 1200 kcal/day is not getting enough calories to fulfill the above four requirements. Consequently, his or her metabolism will cope by lowering its rate and becoming sluggish. This means that eating will become more threatening than ever because weight gain will occur on fewer calories than before.

Most eating-disordered patients are trying to lower weight to feel better. But because most them are eating or keeping down less than the minimum amount of food needed for their body functions, this is not possible. This is where the motivation to get out of this "trap" is so important.

Historically, the "media" have been able to influence eating to the point where 15 years ago people had a normal fat intake but restricted their carbohydrates when they tried to lose weight. It seems like the general population still hasn't got the balance because today the carbohydrate intake is high but among dieters the fat intake is frequently below the medical minimum requirement of 25 grams per day. This, of course, has to do with the notion that a *low*-fat diet is a must for being healthy today. An eating-disordered patient will interpret that as meaning a *no*-fat diet must be the best.

As mentioned above, we've learned that if we eat more than 1,200 calories per day as adults we'll keep the metabolism going. "Metabolism" has become a common concept that people with eating disorders tend to dismiss. In order to motivate patients on this issue we need to give them more information. One strategy that gets their attention (but doesn't do the whole trick) is to break out energy minimums for individual vital organs, such as the heart, kidneys, liver and brain. Figures from the World Health Organization for an adult who requires 1,800 kcal per day put the daily caloric requirements for the brain at 482 kcal, the heart at 338 kcal, the kidneys at 187 kcal, and the muscles at 324 kcal (Guthrie and Picciano, 1995). So, if the patient is only eating a few hundred calories less than 1,200, I usually ask them which organ they fed today and which one they didn't.

Only when patients understand and trust the concept of metabolism and weight gain can they work through this frightening period of eating the required minimum of calories to boost their metabolic rates up to normal. Although patients may initially gain weight during this time, it will be mostly water weight (two to seven pounds).

Through consistent good eating, weight gain will continue until the body reaches normal body weight, or its "set point." When this happens, the metabolism tends to normalize. Reaching the set point is a big moment for both patient and nutritionist. It means that the metabolism has sped up and all calories are being used for bodily functions, not stored as excess fat—the biggest fear of all for anorexics and bulimics.

THE FOOD PLAN

It is important to review how patients experienced the first meeting as well as their understanding of the discussion. Misunderstandings are clarified, and the food plan is discussed again. Was the patient comfortable when we designed the plan on the first visit? Was it too much or too little to eat? No one can follow a food plan exactly, but it's important to create one that patients feel motivated to try.

The plan should be balanced and include choices from the four food groups based on U.S.D.A. dietary guidelines. Again, the *minimum* caloric need to fulfill all bodily functions is approximately 1200–1500 calories daily for an adult and 1500 calories daily for a teenager, divided among these foods:

- Two to three servings of dairy (four servings for teens).
- Five ounces of protein (fish, chicken, meat, or vegetarian equivalent).
- Two fruits and three servings of vegetables.
- Six servings of starch (bread, cereal, pasta, rice, etc.) for women and nine for men.
- Twenty-five grams of fat.

The need to eat a varied diet must be emphasized frequently. A booklet listing examples from the different food groups is a popular and useful handout.

Keeping a diet record helps patients see for themselves how well they are meeting the minimum requirement from each of the four food groups. It is also a helpful tool that enables the nutritionist to gauge the patient's ability to follow the meal plan. If used correctly, the diet record gives room for encouragement and praise. Because eating-disordered patients are likely to be perfectionists, they often have a hard time dealing with their inability to follow the food plan exactly as outlined. By reviewing what their patients have written in their records, nutritionists have the opportunity to help them turn what has been a personal failure into a learning experience.

The meal plan most always includes three meals, with or without snacks, depending on the patient's preference. Breakfast is usually the hardest part, because by eating it patients often think they will be hungrier for the rest of the day. After learning about the nature of hunger and that the body burns more calories if they are spread out over three or more meals, breakfast can frequently become the most enjoyable meal for patients. They learn that hunger is a signal informing us that whatever we previously ate is used up—not stored—and it is now time to refuel.

Often patients will experience some initial gastrointestinal discomfort after eating, but if that has been described and discussed beforehand, they will cope better and understand that this is normal and that their capacity and comfort with food will increase slowly ("Nutrition and Eating Disorders—Guidelines for the Patient with Anorexia Nervosa and Bulimia Nervosa," 1990). Also, it is helpful if the bulk content of meals is kept small because of the patient's sense of fullness or bloating.

ANOREXIA

Nutritional Assessment

For the anorexic, cessation of weight loss has to be the first goal. To achieve this, a nutritional assessment is usually helpful and motivational. Part of the assessment involves measuring the tricep skinfold (upper arm fat fold), the mid-arm circumference, and the hip fatfold. Based on these figures we can estimate the patient's fatfold, muscular mass, and percent body fat and compare them with others of the same age (Grant, 1979). If an individual is below the fifth percentile for upper arm fatfold (which is a trend among the severely anorexic), then he or she has the minimum amount of fat and is malnourished. Less than five percent of the population has so little subcutaneous fat (50th percentile = normal, 95th percentile = overweight/obese). If the person's muscle mass is also low, below the 10th percentile (50th percentile =

normal), he or she can now realize that losing more weight is dangerous because it means loss of more muscular tissue (since there is no more fat to lose). This indicates potentially life-threatening weight loss in all muscular tissue, including such organs as the heart.

From these numbers we can also determine the percentage of body fat. When a female patient looks at the chart, she realizes that normal-thin means having 23–28 percent body fat. When she sees that her own number is below 15 or 16 percent, she may begin to realize why her period has stopped, her hair is falling out, her skin is drying, and she's sleeping poorly.

At abnormally low body-fat levels, the body reverses developmentally and becomes prepubertal. (The ovary shrinks from the size of a pear to the size of a plum.) This reversal brings a woman's body back to the way it was when she was a girl, before she put on the 50 or 60 pounds that paved the way for her to become physically and sexually mature. When she was a child, her body fat totaled about 17 percent. But during the five years it generally takes for puberty to transform her into a healthy woman, her body fat increased to 23 to 28 percent. This happens whether she likes it or not! Menstruation itself may be something a patient believes she can live without, but being healthy and having a normally functioning body *matters*.

Trusting Their Hunger Signals

Anorexic patients usually complain of waking up early (4 to 6 a.m.) and feeling very weak. Actually, they would like to sleep longer but their bodies will not allow it because they are too hungry. Of course, these patients would like to eat. But, as we mentioned earlier, if they give in to eating so early in the day they fear the hunger will increase later on, and they won't be able to make it on the few hundred calories they allow themselves for the rest of the day.

By discussing and clarifying physiological facts such as the caloric needs of individual vital organs, it is hoped that anorexics will be better able to listen to their body's hunger signals and respond to them appropriately.

Once our exhausted patient understands the link between adequate nourishment and healthy functioning, she may realize that eating more will allow her to sleep longer (because she doesn't have to wake up early to search for food). Yet, the positive nature of hunger pangs seems to be one of the hardest truths for anorexics to accept and to follow. Anorexics are known for denying hunger so they can stay thin. Sadly, their strong negative association between eating and weight gain leads many anorexics to prefer even death to becoming fat.

Hunger is our body's way of telling us that it's time to eat; all the food we consumed earlier has been used up for bodily functions. If we don't refuel, the body eventually will compensate by reducing its metabolic rate and make us think about food in an obsessive way. "Well, what if I eat more than I need?" or "How do I know how much I require?" are some of the questions often asked by the worried patient. The answer still remains the same: "If you don't eat enough, you'll be hungry sooner—maybe even within one hour! But if you eat an appropriate amount, there will be a while before you need to eat again. Only the person who eats when *not* hungry will put on excess weight." This is not only hard for eating-disordered patients to understand but also for the 60 million Americans dieting today.

What's so troublesome for anorexic patients is that they are always hungry, but they have become used to suffering and denying it. They consider their state of hunger normal. When they start to acknowledge hunger and begin to eat, they may feel overwhelmed because it may seem they could eat all day long with no bottom to their stomachs. Anorexic patients feel like ravenous animals—as they should—and we nutritionists are glad when they do because it means they can again listen to their hunger signals. Their bodies are simply saying, "Please eat and make up for earlier starvation and deprivation." What is so hard for a patient to trust, however, is that this ravenous hunger will eventually stop when it reaches its set-point weight. Anorexics find it difficult to believe this will happen *before* they put on excess weight.

Body Image and Weight Gain Expectation

All patients should be warned about the possibility of rapid water weight gain (two to seven pounds) when refeeding begins. This results from retention of water through expansion of the extracellular compartment and an increase in depleted liver and muscle glycogen associated with refeeding. If this isn't explained, patients will usually stop eating because they fear they will continue to gain at the same rate. Patients must be reassured that rehydration weight will resolve spontaneously if they continue to follow the prescribed food plan.

Needless to say, anorexic patients must gain weight in order to overcome their eating disorder. But how much? From the nutritional history and assessment we can determine an ideal 10-pound weight range within which normal physiological functions, including menstruation, can be presumed to occur and preoccupation with thoughts of food will decline.

This weight range is central to "set-point theory," which assumes that the ideal weight of each individual is actually tied to a genetically programmed percentage of body fat that the body will actively defend. The set point has been described as a thermostat-like mechanism, revving up metabolism when the body rises above its preferred body-fat level and slowing it down if it drops below. It varies from person to person, which explains why healthy people of similar height often vary so radically in weight. Factors in addition to genetics are believed to affect set point as well, such as age, exercise, pregnancy, years of eating high fat foods, and use of certain drugs (Reiff & Reiff, 1992).

Frequently the ideal weight range as suggested by the nutritionist is unacceptable for the patient, and a lower weight is chosen as an initial goal, with reevaluation of the situation when that goal is achieved.

Usually eating-disordered patients know they are underweight, but they still see themselves as fat. This distorted body image must be addressed frequently so that patients see themselves realistically and are thus motivated to eat. This is easier said than done. It is usually helpful to look at a picture of different body outlines where 1 is emaciated, 2 underweight, 3 normal-thin, 4 normal, 5 normal-heavy, and so forth with 8 as obese. (See Figure 1.) Patients usually think they resemble 3, 4, or even 5 or 6 and would really like to look like 1 or 2. To do so they feel they would have to lose weight. This exemplifies their distorted body image because in reality they often represent a 1 or 2 and have to gain to become normal. If they still cannot see it, it has proved helpful for me to take a full-body photograph of the patient in a bikini. This way she can objectively compare the reality on film with the body outlines as represented in Figure 1.

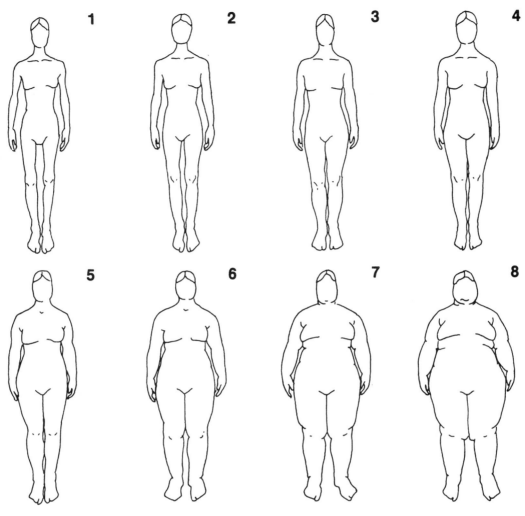

Figure 1. Body image illustrations.

Copyright (permission © 1979 by Profile Associates. Used by permission of Profile Associates, Marcia Mills, R.D.

There is no set pattern for weight gain, but ideally a gain of one-half to two pounds per week is expected. Otherwise, caloric intake should be increased by 200–500 calories per week. This is usually hard to achieve because a person cannot be forced to eat. We frequently have to allow for steps backward, too. What is important is that patients try hard and slowly give up their old habits of denying hunger, which depresses the metabolic rate. When they reach their set-point weight, the ravenous hunger decreases. They can eat less (i.e., a normal amount) and the weight gain eventually stops. The percentage of time they spend thinking and even

dreaming about food drops dramatically. They should now be able to trust their bodies and feel a new sense of control over their lives. They can now see clearly that it's possible to eat at least three times a day, when hungry, without gaining weight.

BULIMIA

Bulimia is characterized by the erratic eating of large amounts of food, followed by self-induced vomiting and/or the abuse of laxatives and diuretics. Since restrictive eating patterns between binges are common, bulimic patients experience many of the anorexic characteristics already mentioned, along with feelings of shame and self-deprecation which negatively influence all aspects of their lives. Although most bulimics are not obese, they, too, misperceive themselves as being overweight and want to weigh less. Treatment must help patients achieve normal weight range goals and maintain them so that they do not remain chronic yo-yo dieters.

Most bulimics exhibit chaotic eating patterns characterized by cycles of fasting or severe dieting followed by bouts of compulsive overeating; sometimes called the "overcontrol-release" cycle. For many, these patterns are so entrenched that the patients have no idea how to eat "normally." They are frightened that if they begin eating regular meals they will gain weight. Patients need to be reassured that establishing a pattern of regular eating is essential in gaining control over binge eating. Initially, eating must become "mechanical." There should be a predetermined and definite maintenance plan that minimizes decision-making. Without such a plan, bulimic patients can easily slip back into a pattern of bingeing and purging, since lower weight is their ultimate goal. They, as well as anorexics, must be warned of possible water retention of two to seven pounds, which is likely to happen when they decide to stop purging and begin to eat normally. This weight gain, which patients often experience as bloatedness and perceive as excessive fat, can happen within a few days and can easily throw them off.

When they eventually resume normal eating and have done so for a while (weeks or even months, depending on how long they have struggled with their eating disorder), their metabolisms will return to normal.

SEPARATING EMOTIONAL EATING FROM PHYSICAL HUNGER IN ANOREXIA AND BULIMIA

One of the most important tasks for anorexics and bulimics is to stop restriction, bingeing and/or purging and to resume normal eating. They need praise and encouragement to go through this painful part of breaking an old habit and to face and deal with their repressed emotions.

Anorexics and bulimics can help themselves stop their eating-disordered behaviors by:

- Realizing what causes restriction or overeating (feelings of anxiety, anger, etc.),
- Deciding on appropriate action, and
- *Never* skipping a meal.

In order to identify what triggers under- or overeating and how those triggers cause them to react, it is critical that patients feel free to talk about their experiences in an accepting, nonjudgmental atmosphere. For the patient to recover fully, treatment often should include therapy—individual and group, as well as nutritional counseling. Therapy can help patients work through underlying thoughts and conflicts that have built high levels of anxiety and low self-esteem and resulted in disturbed eating patterns.

In nutritional therapy, bulimics and anorexics must learn how to separate their thoughts and feelings from eating. They need to learn how to express themselves clearly. Frequently their communication is based on fear of what others will say, so anxiety builds and results in eating. By practicing expressing themselves directly in actual situations, that is, by saying "I feel...because...and therefore...," "I wish you would...," or "I will...," they are on their way to recovery (Faber & Mazlish, 1980).

When patients can identify uncomfortable thoughts or feelings that cause them to restrict or binge, they can then understand that eating-disordered behaviors neither remove the discomfort completely nor solve any long-term problems. Restriction or bingeing eases their discomfort *temporarily* and saves them from having to focus on unresolved emotions.

Eating-disordered individuals who seek treatment generally recognize the need to recover. However, their motivation to actually rid themselves of ingrained behaviors can fluctuate and affect their progress. Reiff and Reiff (1992) suggest dividing the patient's motivation into two opposing categories: one that seeks recovery and the other that would rather maintain the status quo. If 50 percent of her wants to work to get well but the other 50 percent would rather continue her behaviors, the symptoms most likely will persist. If the "sick" part of her grows to 60 percent or more, the symptoms will intensify. But when the patient can begin to trust the therapeutic relationship to the point where she can alter the balance toward wellness, she can start to make incremental changes. At 60 percent "well," she can take small steps away from her symptoms. At 90 percent, she is likely to distance herself substantially from her symptoms and be well on her way to recovery.

While we work on the psychological aspects of anorexia and bulimia we are also teaching patients how to maintain their weight. When they reach their set-point weight (their metabolisms have returned and they're eating 1,800– 2,500 calories a day) they need to practice this new way of eating for at least a month. This way they can trust and respond accurately to signals of hunger and satiety. They can even handle an occasional episode of overeating simply by waiting until hunger returns—a safe signal that all the calories they consumed earlier are now spent.

After maintaining their weight for a month, bulimic patients will be allowed to lose weight if needed. They will not be allowed to eat less than the minimum intake for an adult (1,200–1,500 calories) because that would cause a decrease in metabolic rate. At this point patients frequently prefer not to lose weight. They recognize that eating "normally" gives them more energy and lessens their obsession over food. Therapy, it is hoped, has also helped them like and accept themselves better the way they are.

THINNER MEANS "HAPPIER"

Eating-disordered patients have a distorted image not only of their body size and frame but also of their happiness. They are convinced that only if they get thinner will they be happier. Actually it's the opposite—the more weight they lose the more they are likely to isolate themselves from friends and social activities. They become more miserable and more involved in stricter self-imposed rules about eating.

To reach their goal of becoming thinner and happier, these eating-disordered patients eat very little and quickly burn off what they do eat. Typically, exercise increases, sometimes to the point of workouts during the night when unable to sleep. Energy and emotional tolerance levels become extremely low. That's one reason patients become frustrated by ever-so-small changes—perhaps a different food is served at home, or their schedule is changed, leaving less time for exercise. This can have devastating effects not just for themselves but also for significant others, reinforcing their erroneous belief: "If only I were thinner, things would be better!"

What is known is that the more patients can eat or keep down, the more energy they have. The more energy they have, the easier it is to deal with and accept an ideal body weight with less body-image distortion. It is hoped that they are then more open to therapeutic work.

CONCLUSION

With all this knowledge and these tools, why is it so hard for people to stop hurting themselves when they suffer from eating disorders? There are probably as many answers as there are patients today, but two factors stand out.

First, an eating disorder is the symptom of underlying problems. These have to be admitted and dealt with, and the associated thoughts and feelings have to be separated from eating. Many times it is easier to avoid uncomfortable feelings by focusing on eating or restriction.

And second, today's society certainly sends enough messages telling us that "thin is in." If you're thin you'll be happy, marry the right (upper-class) person, get a better job, and fit into the clothes the models advertise. Less than 2 percent of the population is *naturally* "model thin." The rest of us must learn to like ourselves because of who we are, not because of our size.

REFERENCES

Apfelbaum, M. (1975). Influence of level of energy intake on energy expenditure in man: Effects of spontaneous intake experimental starvation, and experimental overeating. In G.A. Bray (Ed.) *Obesity in perspective.* Washington, DC: U.S. Department of Health, Education and Welfare.

Faber, A., & Mazlish, E. (1980). *How to talk so kids will listen and listen so kids will talk.* New York: Avon Books.

Flatt, J.P. (1980). Energetics of intermediary metabolism. In Ross Conference Report No. I *Assessment of energy metabolism in health and disease.* Columbus, OH: Ross Laboratories.

Grant, A. (1979). Nutritional Assessment Guidelines. Anne Grant, Box 25057, Northgate Station, Seattle, WA 98125.

Guthrie, H., & Picciano, M. (1995). *Human Nutrition.* Mosby-Year Book, Inc.

Nutrition and Eating Disorders—Guidelines for the Patient with Anorexia Nervosa and Bulimia Nervosa. (1990). A Nutrition and the M.D. Publication. California: PM, Inc.

Reiff, D., & Reiff, K. (1992). *Eating Disorders: Nutrition Therapy in the Recovery Process.* Gaithersburg, MD: Aspen Publishers, Inc.

SUGGESTED READING

Siegel, M., Brisman, J., & Weinsel, M. (1988). *Surviving an eating disorder: Strategies for family and friends.* New York: Harper and Row.

Food as Communication: Breaking Through with Experiential Therapies

by Debra Landau-West, M.S.

It has been said many times that food is not the real issue for the eating-disordered individual but that it is only a symptom of the eating disorder. However, to ignore the food issues in an eating disorder would be like waiting out the bacterial infection that causes pneumonia without providing relief for the congestion.

The individual with an eating disorder often uses food as a communication tool. The nutrition therapist sorts through the ritualistic food behaviors and food patterns to read the silent message. Helping patients to understand their behaviors in relation to feelings they may encounter in therapy as well as in relationships frees them to begin the process of change. True recovery involves letting go of any unhealthy food relationship. An individual who has truly recovered is free of guilt, shame, and fear with regard to food and has learned to consider food as an inanimate object used to nourish the body. Many anorexics gain weight but never solve their unhealthy food relationship, leaving them at risk for the development of bulimia or a recurrence of anorexia.

This chapter will review some of the experiential food therapies that have been used successfully in the treatment of anorexia nervosa, bulimia, and compulsive overeating.

EATING BEHAVIOR AS A COMMUNICATION TOOL

All of us communicate with food. In our society food can communicate affection (a mother preparing her child's favorite foods when he or she comes home from college), hostility (never preparing an individual's favorite foods), concern (home-cooked meals), indifference (a freezer full of frozen dinners for the family to heat themselves), anger (sending a child to bed without dinner) and a variety of other feelings. In all communication, the language used, whether verbal or nonverbal, depends on a commonly understood set of symbols. The client with an eating disorder chooses a language often unintelligible to others, leaving many of his or her messages misconstrued or ignored and adding to the feelings of isolation and abandonment he or she often feels (Elbein, 1992).

Clients also diagnosed with dissociative disorder are particularly skilled at communicating with food. Thus, individuals working with these clients must be skilled at reading hidden messages. The prevalence of eating disorders among dissociative patients is high. Torem (1990) found that 77 out of 84 dissociative patients studied exhibited at least one eating-disorder behavior. The dissociative patient's fractured ego often has no verbal means of dealing with painful experiences and memories, and food becomes the perfect remedy (Zerbe, 1993).

Using the eating disorder as a voice, clients usually exhibit one or more of the following: ritualistic eating behaviors; good food, bad food thinking; food rules; or food aversions. Exploring each of these with experiential food therapies helps us to learn an individual's food language (Elbein, 1992).

Ritualistic Eating Behaviors

Clients often communicate shame, guilt, and horrific abuse via ritualistic behaviors that include an inability to touch food to the lips, avoidance of certain colored foods, or the refusal to eat in front of others. Creating a new food ritual is one way of responding to this communiqué. For example, a client's avoidance of white foods may be related to sexual abuse (possibly associated with semen) and feelings of shame and impurity. Creating a food ritual, which the clinician and the client write and perform together, can have a cleansing effect. This might be done by having a client sit with the clinician, taking small amounts of white foods (milk, white bread, white frosting, cream cheese, marshmallows) intermittently and repeating the statement "I deserve to eat this food," or "This food is pure, and I choose to accept it into my body", or "I deserve to enjoy what I choose to put in my mouth." Care should be taken to determine that the client has done adequate therapeutic work prior to this activity so that it does not trigger previously traumatic experiences. Food rituals are particularly successful with clients who have experienced various types of ritualistic abuse.

Good Food, Bad Food Thinking

This belief system can also be thought of as a client's "should and should not" list. It may contain information regarding childhood family and food experiences. Cooking experiences and grocery-store experiences are two methods used to break through this type of belief system. Clients can be taken to a grocery store and asked to walk around the store with items they believe they should not have, or items they consider bad. As feelings related to loss of control begin to manifest, the client and clinician explore other times the client may have experienced similar feelings in their life or with a particular food, whether pleasant or offensive. Cooking experiences may also elicit various memories associated with the smell, touch, or taste of various foods.

Food Rules

Food rules usually make the eating-disordered client feel safe. Unfortunately, they can also leave the client stuck. Providing clients with simple homework assignments to break these food rules usually helps to uncover hidden meanings associated with these rules, as well as to alleviate the compulsion and stress the rules cause in a client's life. Asking a client to eat at a fast-food restaurant with the clinician or changing the time of a meal are examples of simple techniques that can help eliminate the need for food rules. If experiences are done without the clinician present, the client should journal all feelings associated with them and share these journal entries with the clinician at the next session.

Food Aversions

Very often food aversions are related to sexual trauma. Care should be taken during experiential work not to retraumatize the client, for whom contact with certain foods might trigger uncomfortable memories. Aversions are often related to food textures, smell, or color. Clients might be asked to sit with a particular food and draw the feelings that come up, or to draw what it might feel like to eat that food. Desensitizing the individual to a particular food is accomplished by reclaiming power from that food. Clients may accomplish this through psychodrama, actually reclaiming the food and taking it back from the abuser, or through food rituals.

ACCESSING AND REMEMBERING PLAYFULNESS

Individuals with eating disorders often present as responsible, perfect, and overachievers. Often, they were asked to grow up too fast, leaving childhood playfulness behind at a very early age. The memory of how to play and be childlike is frequently forgotten, buried away in the subconscious mind, waiting to be found and awakened. Food play can access that aspect of the client's self and can be particularly useful when the client is having difficulty accepting inner-child work prescribed by the therapist. Inner-child work serves to establish adult self-care, which includes appropriate food intake and proper nutrition.

Food play can be done on an individualized basis or in a group setting. When done in a group, individuals must establish certain boundaries, such as not throwing food at one another, unless such behavior is accepted by all. Food play should be fully explained so that the clients understand the goals of the experience. Clients should be asked to imagine what a child might do if left in the room with the foods presented to them, with no utensils and no parent to critique their behavior. Foods that would be easy for a child to play with include canned frosting, whipped cream, sour cream, sprinkles, graham crackers, peanut butter, and syrup. Foods that an individual typically avoids may be used as well to help overcome fear. Keep in mind that if repressed childhood sexual abuse is present, an individual may have difficulty with some of these foods. Such difficulty is another communication tool, one worth exploring at a later session.

Clinicians should allow clients to build houses, wear the food on their face, create designs, mix everything together, or have fun in any imaginable way. One hopes that after the food play a client will have less fear surrounding certain foods, and be willing to at least try some of them. Following this experience many clients will make commitments to their inner child with regard to consuming more fun foods. Clients should explore methods of play long since forgotten or abandoned and begin to add these to their daily or weekly routines.

THE GENTLE EATING EXPERIENCE

Our society teaches women not to enjoy food too much. You rarely see women eating with gusto; men seem much freer with food, particularly in public places. The guilt associated with the eating experience adds to the scenario of shame and body-image distortions commonly found in the eating-disordered client. Gentle eating can help a patient to avoid dissociation from the eating experience and to identify body-image problems. It can also lessen the guilt associated with food enjoyment, an important step in recovery from bulimia, anorexia, or compulsive overeating.

Gentle eating experiences incorporate relaxation techniques and increasing awareness of the food being consumed. Clients are asked to focus on appearance, flavor, and texture to increase the pleasurable experiences associated with eating a meal. The gentle eating technique is also used to access true feelings of hunger and fullness.

In the dissociative client with multiple personality disorder, gentle eating experiences allow altered selves to share the experience of food. In this way clients learn to share body experiences, as well as other experiences, whether from the past or present, among the system of altered states.

THE NUTRITION THERAPIST

A registered dietitian with eating-disorders experience should be versed in the types of experiential work outlined in this chapter. It is important that the search for a nutrition therapist produces someone willing to communicate with other members of the treatment team (Reiff 1992). Many clients fear that the only role a dietitian will play in their treatment is to "make them gain weight" or " follow a diet." The road to recovery is long, and major behavior changes take time (Reiff 1992). Dietitians working with clients often become frustrated while trying to cajole them into increasing or changing food intake. The nutrition therapist can maintain a working, therapeutic relationship with a client who may not be ready to make significant changes in eating patterns by educating and by using some of the experiential methods outlined here. In this way, the relationship can be maintained and strengthened, fostering safety when the client is ready to change nutrient intake.

REFERENCES

Elbein, Richard. (1992). *Eating behavior as a communication tool.* Presentation at the Fourth Annual National Conference on Eating Disorders, Houston, Texas.

Reiff, Dan, & Reiff, Kim Lampson. (1992). *Eating disorders nutrition therapy in the recovery process.* Gaithersburg, MD: Aspen Publishers.

Torem, M. S. (1990). Covert multiple personality underlying eating disorders. *American Journal of Psychotherapy,* 357–68.

Zerbe, Kathryn. (1993, Summer). Selves that starve and suffocate: The continuum of eating disorders and dissociative phenomena. *Bulletin of the Menninger Clinic,* 319–27.

Drama Therapy: A Powerful Adjunct in the Treatment of Eating Disorders

by Jan Rothman-Sickler, M.A.

Drama therapy is a valuable therapeutic tool to help individuals with eating disorders overcome their fear of danger and change. Such individuals are trapped in a physical metaphor for their emotional pain, making drama therapy a "bridge to expanded possibilities" (Wiener, 1994, p. 16) because it offers these people a metaphorical voice with which to explore and express themselves (Wiener, 1994, p.16). Drama therapy is an important adjunct to traditional psychological treatment because of its ability to remove the intellectual defenses that clients often erect in conversations with their therapist or group. Through its use of physicalization and role-play, drama therapy has the potential to enlarge the scope of communication techniques between a client, therapist, or group, and help the individual to grow and function creatively in life.

SPONTANEITY, GROWTH, AND CREATION

Creativity is a necessary component for a healthy human being to experience life fully, attain his or her potential, and take risks. Yet, in our success-driven and product-oriented society, creativity is often seen as a special gift bestowed only on artists who can produce a "work of art." In my work I maintain that creativity can exist in individuals as an attitude separate from any artistic achievement. Creativity belongs to every healthy human being and can be a part of anything we do. Maslow states that the concepts of creativity and self-actualization are so closely linked that they may be the same thing. According to Maslow, the creative process consists of two phases. The first or primary phase is purely inspirational. It is the phase in which all options are possible, our imagination runs free, and ideas flow. The secondary phase is the "working out and development of inspiration" (1971, p. 57). It is the product-oriented phase. Maslow's concept of self-actualization makes no value judgment based on a finished product. He is in agreement with Winnicott, who warns that the concept of creativity should not "get lost in the successful or acclaimed creation" (1971, p. 65). A creative product is not a substitute for a sense of self. Consider the German word, *funktionlust*, which means "the pleasure of doing. . . . The focus is on PROCESS, not PRODUCT" (Nachmanovitch, 1990, p. 45).

Acquiring and maintaining a creative attitude is an important challenge for every individual. A creative attitude means that when faced with any challenge, creative individuals are able to listen to their inner voice and at the same time logically consider the external circumstances and the possible consequences of their choice. Most eating-disordered clients are so busy protecting themselves from insecurities and depression

through compulsive behavior that they have lost touch with the basic elements of creativity: imagination, originality, and, most important, spontaneity. "Through spontaneity," Viola Spolin says, "we are re-formed into ourselves" (1963, p. 4). Once spontaneity is discovered, original and imaginative thinking has no need to change others, fulfill social needs, or be judged. Imagination adds the capacity to symbolize and project options and alternatives, which can be used to shape and color the creative process.

In summary, creativity can be viewed as an attitude that allows us to employ spontaneity, originality, and imagination to create an artistic product and essentially to re-create ourselves.

COMING FACE TO FACE WITH ONE'S CREATIVITY AND SELF

How do we access creativity in a population that is rigid and resistant to change? We play! Play is a familiar yet mysterious phenomenon usually relegated to childhood. Perhaps because it is difficult to define, ephemeral in nature, and imprecise as a scientific tool, play has always had a tenuous place in psychology. Yet the benefits of playtime are worthy of serious consideration. In play, we can let our defenses down, be authentic, and truly engage one another.

Do not confuse play with sports or the arts. Play has no defined set of rules, requiring only a place and time. It encompasses a unique combination of internal and external environments. Winnicott designates this human state for play as the "Potential Space" where the "doing of playing takes place" (1971, p. 41). In this Potential Space is no past or future, only an endlessly improvisational present where an individual can "make do" with any material at hand. Nothing is planned, everything is possible. Through play, one cannot avoid one's own spontaneity, originality, or imagination. One must come face to face with one's creativity and, ultimately, one's self.

CONDITIONS INFLUENCING PLAY

Almost all adults need help in overcoming their inhibitions about freeform play or the structured improvisational play offered in a therapeutic situation. If the average adult is normally inhibited about playing, imagine the reaction of an individual whose energy and creativity are rigidly invested in the obsessive-compulsive behavior of maintaining, concealing, and disguising an eating disorder.

Special settings and conditions help all adults acquire a comfort level in which play is possible. The setting must be reliable and predictable. Certain essentials are necessary to make relaxation possible, including trust, safety, friendliness, cooperation, and creative, physical, and mental activity, as well as processing of the experience to form a better sense of self (Winnicottt, 1971).

Singer and Singer (1990) point out that not only is it important to create a safe space to play, but the therapist should also guide the participants through acceptance of their activities by modeling desired behavior. In experiential therapy, the role of the therapist is more directive and more involved. The therapist models comfort with play by becoming a participant and joining, as well as leading, the group activity.

Another important feature of play is that it is "relational in nature" (Grainger, 1990, p. 24), a "meeting place of selves" (Grainger, 1990, p. 12). It is a place in which people can experiment with rules, roles, thoughts, words, objects, images, and situations that they would otherwise be unable to experience. It is truly a world of "expanded possibilities."

The use of play in therapy requires special conditions, exercises, and training for the therapist. Therapists who specialize in arts-based experiential therapy are often trained first in their art and then learn to apply it to their work as a therapist.

DRAMA THERAPY

Drama therapy is a broad-based practice drawing on many sources: dramatic play, role-play, theater, psychodrama, and dramatic ritual. Renee Emunah (1994) outlines a five-phase drama therapy model, which is the practical and therapeutic application of the theoretical elements. I have found this model to be extremely effective in my own work. The model features: (1) dramatic play, (2) sustained improvisation or scripted scene work, (3) scene work/role-play from the patient's life, (4) psychodrama, and (5) ritual.

Phase 1: Dramatic Play

Dramatic play is structured improvisation with simple rules, few objectives, and no products. The individual can explore, express, and practice certain behaviors and attitudes. A core concept of dramatic play is the paradoxical "as if": We can act *as if* a situation is real even though we know it is not. What is best about this imaginative reality is that one benefits from the experience, while being exempt from the consequences.

Emunah (1994) stresses that dramatic play lays the groundwork for all subsequent phases. A nonthreatening, playful environment is established through processes that include creative dramatics; improvisation; playful, interactive exercises; and structured theater games. Many of these techniques are physically active, and most are socially interactive.

One of my favorite exercises (and usually the group's favorite as well) is the "Machine." Building on sound and movement exercises, the group works together to create an abstract machine. One person starts a repetitive sound and movement. One by one, group members join in to become integral parts of the machine. Everyone is a cog in the movement machine. Group members are encouraged to take risks by using their whole bodies rather than just their arms. Sounds become wild as people express the movement. After one of my workshops, a participant commented to me,

> What was the one with our bodies? The machines! That thing! That was hysterical for all of us. I think it was one of the most joyful times I've spent in a long time. Seeing all of us together, in those weird positions, trying not to hit one another, and still fit together like a mechanism . . . the silliness . . . the machines. The ridiculousness of these grown women getting together in these stupid stances, making weird noises was just hysterical. It was so loving and giving.

Phase 1 is based on a health model in which the strengths and healthy parts of the clients are elicited.

Phase 2: Sustained Improvisation

Sustained, improvised scenes are composed of roles and characters. The theatrical concept of working with different roles is the most distinguishing feature of drama therapy. Role-play is an extension of dramatic play and can result in fictional, fantasy, or real-life role-playing situations. In role-play, people can "try on" alternative sets of beliefs and behaviors. They begin to see the transitory and ambivalent nature of roles. With ambivalence comes options, and as a role player, one is armed with the theatre's "magic if." Readiness is central to the goal in drama therapy of helping the client become aware of, rehearse, and expand his or her role repertoire for life.

An excellent exercise to begin work with role-play is called "Accepting Offers." A volunteer is asked to move around freely until told to FREEZE. (As you can see, a great deal of physical freedom must already be established through dramatic play to accomplish this exercise.) Another volunteer then joins her and accepts the physical offer by beginning a scene. For example, if someone is frozen in a position where he or she is holding out his or her arms, the other volunteer might come up and say, "Here, let me help you carry that sheet of glass upstairs." The person who is frozen would accept this offer and join in the scene verbally and physically. This activity helps participants not only create roles, but support one another, be spontaneous and flexible, and use their imagination and their body to communicate. Once people start accepting offers, they usually want to play out longer scenes.

Phase 3: Scenes from Life

Phase 3 marks the shifting of the dramatizations from the imaginary to the actual. Clients begin to use the dramatic medium to explore situations in their own lives. Once again, the primary process is role-play. I begin by simply asking a client to choose a recent event that was challenging or upsetting. In setting up a scene for the group to act out, members must choose people to act out the characters. They need to describe their relationships with the characters, their objectives, and their emotional state. They must describe the place where the event occurred and what, if anything, was special about the place. In doing so, they are exploring self-concept and identity as well as relational values. They can even rehearse new behaviors (such as assertiveness) for real life. One group member commented that it was hard for her to act out emotions. She said,

> I think it helped me because I noticed the more we worked with emotions, the more outside of the group I started showing the emotions. If I was angry, I would tell somebody. . . . I actually knew what I felt and I could see how other people were showing emotions; and I could pick up on that. Before, I wouldn't want to know.

Phase 4: Psychodrama

Phase 4 marks a shift from present-day, concrete issues to more core issues in one's life. The primary conceptual source of Phase 4 is psychodrama. Dr. Jacob Moreno (1889–1974), the founder of psychodrama, defined it as the exploration of the human psyche through dramatic action (Goldman & Morrison, 1984). The basic assumption of psychodrama is that individuals learn more effectively when they act out a scene from their life than if they simply talk about it. The psychodrama experience involves "insight in action" (Yablonsky, 1976, p. 13) in which a protagonist reenacts, in scene-like fashion, emotional issues from his or her life. Psychodrama involves the entire group as actors and audience, but its focus is on one person to sculpt others to represent various aspects of himself or herself. This person physically moves all of the participants, placing them in postures and positions as well as in relation to one another. The protagonist describes each part and tells each participant what to say. The sculpture literally come alive and moves and talks to the protagonist. By embodying each of the protagonist's own aspects, the exercise allows him or her to finally confront each of them. This is a powerful, emotional, and very personal exercise.

Phase 5: Ritual

Ritual has always been historically linked with drama, religion, and healing. It is used throughout the group work in the opening and closing circle for warm-ups and sharing. At the completion of a drama therapy workshop, it is incorporated to help individuals review what they have done, evaluate their progress, experience the rewards of accomplishment, and express sadness and joy. Group members can co-create one major ritualistic experience. In my groups, I have asked each group member to create a simple ritual of closure to share with the group on the final day. One member brought a different and special flower for each individual in the group. Another woman brought in small rose quartz gemstones, which symbolize femininity and health, for each woman. Yet another woman wrote a poem about our group which she shared with us. The simple rituals provided a moving closure for this 12-week drama therapy workshop.

The amount of time spent on each phase of drama therapy is up to the group leader. In my work, I find most groups need more time and emphasis on Phase 1: Dramatic Play. Once they become comfortable with physical and nonverbal self-expression, enjoy their own spontaneity, and establish group trust, they can move more easily into the verbal and more realistic aspects of role-play.

THEATRICS OR THERAPY?

For those who believe therapy based on theatrics is not integral to the psychological treatment model, remember that drama therapy is informed by the three major forces in psychology: psychoanalysis, behaviorism, and humanism. In psychoanalytic terms, drama therapy shares an appreciation for the history, inner, and unconscious experiences of the client. In behavioral terms, drama therapy is action oriented, and change seeks to break old habits. Humanism contributes the most to drama therapy in terms of values and a therapeutic stance. Drawing from humanistic psychologists such as Maslow and Rogers, drama therapy underscores the belief that humans want to reach their true potential (Maslow, 1971; Rogers, 1961). It is similar philosophically to Gestalt therapy, which also strives for wholeness and integration of thinking, feeling, and behaving, and like drama therapy, works on direct experience rather than merely talking about feelings (Corey, 1991). Ultimately, the therapeutic goals of drama therapy are goals shared by all three major forces in psychology: emotional expres-

sion and containment, the development of the observing self, expansion of role repertoire and self-imaging, and enhancement of interpersonal relationship skills (Emunah, 1994, p. 33).

In conclusion, the elements and goals of drama therapy form a powerful experiential package that allows individuals to explore themselves through laughter, tears, and intimacy, as well as their own autonomy. In the safe environment of the drama therapy workshop, individuals can find the freedom and courage to build their own bridge to the expanded possibilities of a life in which one thinks and acts creatively.

REFERENCES

Corey, G. (1991). *Theory and practice of counseling and psychotherapy.* Pacific Grove, CA: Brooks/Cole.

Emunah, R. (1994). *Acting for real.* New York: Brunner/Mazel.

Goldman, E., & Morrison, D. (1984). *Psychodrama: Experience and process.* Phoenix, AZ: Eldemar.

Grainger, R. (1990). *Drama and healing.* London: Jessica Kingsley Publishers.

Maslow, A. H. (1971). *The farther reaches of human nature.* New York: Penguin.

Nachmanovitch, S. (1990). *Free play.* Los Angeles: Jeremy P. Tarcher.

Rogers, C. (1961). *On becoming a person.* Boston: Houghton Mifflin.

Singer, D. G., & Singer, J. L. (1990). *The house of make-believe.* Cambridge, MA: Harvard University Press.

Spolin, V. (1963). *Improvisation for the theater.* Evanston, IL: Northwestern University Press.

Wiener, D. J. (1994). *Rehearsals for growth: Theater improvisation for psychotherapists.* New York: Norton.

Winnicott, D. W. (1971). *Playing and reality.* London; New York: Tavistock/Routledge.

Yablonsky, L. (1976). *Psychodrama.* New York: Basic Books.

Combining the Creative Art Therapies and Rubenfeld Synergy as a Means for Healing for Eating Disorders
by Cappi Lang, Ph.D.

Seven and a half years ago I was working as an art therapist in an inpatient program for eating disorders in Phoenix, Arizona. I was frustrated

with what I saw as the sometimes limiting effects of the verbal therapies and the art therapies. I observed some good work occurring using both modalities, yet I had a sense that to add another dimension, that of body work, might be even more helpful to these clients in their healing process.

In what is to follow I will describe both art therapy and Rubenfeld Synergy, a form of mind/body integration, along with the conjunction of these two modalities and case examples that illustrate both the process and effects of this work.

ART THERAPY

Art therapy uses art, the process of creating with unstructured art materials such as paint, pastels, clay, and collage, as a way of understanding and healing oneself. It is a communication from the self. Movement, drama, and poetry are also a part of the art therapies and can be used interchangeably. In the artistic process several things occur. One, what is inside the person is projected outward into a form that can be experienced and explored, experimented with, and reworked if desired. A bridge is formed that brings psychic material and energy from the unconscious into conscious awareness. It is a bridge from the inside to the outside, from the past to the present and into the future. It is a means to bring about connection. The art form itself and the process become a mirror into the self.

Two, art communicates in symbols and metaphors much as in dreams. Symbols and metaphors are attached to energy held in the body. As the symbol or metaphor is released in the art form, the energy is also released and activated, allowing for movement and awareness and change to occur. To summarize, through the art process the person is able to release pent-up feelings through symbolic communication, projecting what is inside into a form that releases energy for experimentation, creative expression, and play. This forms a bridge from one state to another, bringing awareness, integration, and healing. This space between states and between therapist and client is often referred to as the transitional space where transition and change can occur.

RUBENFELD SYNERGY

In Rubenfeld Synergy, its founder, Ilana Rubenfeld, combines principles of Gestalt therapy, Feldenkrais work, and the F. M. Alexander Technique, plus the work of Milton Erickson, to bring about the integration and balance of body,

mind, heart, and spirit of the person. This synergistic multimodal approach offers a way to sustain change and to help clients integrate previously unassimilated traumatic experiences that are still active in subtle and not so subtle ways. In other words, the system's purpose is to express the unexpressed.

The work is based on the theory that the body, mind, emotions, and spirit are dynamically interrelated. The uniqueness of each individual is respected. There is the belief that each person has a natural capacity for self-healing.

According to Rubenfeld, her work is a four-stage metaprocess consisting of awareness, experimentation, integration, and reentry. Awareness is the first step to change. Unconsciously held habit patterns are brought into awareness through touching the client in a specific way. The client then has the opportunity to explore alternative choices and opportunities for psychological change. Touch during this process acts as a bridge from the outside in bringing material from the inside out.

As this happens, the second stage of experimentation occurs, which supports a heightening of awareness. At times there is confusion, which Rubenfeld believes is essential to create the possibility for change. During experimentation, touch is communicating and inviting a learning exchange through the client's system to each individual cell. Touch becomes an entry point to the whole person. Touch both "listens" and "talks." Noninvasive and intentional touch in the Rubenfeld Synergy process creates a dialogue with the unconscious mind. This produces an altered or trance state bringing into awareness what is needed for healing in the present moment. The conscious mind selects from the unconscious mind what is necessary for healing and growth in the present. Humor is an essential part of the process, easing the emergence of sometimes painful and traumatic experiences.

Rubenfeld asks clients "to send their metaphoric and poetic mind into my hands while using various images to loosen different places in their bodies." Themes and meta-themes emerge in this body and voice dialogue. A bridging occurs between inside and out; past, present, and future and body, mind, heart, and spirit. The client communicates in a symbolic metaphoric language. The client receives the message that all parts are connected and the third stage of integration begins. During this phase the client becomes aware of both his or her tension and energy, each essential for growth and change. At the end of the session the client brings the shared experience back as he or she reenters the everyday world of reality.

ART THERAPY AND RUBENFELD SYNERGY

In both art therapy and Rubenfeld Synergy the client's story unfolds. There is a releasing of energy plus a telling through the symbolic language of symbols and metaphors. Touch releases energy just as the symbol does when externalized in the artwork. The trance state is an important component of both modalities in opening up the channel from the unconscious mind to the conscious mind. In both modalities the process of awareness, experimentation, integration, and reentry occurs. The dialogue is important for both to provide a safe place with boundaries. Both incorporate play and humor. The difference between art therapy and Rubenfeld Synergy lies in the fact that in art therapy what is released or communicated is projected into a concrete form through the artwork, which is a visual and/or tactile image; in Rubenfeld Synergy what is released and communicated is done through the body through touch. In both cases the therapist/synergist communicates with the patient using his or her own modality, thus forming a bridge or interface.

EXAMPLES

To illustrate the effects of these two modalities used in combination, the work of two clients is presented below. Personal reflections of the patients are included.

"Lisa"

I first met Lisa at an inpatient treatment center for eating disorders where I was working as an art therapist. She was in her early 30s at that time and had been both anorexic and bulimic since she was 16. She was also a shoplifter. She was referred to me by her therapist in the hope that art therapy and Rubenfeld Synergy might facilitate her therapeutic process. Specifically, the goals were to help Lisa get in touch with childhood abuse issues that might be causing her to remain stuck, to help her replace her destructive behaviors with more constructive ones, and to provide a healing. Thirteen sessions occurred at this time.

During Lisa's first session she talked about her feelings of depression and her inability to get away from these feelings. Rubenfeld Synergy work is done on a table. The client lies down on his or her back, fully clothed except for shoes. At this point I asked Lisa to lie down on the table. I touched her head lightly and observed her body to be extremely tight. When I touched her foot, she pulled back. We discussed what would feel comfortable to her and we decided that in the next several sessions I would work only with her head and shoulders. After the body/mind session, Lisa did a drawing. (This would be the format of the sessions; first Rubenfeld Synergy and then the expression of the session through art.) The drawing showed Lisa walking on a sidewalk in a dress with a ruffled skirt. A large dark cloud approaches her on the right. This, she says, is the size of her depression as illustrated by the cloud. There is also an indication of anxiety and a wish to cover the pelvic area (the ruffles).

In Session 2, Lisa describes three parts of herself: (1) Sara, age 4, who is scared and helpless and is picked on by her brothers, who are much older; (2) Tomboy, age 6, who is tough, can take care of himself, and steals; and (3) Amelia, the helpless adult who tries to deal with Sara and Tomboy. These parts have the opportunity to dialogue as treatment progresses. Lisa asks to turn onto her side for this session. This position is often a childlike, protective position. I cradle her head in one hand for support and comfort and put my other hand on her upper back and shoulder. The drawing for this session is the three parts described. It is noteworthy that in the drawing, none of the figures has a body below the waist. This is another indication of anxiety and possible trauma to that area, often reflecting helplessness or an inability to move. Lisa describes depression around Sara and anger around Tomboy.

In Session 3, Lisa says she is afraid to be touched. She lies on her side, curled up, I sit in a chair next to her, and we talk. She says she wants nurturance but that she does not deserve it because she steals. She describes a cycle of wanting nurturance, being denied it, becoming angry and stealing, and then punishing herself by denying herself food and company. The three parts—Tomboy, Sara, and Amelia—begin to speak, and Lisa's story emerges: of an alcoholic and abusive father who leaves when she is 5, a mother who goes to work to support the family and has no energy to give to this small child, and two older brothers (her caretakers) who tease her, abuse her physically, and taunt her. The drawing depicts this experience of reaching out for nurturance, being denied and abused, then becoming angry and tough and eventually hopelessly going into the corner to hide. The position on the table, curling into a ball, reminds her of this.

Lisa brings a drawing to the next session. It is a drawing she had done a year ago. It depicts fighting adults and a scared child. I suggest how abusive this must have been. She denies it, saying it was not that bad. During the Rubenfeld Synergy she curls up on the table and describes her feelings of despair and pain. She describes how her brothers called her ugly and teased her relentlessly. She feels helpless. I place one hand gently on her back, the other on her head. She reaches out to me. I take her hand and hold it. In her drawing she depicts herself starving, cut off from a large bowl. She titles this piece "Her Soul Murdered, Her Power Taken."

Session 5 makes a breakthrough. Lisa lies on the table stating that she is a big baby afraid of touch, of life. She reaches her hands up toward me. I am standing by her head. I take them. She grabs and releases, saying she is afraid she will grab on too hard and frighten me, use me up. I say I will tell her if she does. I take her hands, she holds on. She hardly breathes. I put my hand on her heart. She says it feels like a ton. The story of her brothers sitting on her emerges. She can't breathe or speak. She is desperate. She holds onto my hands. The drawing of her with a 5,000-ton weight on her chest, an empty goblet, an injured heart and hands reaching depict the session. She says that there is a little part of her heart that can now feel.

In Session 6 Lisa says she is beginning to feel her body, especially her anus holding and controlling. She feels anger, release, and then black coming. She allows me to release her shoulders, then turns on her side and asks to be covered with a blanket. She clutches my hands and keeps clutching them, saying, "I am scared you'll go away." She turns on her back, and I gently work with her head. She then sits up and says, "That's enough, just sit with me," which I do. Her drawing is of a huge black cloud on the left, taking up three-quarters of the paper. She is very small in the drawing. There is a barrier between her and her heart on the right. She is trying to get to the heart, which is love and nurturing.

In the next session, Lisa comes in and says she wants to die and she cannot relax. She is feeling scared. Her body is like a rod. She says I can work with her shoulders and head. She talks of the black coming and remembers her mother and brothers calling her bad. I feel her shoulders relax and release. She sees the black breaking up. I place my hands on either side of her head. She says, "My mother said I cost too much and I'm bad." She rolls onto her side and clutches my hands, asking me not to leave her. Later she releases them and asks me to hold her. Her drawing shows the black breaking up and colors emerging from behind it.

The theme in Session 8 is abandonment. I am going on a trip, and she feels that I will not return, that I will die. She lies on her back and asks me to touch her feet. I gently move her feet from side to side and then move to her head. She reaches for my hand. I roll her head gently from side to side and then place her hand under mine, which is on her forehead, and we roll her head together. I take away my hand, and she continues the head roll from side to side. She says she feels calmer. I see her body relax. She has learned a way of nurturing herself. She asks to take home one of my stuffed toy bears. Her drawing shows me holding her down by her feet, keeping her from floating off into depression.

In the next session she says she really wants to do the body work, to try it. She says she is feeling something more than depression. She feels an energy that is good. I work with her head and feet and release her hips. She begins to feel anger and wants to fight. She kicks her feet. I give her a towel to twist. She twists it and kicks, then turns on her side and scratches at a pillow. She relaxes and lets go and says she is Sara. I soothe her. Tomboy then comes and appears tough. Sara then asks for a song. I sing "Lavender Blue, Dilley, Dilley, Lavender Green." She likes this. Tomboy also likes it and asks for a hug. I hug her. Lisa's drawings are of rage and then me sweeping her up into a form.

Session 11 finds her describing a yelling in her head, saying, "Get it out, just tell." She says she feels as if she is a shattered vase. She rolls onto her side and then onto her back. She asks me just to support her. I roll her head and then put my hands under her shoulders. Her shoulders relax and release. Her drawing is a shattered vase. I tell her it has a base. She says I am helping her to glue the vase back together and that this work is powerful glue.

In Session 12, she comes in to tell me that she has found out that her primary therapist has sexually abused two clients. She pounds the table with her fists, expressing feelings of betrayal, hurt, and abandonment. She decides to leave her therapist and asks if I will continue to see her. I agree. Her drawing shows her enraged female parts and the questioning of whether she herself had ever been sexually abused.

In the next session, she says she feels comfortable with the Rubenfeld work. I observe some stiffness in her body, but gradually she relaxes. We talk a bit about our future work together and her recent termination with her previous therapist. She jumps off the table at the end of the session and says she wants to draw and to play, to let Sara and Tomboy do a drawing together. She chooses the scented markers and says that Sara and Tomboy like the smell. She laughs. They (Sara and Tomboy) decide to do a drawing of fruit; the fruits of Lisa's labor.

At this juncture in treatment Lisa and I review the drawings that she has done and the content of the sessions. We then each write our own responses to the work done so far.

My Story of Lisa

Once upon a time there was a family where a small child was abused by the father and brothers. The parents fought; the brothers fought. The mother used the child for her own nurturance as her first husband, a raging alcoholic, left and her second husband, the abuser, died. The mother was so drained by supporting the family and being abused that she was empty, having nothing to give. She became angry at the little girl, whom she experienced as wanting too much and never being satisfied. She said "grow up," "quit sniffling." When the mother went to work, the brothers wrestled with, teased, and molested the small child. She fought back and acted tough (Tomboy) as they called her "baby" and "brat." She tried to call her mother, but they prevented her. She raged and was only hurt more, so she retreated to the corner, where she was scared to move, make a sound, or even breathe. She became hopeless and shattered. However, inside was a strength, a light, a heart she experienced from time to time. She reached toward that place. Then began to pull. She reached toward this light and this heart with all her strength and was pulled back. She did not give up. She kept on reaching. She had a mind. She had strong legs. In between she felt emptiness, yet a voice

called out, "Tell!" With touch, awareness, experimentation, and love, she is beginning to tell and to put together her shattered self, to integrate her shattered parts. She reaches out. I take her hand. I remain present and patient. We play together. She learns to touch, nurture, and hold herself. The journey continues.

Lisa's Personal Reflections

This has been an emotional journey that has oftentimes been unpleasant; a process of unlocking various doors that only emit glimpses of light often in cryptic form. When the information revealed is overwhelming, the defensive parts of me effectively (but unfortunately) slam the doors shut out of fear. The Rubenfeld body work, art therapy, dream work, and analysis of transference issues have deciphered the messages. Yet this is a painstaking process which one would easily give up if there were not a companion/witness/guide/safety net to accompany one along the path.

Because my body has so much protective armor, I was not even aware of the many emotions buried beneath the skin until the Rubenfeld body work facilitated their release. The gentle touch of Cappi evoked sadness and longing for the nurturance lacking in childhood along with terror that she might hurt me with that same physical contact. However, because she did not touch beyond my comfort level at various stages of the process, I was able to slowly develop trust that provided me the safety in which to experience the terror, express the anger, and accept the comforting offered. The Rubenfeld Synergy work evoked images which I was unable to access previously via hypnosis alone. Also, it gave permission to the various aspects within me to dialogue with each other so that they now understand each other better and, therefore, can eventually interact more harmoniously.

The art therapy, which included symbols from dreams, served to bypass my intellectualization. It gave Cappi information via symbols that I could not put into words because, once again, I was not even aware of the information regarding early trauma that was stored within me at a preverbal level. In addition, the artwork was visual evidence of aspects of my life that I could not rationalize away as easy as I did with straight "talk" therapy.

Finally, the permissiveness and genuine concern which encompasses both processes allowed me to express my feelings toward Cappi without fear of judgment, abandonment, or retaliation. This provided a corrective parenting experience. I now understand those were transference feelings which I could not safely express in my family of origin.

The journey continues as the enigma of the past slowly unfolds in treatment with someone to hold my hand for support and clarification as we move toward the light of healing.

"Debbie"

I also met Debbie at the treatment center where I worked with eating-disordered patients. I worked with Debbie for six sessions. Debbie compulsively overeats and has a history of severe sexual and physical abuse. She was referred to me by her therapist. I include this particular case to show how Rubenfeld Synergy and art therapy touch the soul.

In the first session, Debbie described her drawing as showing the unity she felt on the table during the Rubenfeld Synergy. In contrast is a drawing describing how she felt in the past. In the second session she talked about a stressful situation with her tenant who had moved out and how this situation relates to the abuse of her childhood and feelings around men. One of the things that releases her stress and tension is the ocean. She visualized this on the table, and as she did, her body released. Her drawing of the ocean shows the visualization. I suggested she hang it up in her home to remind herself of the feeling of peace that the drawing brings her.

In Session 3 she visualized herself on earth and was able to get in touch with a part in her heart that no one could hurt or abuse or make feel bad or dirty. It is her essence, still beautiful and intact. This reminded me of the Eastern description of the soul. She said she agreed with this interpretation. Her drawing of a desert with stars depicts this image and feeling.

Session 4 was very special and profound for both of us. In the session, while I was supporting her shoulders with my hands under them, Debbie said she smelled smoke. I did not smell or see smoke. She visualized the experience, which she later painted with watercolors, of herself on the table surrounded by white light and her Indian guides with two wolves under the table protecting her. She said her soul was pure gold and no one could violate it.

In Session 5, she was able to work more on her sexual abuse issues. Her drawing shows the violation of her body. She felt that the previous body work enabled her to get in touch with her

unsoiled and perfect soul and at the same time enabled her to get in touch with her abuse issues. Debbie left her painting for me to hang on my studio wall so that others could realize that, no matter what their experience has been, no one can ever touch their souls of pure gold.

CONCLUSIONS

It appears from the work I have done with clients over the last seven years that both art therapy and Rubenfeld Synergy access places that verbal therapy cannot. The art seems to build a trust and facilitates visualization. There is continued expansion and awareness as patients engage in the art process. Art facilitates experimentation and integration in a different way than verbal therapy. In art therapy, what is inside a client takes a form that can be referred back to and can anchor the experience of the Rubenfeld work. A visual journal is produced that, when reviewed, gives new insight. Art therapy also adds playfulness, which is much needed for these patients.

Rubenfeld Synergy takes clients deeper into the trance and relaxation state than verbal therapy or art therapy, enabling them to access more deeply buried material and energy. Touch is both healing and pleasant and facilitates the therapeutic and healing processes. Both modalities amaze the participants with their gentleness and ability to open them up to memories (and feelings associated with them) in a safe way. Both modalities facilitate the reframing process.

It has been a profound experience and a true gift to work with both of these clients using Rubenfeld Synergy combined with art therapy. To me, this work not only integrates body, mind, heart, and spirit but also touches and reveals the very soul. According to Hornbacher (1998), this is a place that the eating-disordered patient hungers and starves for, a place much neglected in our technological and mechanistic culture. It is the quadrant neglected not only in many modern families but in the field of psychology and therapy. It is where starvation runs rampant.

REFERENCES

Bartenieff, I. (1980). *Body movement coping with the environment.* New York: Gordon & Breach.

Bernstein, P. (1979). *Eight theoretical approaches in dance-movement therapy.* Dubuque, IA: Kendall/Hunt.

Bollas, C. (1987). *The shadow of the object.* New York: Columbia University Press.

Browning, N. (1985). Long term dynamic group therapy with bulimia patients. In S. W. Emmett (Ed.), *Theory and treatment of anorexia nervosa and bulimia*. New York: Brunner/Mazel, 30–41.

Bruch, H. (1978). *The golden cage: The enigma of anorexia nervosa*. Cambridge, MA: Harvard University Press.

Crowl, M. (1980). Art therapy with patients suffering from anorexia nervosa. *The Arts in Psychotherapy 7*, 141–51.

Emmett, S. W. (1985). *Theory and treatment of anorexia nervosa and bulimia*. New York: Brunner/Mazel.

Geist, R. A. (1955). Therapeutic dilemmas in the treatment of anorexia nervosa: A self-psychological perspective. In S. W. Emmett (Ed.), *Theory and treatment of anorexia nervosa and bulimia*. New York: Brunner/Mazel.

Gendlin, E. (1986). *Let your body interpret your dreams*. Wilmette, IL: University of Chicago.

Giovacchini, P. (1986). *Developmental disorders*. New York: Jason Aronson.

Hornbacher, M. (1998). *Wasted, a memoir of anorexia and bulimia*. New York: HarperFlamingo.

Horner, A. (1979). *Object relations and the developing ego*. New York: Jason Aronson.

Kramer, E. (1972). *Art as therapy with children*. New York: Schocken Books.

Jung, C. G. (1964). *Man and his symbols*. New York: Doubleday.

Jung, C. G. (1974). *Dreams*. Princeton, NJ: Princeton University Press.

Leonard, L. (1983). *The wounded woman*. Boston: Shambhala.

Levenkron, S. (1982). *Treating and overcoming anorexia nervosa*. New York: Warner Books.

Levenkron, S. (1985). Structuring a nurturant authoritative psychotherapeutic relationship with the anorexic patient. In S. W. Emmett (Ed.), *Theory and treatment of anorexia nervosa and bulimia*. New York: Brunner/Mazel, 15–27.

Lowen, A. (1976). *Bioenergetics*. New York: Simon & Schuster.

Mahler, M., Pine, F., & Bergman, A. (1975). *The psychological birth of the human infant*. New York: Basic Books.

Mahoney, F. (1966). *The meaning in dreams and dreaming*. New York: Citadel Press.

Mindell, A. (1985). *Working with the dreaming body*. Boston: Routledge & Kegan Paul.

Mitchell, D. (1981). Anorexia nervosa. *The Arts in Psychotherapy 7*, 53–60.

Perls, F. (1988). *Gestalt therapy verbatim*. New York: The Center for Gestalt Development.

Rhyne, J. (1984). *The gestalt art experience*. Chicago: Magnolia St. Publishers.

Rizzuto, A. (1985). Eating and monsters: A psychodynamic view of bulimarexia. In S. W. Emmett (Ed.), *Theory and treatment of anorexia nervosa and bulimia*. New York: Brunner/Mazel, 61–75.

Robbins, A. (1980). *Expressive therapies: A creative arts approach to depth oriented treatment*. New York: Human Sources Press.

Robbins, A. (1994). *A multi-modal approach to creative art therapy*. London: Jessica Kingsley Publishers.

Rosen, S. (1991). *My voice will go with you: The teaching tales of Milton H. Erickson*. New York: W.W. Norton.

Rubenfeld, I. (1988, Spring/Summer). Beginner's hands: 25 years of simple: Rubenfeld Synergy, the birth of a therapy. *Somatics* 15–21.

Rubenfeld, I. (1990, July). The Rubenfeld Synergy method: a journey of integration. AHP, 6–11.

Rubenfeld, I. (1990-1991, Autumn/Winter). Ushering in a century of integration. *Somatics*, 59–63.

Rubenfeld, I. (1995, June). Sing the body electric. *Changes*, 30–35.

Rubenfeld, I. (1997, September/October). Listening hands. *Family Networker*, 20–26.

Sandel, S. L. (1982). The process of individuation in dance movement therapy with schizophrenic patients. *The Arts in Psychotherapy 9*, 11–18.

Spegnesi, A. (1983). *Starving women: A psychology of anorexia nervosa*. Dallas, TX: Spring Publications.

Winnicott, D. W. (1971). *Playing and reality*. London: Tavestock Publications Limited.

Wolf, J. M. et al. (1985). The role of art in the therapy of anorexia nervosa. *International Journal of Eating Disorders 4*, 185–200.

Woodman, M. (1980). *The owl was a baker's daughter*. Toronto: Inner City Books.

Woodman, M. (1982). *Addiction to perfection: The still unravished bride*. Toronto: Inner City Books.

Overcoming Eating Disorders: 12 Steps to a Behavior Contract

by Margo Maine, Ph.D.

Recovering from an eating disorder is probably the most difficult task you will ever face. At times it may seem impossible to you. Recovery demands every resource and every bit of courage you can muster. Unfortunately, wanting to get better is not enough. You must change both your mind-set and your behavior: One without the other is not enough. And you must face the substance that represents so much to you and frightens you the most: food.

Unlike other problems like alcohol or drug abuse, you have to meet and integrate the enemy—

you cannot abstain or avoid it. Food is essential to life. Furthermore, because of the impact of nutrition on our ability to think, concentrate, and handle stress and emotion, you must eat to feel better. Also, without adequate calories, especially in protein and fat, medications that you take to help you with anxiety or depression will not work. They simply cannot be absorbed unless you eat appropriately. Despite how scary this may be, changing how you eat, and how you treat your body, is essential.

FIRST THINGS FIRST: INSIGHT OR BEHAVIOR CHANGE?

For most of you, it will take years to figure out what your eating disorder is about. Certainly it is a way to deal with painful feelings that you have been unable to face or express any other way. The insight you need to understand all the complicated reasons for your difficulties with food, however, is unlikely to emerge when your symptoms are severe. Instead, starving, bingeing and purging, or excessively exercising will control your consciousness. When you are extremely depleted or uncomfortably full, your discomfort with your body is all you can think about. Nothing else is important enough to overshadow these feelings. So, you miss a lot of life.

Eating disorders are a true paradox. Initially, they are a means of dealing with problems you cannot face directly. But, soon, the eating disorder becomes bigger than the original problems. Eating disorders can ruin your health, eventually affecting every organ and system in your body, and, simultaneously, they can destroy your relationships. The eating disorder becomes so powerful that nothing else matters. You can no longer hear, see, feel, touch, or taste things you used to love, so you may believe there is no reason to get better. In fact, until you begin to change your behavior, you may not even remember why you should want to be better.

Eating disorders lock you in a prison of self-doubt, inadequacy, isolation, and depression—not a place where insight abounds. So, waiting until you understand and resolve all the problems that led to your eating disorder will not work. You must change your behavior first. Insight, and the peace and fulfillment it brings, will follow.

THE PROCESS OF RECOVERY

For long-term recovery, understanding the problems, feelings, and issues that led to your eating disorder is essential. The first phase of recovery, however, requires that you just decide to be kinder to yourself. Stop beating your body with abusive behaviors: not eating, eating too much, doing anything you can to lose weight, exercising until you ache. Once you begin to take better care of your body, you will gradually be able to understand more of the reasons for your behavior. Initially, this will be scary: You have had good reason to avoid these feelings, and they will be disorganizing and sometimes startling to you. Soon, however, you will feel less out of control, less crazy, and more accepting of yourself. Psychotherapy can help you deal with these feelings, as can sharing them with others with similar problems. Do not try to do this alone. Early in recovery, a behavior contract can help because it breaks a long process down into manageable steps. Instead of trying to recover perfectly and immediately, you will establish a progression of goals. The contract may help you to be more reasonable with yourself and counter your all-or-nothing, black-or-white thinking.

A behavior contract is basically an agreement with yourself that you are going to try to get better. As a statement of commitment to your recovery, it also should involve others because you cannot do this alone. A contract will not only help you but also will help your loved ones, for it gives them clarity about how to support you. This can be very useful, as your suffering bothers them, too, and they may not always handle their anxiety well. A contract clarifies their role, as well as your goals, for the time being.

12 STEPS TO A BEHAVIOR CONTRACT

The wisdom of the 12-step programs for alcoholism, drug abuse, and other addictions also applies to some of the challenges in overcoming an eating disorder. Thus, borrowing some of their language, here are 12 steps to help you develop a behavior contract so that you can gain control over your eating disorder. As you approach the idea of a contract and of recovery, keep in mind the Serenity Prayer, the guiding philosophy of Alcoholics Anonymous:

God grant me the serenity to accept the things I cannot change, courage to change the things I can, and wisdom to know the difference.

In every phase of recovery and every aspect of life, those words can help us to risk change and to accept reality.

Steps 1-5: Getting Ready to Let Go

Step 1. Admit you have a problem. Although this sounds easy, it often is the hardest step. Why is it that everyone else can see what's wrong, but you don't believe them? Are all those people who love you wrong? No. Your solution to painful feelings has been to control your body through your eating disorder. Now your eating disorder controls you. Admit it: Your life is out of control.

Step 2. Believe two things: "Change is possible" and "I deserve to have a better life." Repeat these two statements to yourself, especially the one concerning a healthier, happier existence.

Step 3. Make a decision to change. Decide to tolerate whatever feelings come up if you begin to change your behaviors surrounding food and your body. With the right support and the benefit of time, you will be able to tolerate the uncomfortable and unpredictable feelings that accompany change.

Step 4. Make an inventory of the problems you need to address. Be honest about the things you do to hurt or punish yourself. Write down every symptom, from how you eat, to how you exercise, to how you punish yourself for eating, to how you try to lose weight, and to how you degrade and criticize yourself and try so hard to be perfect and need no one. All of these are behaviors you need to change. Again, be painfully honest about how you treat yourself—this inventory will help guide later steps to recovery.

Step 5. Share your inventory with someone who can help you. In other words, come clean! Admit your problems and imperfections—people will still care about you. In fact, doing so may draw you closer to others, as they will begin to understand the agony you have been living. You won't have to "act" all the time, and you can concentrate on being yourself. Just be sure that the person you share this with really can help. Your doctor may be a good person to start with, but a therapist or dietitian can help you formulate an exact plan for the next steps.

Steps 6-12—Giving Up the Game

Step 6. Develop a plan, but keep it simple. A contract needs to include attainable goals and not be overly ambitious or complicated. Otherwise, it will be overwhelming, just as your eating disorder is. Identify one problem and work on that. Do not set yourself up for failure by trying to change everything at once. The plan can include other people. Especially if you are young or living with your family, involving them can help. If they have a clearly defined role in your recovery, they may not get as frustrated and you can all live together more peacefully. An eating disorder is hard on everyone.

Step 7. "Fake it till you make it." Changing any behavior is difficult and takes time before you feel better. Sometimes you have to do something for a long time before you sense a change. Try to believe that you're going to feel better, that the anxiety you feel as you take better care of your body will eventually disappear. Gradually it will, but obsessing over it and avoiding change only makes it worse.

Step 8. Take life "one day at a time," or even "one meal at a time" or "one hour at a time." If you have trouble meeting your goal, start again. Give yourself another chance. You have probably had your eating disorder for a long time, and the problems leading up to it have been with you even longer. So be patient. Remember: "Rome wasn't built in a day"; "No pain, no gain." Come up with some other sayings that will help you be more patient with yourself. Very few people can climb straight up a mountain.

Step 9. Build in some rewards for your efforts. Recovery is hard work. Be sure to take care of yourself by indulging in things that will make you feel better. Find ways to soothe yourself. Reading affirmations, doing relaxation exercises, participating in favorite activities that are easy on your body will all help your spirits. List these rewards and allow yourself one of them every day.

Step 10. Talk about how you feel as you make changes in therapy, in support groups, or in your interactions with trusted friends and family. As you change your behavior, more feelings will surface. To understand how these feelings contributed to your eating disorder, you need to talk, talk, talk. Writing in a journal each day can help you to remember the issues you want to discuss with your therapist. Remember: You can't do this by yourself.

Step 11. Keep on changing. Each week take a look at your contract and decide if it is helping you now. Many people with eating disorders have multiple behaviors to change, so take a look at your inventory and decide which problem to attack next. However, it is also sometimes helpful to stay in the same place awhile. If you have worked hard and don't think you can do anything more right now, simply try to maintain the change you have made before moving on again.

Step 12. Believe in yourself and give yourself some credit. Acknowledge what you have accomplished, then, when you are ready, refer to your contract and repeat the steps you have accomplished to reinforce your program. Because eating disorders are so complicated and you had to keep your contract simple, it is now time to review your progress and identify another behavior from your inventory to work on.

Remember: Recovery is going to take time, and you will need help. Share this chapter with your therapist, dietitian, and doctor so they can help you.

SAMPLE CONTRACTS

For an Underweight Anorexic Living at Home

I will

- gain a pound a week;
- follow my doctor/therapist/dietitian's guidelines for exercise and food intake;
- record what I eat each day and share it with the dietitian.

Parents will

- ask what food I need and make it available;
- measure my food if I request it;

- ask me if I need to talk or do something else after meals;
- come for family therapy.

For an Underweight Anorexic Making Adequate Progress with Weight Gain and out of Medical Danger

I will

- continue to gain weight;
- be allowed to exercise/play sports as discussed with dietitian/therapist/doctor;
- increase my intake as prescribed on the days I exercise;
- not be allowed to exercise if I lose weight but can resume it after I regain the lost weight;
- abide by decisions made each week about sports/exercise.

Parents will

- ask what food I need and make it available;
- measure my food if I request it;
- ask me if I need to talk or do something else after meals;
- come for family therapy;
- enforce the exercise restrictions.

For a Bulimic Adult

I will

- decrease my [purging behavior] to [frequency];
- record my food intake;
- journal about my feelings;
- honestly report my feelings to my therapist and dietitian;
- comply with medical follow-up;
- do something that feels good and is healthy every day;

Family members will

- ask if I need help or want to talk;
- participate in therapy or support group to address their own anxiety and worries.

More Than Anorexia: An Example of Integrated Treatment for Adolescents with Eating Disorders

by Alexandra O. Eliot, Ph.D.

Eating disorders such as anorexia, bulimia nervosa, and binge eating continue relatively unabated despite vigorous and varied treatment approaches. Efforts aimed at prevention through the psychoeducation of potentially vulnerable young people have yielded rather disappointing results. Although clinicians coming in contact with this population are more knowledgeable than before, there is still no established road to recovery from dysfunctional eating. Overall, one in five adolescents has a serious physical or emotional problem that may interfere with a healthy and smooth transition to adulthood (Brindis & Irwin, 1994). Snyder (1989) noted in a policy paper developed for the American College of Physicians that eating disorders were among the nine most serious problems confronting adolescents. Almost all epidemiological studies suggest that the incidence of eating disorders has increased, occurring primarily in females between the ages of 15 and 24 in the developed countries of the world (Hsu, 1990). Data compiled by me and other authors note that age of onset for anorexia nervosa has decreased so that it is not uncommon to see patients as young as nine years of age. There is also a higher incidence of dual diagnoses among these patients; in particular, obsessive-compulsive disorder and a history of sexual abuse.

PROBLEMS OF ACCESS TO CARE

Providing comprehensive and specialized care to adolescents is a challenging task, one further complicated by the recent economic constraints of managed care and inadequate or totally absent health insurance coverage for them. The Children's Defense Fund (1997) estimates that in 1995 10 million children were uninsured, a number that has increased since the enactment of welfare reform legislation. Other factors jeopardize access to care for adolescents. Despite serious acute and chronic problems, adolescents have the lowest utilization rate of health care services of any age group in the United States (Brandis & Irwin, 1994). Lack of experience in negotiating complex medical systems and a desire for independence and freedom from authority, combined with denial that there is a problem with over- or undereating, make it highly unlikely that the teenager will seek appropriate treatment on his or her own. Sustained concern and support from parents and other referring agents are necessary to ensure that adolescents receive care that is acceptable to them as well as in their best biopsychosocial interests.

OUTPATIENT EATING-DISORDERS CLINIC

An outpatient eating-disorders clinic (EDC) at one of Boston's teaching hospitals is described here. The clinic began in 1981 as a collaborative effort between the departments of psychiatry and adolescent/young adult medicine. Its purpose is to deliver treatment to males and females with eating disorders between the ages of 12 and 21 (and recently younger), within the framework of their general care as developing adults. Thus, the reason for referral (seldom by the identified patient) may be anorexia or bulimia nervosa, but during the initial evaluation, equal attention is paid to other concerns that may be raised by the adolescent or physician, such as physical and emotional complaints, substance use, sexually transmitted diseases, academic issues, and interpersonal or family problems.

Since its inception, EDC has seen just under 1,400 patients and their families, in varying degrees of intensity, depending on the severity of illness and insurance authorization.

Of this number, approximately 60 have been males. Many changes in the management of these patients have occurred, but the basic commitment to treat eating-disordered adolescents holistically instead of as disease entities such as "anorectics" or "bulimics" has remained at the core of the clinic's philosophy.

EVALUATION PROCESS

EDC is no longer headed jointly by a psychiatrist and a social worker. Its director is a physician in the adolescent/young adult medical practice, reflecting the fact that many health maintenance organizations have their own mental-health providers and thus do not wish to contract with the hospital for psychiatric services. A psychiatrist from the department of psychiatry is involved almost exclusively, if at all, for psychopharmacology consultation. Ironically, this arrangement has led to greater fragmentation of care, challenging the original mandate of EDC to deliver integrative services to eating-disordered adolescents. It has also complicated the maintenance of close communication among members of the treatment team.

A social worker completes all the phone intakes, averaging six or seven new patients per week. Demographic information and a brief summary of the problem are recorded, after which the initial medical appointment for the patient and psychosocial assessment for the family are scheduled. There is a two- to three-week waiting list, but "fast-track" appointments can be accommodated.

Patients begin the evaluation process by being weighed and measured, having their blood pressure monitored, and taking an eye screening test; a nursing assistant administers these procedures. While the parents meet with the physician to give a developmental history, the patient completes a standardized questionnaire. This includes the Beck Depression Inventory (Beck, 1967) adapted for adolescents, "anorexia" questions developed by Rollins and Piazza (1978); and the Eating Attitudes Test (Garner & Garfinkel, 1979). These instruments have contributed useful data for several follow-up studies (Eliot, 1988, 1989, 1991). The adolescent then undergoes a complete physical exam and has the opportunity to discuss his or her concerns without parental interference. Concerns may range far afield from the anorexia or bulimia. In the meantime, parents meet with the social worker for psychosocial evalua-

tion and a chance to share their concerns and learn about the treatment process in greater depth. This meeting is important because parents generally arrive at the clinic highly anxious and distressed. In addition, the social worker's advocacy and supportive roles provide a critical perspective to parents and other members of the treatment team because parents, especially mothers, often feel that they are to blame for their child's dysfunctional eating. Unfortunately, this notion is sometimes reinforced by family, friends, and even other clinicians who too readily identify with the teenager's negative characterization of the parents (Eliot 1996). Mothers and fathers are encouraged to be active collaborators in their children's treatment and recovery process, while respecting their healthy drive for autonomy and privacy. They are often relieved when they realize that they can begin to share responsibility for their child's care with the EDC staff and thus distance themselves somewhat from day-to-day management. If circumstances and time permit, the adolescent may also be evaluated by an EDC social worker or psychologist. Finally, recommendations are shared with parents and patient, and subsequent medical and nutritional appointments are scheduled.

Under the rubric of generic care for the eating-disordered patient are several possible interventions considered by the team following the medical workup and psychosocial assessment. These may include continued outpatient medical monitoring; nutritional counseling; family, group, or individual therapy and/or support groups; medication; cognitive-behavioral techniques, and emergent inpatient admission.

In recent years the necessity for immediate admission has increased because patients' illnesses are more advanced by the time the patients are referred to EDC from other facilities. These medical admissions tend to be very brief, lasting only long enough for vital signs to stabilize, whereupon the adolescent is usually referred back to the outpatient clinic. Admission to the inpatient psychiatric facility is briefer by far than in years past. Driven by economics, referrals are made to residential ("step down") or day programs elsewhere in the community if the patient is not well enough to resume outpatient status.

As a result of such financial considerations, the majority of EDC's efforts have shifted from extended treatment and longer-term follow-up care to shorter-term evaluation and consultation.

Consequently, its population is more severely eating-disordered because initial treatment occurs with outside primary care providers who may have less expertise and resources at their disposal than EDC. Relatively few patients receive long-term psychiatric care within the clinic, and no therapy or support groups are offered, although several exist in the Boston area that are suitable for adolescents and families.

CONCEPTUAL FRAMEWORK

A variety of opinions expand on the etiology and optimal treatment for anorexia and bulimia; Hsu (1990) asserts that even the distinction between the two conditions is unclear. Some scholars believe that anorexia represents a psychobiological regression from the demands and changes inherent in normal-weighted adolescence and adulthood (Crisp, 1980; Palmer, 1980). Bruch (1973) believed that self-starvation was the result of the "desperate struggle for a self-respecting identity." The current obsession with idealized body image fueled by the media certainly strains the ability of young people to focus on internal, rather than external, attributes (Brumberg, 1996; Orbach, 1986).

In the EDC group, a correlation appears to exist between onset of the eating disorder and various family issues such as losses and financial or psychological disruptions that result in a need to regain a sense of control through the manipulation of food intake. Families appear generally very stressed, with mothers and fathers working as well as parenting. Family members are more overtly preoccupied with worries about being fat and getting enough exercise; in short, they are influenced to an unhealthy extreme by sociocultural forces. It is the exception rather than the rule that such families enjoy a meal together.

Obviously, for the young person with anorexia nervosa, remaining very thin is of enormous importance. For the bulimic or binge eater, obtaining, eating, and/or purging vast amounts of food consume the majority of his or her physical and psychic energies. Both avoidance of normal weight as well as excessive caloric ingestion become addictive and beyond individual control. Interference with these behaviors can be so threatening that the patient seeks to withdraw from treatment altogether. The initial task of the treatment team, therefore, is to "help the patient become a patient" (Crisp, 1986); that is, to introduce the idea that there is a problem that needs to be acknowledged and

dealt with instead of denied. The adolescent and the family need to understand that uncontrolled self-starvation and binge/purge behavior are incompatible with survival.

In treating anorexia, the fundamental commitment to weight restoration must be maintained, but choices among various treatment strategies, such as amount of permissible exercise or use of supplemental feedings, may be offered within the basic framework. As the patient reassumes responsibility for self-nourishment, the degree of participation by the patient in decision making can increase. Collaboration between the patient and members of the treatment team calls for "negotiated moderation" (Levenkron, 1985), rather than abrupt changes, to facilitate integration of more normalized behaviors.

Along with careful attention to the pertinent developmental needs of the adolescents, this cognitive-behavioral approach serves regressed patients as well. For example, concrete, clearly outlined guidelines about eating meals or limiting binges can be negotiated: "This is the number of calories you need or may have for lunch, but you can make some choices from the menu," or, "You may decide it is too difficult for you at this time to make choices; if so, we can make them for you," and finally, "If it is too frightening at this stage to eat regular food, we can help by prescribing supplemental feedings until you feel stronger and safer."

Many years, and a number of changes later, this clinic's sustained effectiveness and rate of recovery or substantial improvement from eating disorders (between 77 percent and 83 percent; Eliot, 1988, 1989, 1991) supports the view that it is important to treat adolescents in a setting where all their medical and psychosocial concerns can be addressed. It is equally critical that those treating them be aware of the disruption or arrest in normal adolescent development that occurs as part of the natural course of anorexia and bulimia. They need to be able to relate to patients whose intellectual and emotional views of the world are not commensurate with their chronological age. The tasks of adolescence, especially the social ones, may need to be mastered at a slower pace using a different timetable. This approach offers the best hope that, ultimately, restoration to normal health and activity will compensate for the loss of self-perceived, illusive power and control that the eating-disordered adolescent experienced while within the eye of the anorectic or bulimic storm.

REFERENCES

Beck, A. (1967). *Depression: Clinical, experimental, and theoretical aspects*. New York: Harper & Row.

Brindis, C., & Irwin, C. (1994). *Promoting adolescent health: Policy recommendations for health care reform*. Proceedings from the working seminar on adolescent health and health care reform. National Health Information Center, San Francisco.

Bruch, H. (1973). *Eating disorders: Obesity, anorexia nervosa and the person within*. New York: Basic Books.

Brumberg, J. (1996). *Body projects: The changing experience of American girls*. Proceedings of the Seventh International Conference on Eating Disorders, New York, NY.

Children's Defense Fund. (1997). *The state of America's children*. Washington, DC: Author.

Crisp, A. (1980). *Anorexia nervosa: Let me be*. London: Academic Press.

Crisp, A. (1986). *Prevention of eating disorders*. Proceedings of the Second International Conference on Eating Disorders, New York, NY.

Eliot, A. (1988). *Disorders of consumption: A follow-up study of the anorexia nervosa and associated disorders clinic*. Unpublished doctoral dissertation. Boston: Simmons College School of Social Work. (Printed in 1994 by U.M.I. Dissertation Services, Ann Arbor, Michigan).

Eliot, A. (1989). *Paths to recovery: A follow-up study of outpatients with anorexia and bulimia nervosa*. Unpublished

master's research project. Boston: Simmons College School of Social Work.

Eliot, A. (1991). *What makes the difference? Outcome and follow-up evaluation of adolescents with anorexia and bulimia*. Unpublished master's research project. Boston: Simmons College School of Social Work.

Eliot, A. (1996, Fall). Maternal stressors and eating disordered adolescent girls. *Simmons School of Social Work Alumni Newsletter*, 6–8.

Garner, D., & Garfinkel, P. (1979). The eating attitudes test: An index of the symptoms of anorexia nervosa. *Psychological Medicine 9*, 273–79.

Hsu, L. K. (1990). *Eating disorders*. New York: Guilford Press.

Levenkron, S. (1985). Structuring a nurturant/authoritative psychotherapeutic relationship. In S. Emmett (Ed.), *Theory and treatment of anorexia nervosa and bulimia* (pp. 234–45). New York: Brunner/Mazel.

Orbach, S. (1986). *Hunger strike*. New York: W.W. Norton. Bungay, Suffolk, England.

Palmer, R. (1980). *Anorexia nervosa: A guide for sufferers and their families*. Bungay: The Chaucer Press.

Rollins, N., & Piazza, E. (1978). Diagnosis of anorexia nervosa: A critical reappraisal. *Journal of the American Academy of Child Psychiatry 17*, 126–37.

Snyder, L. (1989). Health care needs of the adolescent: Position paper. *Annals of Internal Medicine*.

The Importance of Self-Help Groups in Recovery from Eating Disorders

by Jeanne Phillips, M.A.

WHY SELF-HELP?

The major goal of a self-help group for people with eating disorders is to provide support and communication between individuals who are at different stages of recovery, create self-awareness and insight, and give members an opportunity to increase communication and problem-solving skills. For teenagers and young adults, self-help group meetings allow for safe formats in which members can express an opinion that is often opposite to that expressed within their peer group and culture—and still remain a part of that culture. As members become comfortable with one another and more self-assured in expressing feelings and concerns that do not necessarily support the cultural preoccupation of thinness and per-

fectionism as the ideal, they are practicing skills of independence and autonomy, possibly for the first time in their lives.

The teens and and early 20s are an especially frightening, confusing time with tremendous pressure from our culture that dictates how one must look and feel about themselves. When a group becomes cohesive, and people begin sharing and bonding, they are able to let go of some of the cultural stereotypes, shame, and guilt associated with eating disorders. Sharing one's experiences and being supportive to others undergoing similar experiences is an important part of how a group empowers its members. The group provides a safe environment in which to feel close to one another; take risks;

and share feelings about home life, emancipation, relationships, fears of intimacy, sexuality, and fears of disappointing family. Unique relationships often develop through these meetings. Members are encouraged to respond to their real feelings, rather than to be the "perfect person" one thinks he or she must be in order to be accepted. A support group allows for an opposite stand without the fear of rejection or abandonment and enables one, for the first time perhaps, to gain a feeling of being authentic.

WHAT TO EXPECT

The group is typically led by an individual who has recovered from an eating disorder. In this way it differs from structured group therapy which is led by a professional. The group provides support at no cost or a minimal fee, thus making a resource available for those who might not be able to afford professional care. A support group also can provide names of reputable professionals for more formal treatment. The group is constantly in transition and can be attended as needed, and it is ongoing, with participants not having to make a commitment to join as opposed to structured, time-limited group therapy. In this informal fashion, the group provides individuals the opportunity to begin sharing when they feel comfortable and the ability to identify with someone who has gone through similar experiences. They may also come to see that an eating disorder need not be a lifelong disorder and that, indeed, recovery is possible.

It is important for the group leader to model honesty and be open with the members, sharing the story of his or her own recovery, giving direct feedback, letting people know that recovery is, indeed, a process, and, most importantly, that trying to do it perfectly (recover) is another set-up for failure.

Coming to a self-help group is a major step for someone who is eating-disordered. It is an awakening to the fact that they are not "terminally unique" but have things in common with other members. The purpose in opening these meetings only to individuals struggling with the disorder is to provide anonymity as well as to support each other in taking responsibility for one's own recovery. Individuals with eating disorders not only have a strong desire to be taken care of, but also have issues of perfectionism and fear of change. Being able to speak one's truth instead of relying on family or friends to do so is important to the

recovery process. With this model, there is no doubt who is responsible for changes being made.

Joining a group can create feelings of anxiety and apprehension. In order to alleviate these fears, the group process is explained either prior to the meeting or at the beginning of each session. Members are asked to share when they feel comfortable in doing so. It is explained that all one must do is sign in. Often during a meeting, an individual who has just joined will hear what other folks are going through and begin to identify with other group members. At the end of the meeting, the individual may be asked by the group leader how it felt to be there and often the response is, "What was discussed were many of the things I am going through or have gone through. It feels good knowing I'm not so alone," or, "I thought I was the only one who had those feelings," thus enhancing the feeling of not being alone.

Some individuals come to group expecting to attend just a few times and to recover from their eating disorder. This type of thinking is common. Upon joining a self-help group, one learns quickly that recovery is a process and takes time. Individuals with eating disorders tend to place very high expectations on themselves and become impatient in the process. Members with more recovery take pride in sharing their process, thus giving others realistic expectations and modeling healthy behaviors. Myths are dispelled regarding food, weight, and body image, lending the freedom to work on underlying issues of low self-esteem, people-pleasing, and perfectionism. The length of time spent in a self-help group depends primarily on one's willingness to take risks and make the necessary changes to start feeling better about oneself.

Often, people come to a group meeting believing that their problem is only with food and fear of weight gain, and they just need to learn how to eat normally. It is important to shift the focus from food and weight to feelings. Discussion topics in a self-help group may include: issues surrounding poor self-esteem, perfectionism, people-pleasing, setting realistic goals and expectations, the desire to be special, control issues, the desire to be accepted and loved by everyone, the purpose and function of rituals, the meaning of thinness and fatness, fear of intimacy and sexuality, fear of inadequacy, fear of anger, emancipation and separation from family, fear of rejection and abandonment, feelings of guilt and shame, and cultural attitudes towards fatness and thinness.

When a person finds others who share their same feelings and fears and have gone through similar experiences and feelings, that person often experiences a tremendous sense of relief. When group members together identify what triggers their eating-disorder behavior (anger, shame, guilt, loneliness, boredom), they usually begin to identify with each other as well, thus establishing a sense of camaraderie.

The group provides a safe place to do some role-modeling and risk-taking, to be honest in feelings and feedback in terms of what others are doing regarding their recovery, and to receive honest feedback with one's own issues. One can expect anonymity; a networking and support system. Thus one no longer feels so alone or different.

SUPPORT GROUPS BASED ON 12-STEP MODEL

Another type of support group is based on the Alcoholics Anonymous (AA) Twelve Step Model. It is based on the AA concept of alcoholism as a progressive lifelong illness, which must be controlled by abstinence from the substance to which the individual is "addicted." This model views someone with an eating disorder as having a disease rather than a disorder. These people are viewed as suffering from a compulsive illness which cannot be cured, but rather arrested.

In these groups people believe that they are powerless over food, with emphasis being placed on abstinence rather than normalizing intake and on addressing underlying issues. This model does not explain the behavior, but redefines it with terms such as "compulsive" or "addiction"; thus, the individual must struggle with the disease over his or her lifespan. Members are encouraged to find a sponsor whom they can call when they need help abstaining from bingeing or purging. The sponsor, someone who is at a later stage of recovery, is available to people first entering the program.

SELF-HELP GROUPS NOT FOR EVERYONE

Support groups are not usually recommended for individuals who are severely restricting their food intake and unable to relate well enough to others to benefit from the interaction. In addition, these individuals may be competing so intensely to be the thinnest that they are unable to experience the good feelings one gets after sharing problems and the mutual support, trust, and respect that occurs in this kind of setting.

A PERSONAL NOTE

It is the opinion of this author that one can recover completely from a eating disorder. It is my belief that an eating disorder is a behavior that is learned and can be unlearned rather than a disease; that one is not powerless over food but has become powerless over one's feelings and must learn to take responsibility for feelings and behaviors. To accomplish this, one must begin realistic goal-setting, be willing to take a risk without being absolutely certain of the outcome, ask others for help and support, take the words "should" and "can't" out of their vocabulary, realize that recovery is a process and cannot be done perfectly, avoid isolating and withdrawing, not presume to know what other people are thinking, or gauge one's feelings of specialness on external symbols of success, (i.e. thinness or clothes size), and begin to establish an identity apart from being bulimic or anorexic.

Information about support groups may be found in local telephone directories, Information and Referral, mental-health facilities, newspapers, county social services departments, or self-help hotlines. Also, please see the directory of non-profit organizations in Part VI of this volume.

How to Find Treatment for an Eating Disorder

by Nancy Ellis-Ordway, A.C.S.W.

Most individuals with eating disorders need some sort of treatment to recover. Although some people get better on their own, most people need to be under the care of trained professionals. The longer treatment is delayed, the greater the risk of serious complications, and the more entrenched the illness may become. People treated early in the course of the illness tend to get better more quickly and spend less time in treatment.

Once the decision has been made to enter treatment, an equally difficult decision must be made concerning where to go for help. Good treatment is much more available than it was a couple of decades ago, but it still must be sought out. Ideally, an individual will research all the options and make a calm, considered decision. More often, however, the decision is made in the midst of a crisis, or the person with the disorder is too overwhelmed to carry out the task of finding and inquiring about programs. An interested family member or friend can be of great help at this point by making phone calls and following up leads, when possible, to discover what options are available.

KINDS OF TREATMENT

Treatment can include individual psychotherapy, group therapy, family therapy, medication, nutritional counseling, support groups, self-help groups, and classes. Most people need some combination of approaches at different points in recovery. All of these can be provided on an inpatient or outpatient basis. Professionals who treat individuals with eating disorders include psychiatrists and other physicians, psychologists, psychotherapists, social workers, dietitians, nurses, counselors, music therapists, art therapists, and pastoral counselors.

Inpatient Treatment (Hospitals and Special Eating-Disorder Units)

There are advantages and disadvantages to both inpatient and outpatient treatment. Inpatient treatment is, obviously, more disruptive to school, work, and family life, and it is also more expensive. On the other hand, a specialized inpatient unit can provide much more structure and safety for the person with a significant eating disorder. Inpatient treatment provides a more intensive psychotherapeutic experience in that therapy can continue on a 24-hour basis, as opposed to starting and stopping for an hour at a time once or twice a week. Some people also need the close medical monitoring that can only take place in the hospital.

There are several reasons to consider in-patient treatment. A person who is significantly underweight will have a hard time eating enough to gain weight without a great deal of structure around food intake. Because of metabolic abnormalities, such individuals usually require a huge number of calories to restore the metabolism to normal before they even begin to gain weight. For a person with a terror of food, this can be a seemingly impossible task. In addition, certain medical risks associated with weight gain should be monitored. Malnutrition can cause depression, inability to concentrate, moodiness, and a decreased ability to think clearly. All of these symptoms impede the success of outpatient treatment. Even people of normal weight can benefit from inpatient treatment if they are feeling out of control with food as it is possible to be malnourished even at a normal body weight.

Among the numerous medical reasons for inpatient treatment are to monitor, control, or prevent fainting, dizziness, abnormal electrolyte levels, dehydration, persistent muscle cramps, uncontrollable or spontaneous vomiting, vomiting of blood, and chest pain. Suicidal thoughts, plans, gestures, and attempts are other reasons to choose inpatient treatment.

Sometimes inpatient treatment for an adolescent can be helpful if the family is feeling overwhelmed and out of control. The time away can give family members a chance to calm down and reevaluate their roles in the problem. Adolescents who deny having an eating disorder may need inpatient treatment to help them confront their problems.

People with eating disorders tend to get better faster on specialized inpatient units. Some units just treat people with anorexia and bulimia; some also treat compulsive overeating. Many hospitals treat eating disorders on a general unit, housing patients with diagnoses ranging from depression and stress to chemical abuse, mood disorders, and psychosis. Some specialized treatment programs for problems such as stress and personality disorders see so many patients with eating disorders that they have developed treatment protocols especially for them. In other words, the title of the program may not tell you everything you need to know.

Following are some questions to ask about an inpatient eating-disorder program.

How specialized is it? How do you feel about being on a unit with people undergoing treatment for something other than an eating disorder? Will you have enough in common with them to benefit from group therapy?

What is the age range of the patients? If all the patients have similar diagnoses, a mix of adolescents and adults may do well. However, being the only adolescent on a general adult psychiatric unit or the only adult on a general adolescent unit may be difficult.

How individualized is the treatment? Some people get better quickly; some get better slowly; some require more than one hospital stay. A program with a fixed number of days does not necessarily allow for such variance. A program that recognizes individual differences will be more likely to be flexible about the length of stay.

How is food handled on the unit? The goal should be to allow patients a sense of safety and structure until they are able to eat normally and then to allow them to gradually take more responsibility for making good decisions about food. Too often general psychiatric units have food sitting out for snacks throughout the day, a terrifying prospect for someone with an eating disorder and one that makes it difficult to eat at all.

How much is the family involved? Family involvement in treatment is often critical, especially with younger patients. Programs may offer treatment for the immediate or extended family, classes and educational programs, group family therapy involving members of several families, and/or support groups.

What kind of follow-up is available? No one is cured when he or she leaves the hospital. Aftercare can include group, individual, and family therapy; ongoing nutritional counseling; weight monitoring; and partial hospitalization or "day treatment."

What is the training and experience of the staff? Professionals can obtain ongoing training in this field by keeping abreast of current research providing new information about the problem as well as effective treatment approaches.

How long has the program been in existence? If the program is new, it is important to ask about the qualifications of specific staff members. Asking about the program's "success rate" will not tell you very much. First, "success" is very difficult to define in the field of eating disorders; therefore, any statistics quoted are suspect. Second, a program widely known for excellent treatment tends to draw more patients who are very ill or have been involved in the illness for a long time, and thus will achieve poorer "success rates" than a program with less expertise.

May I tour the unit? In a sense, allowing tours of the unit is a violation of the privacy of the patients already there. For an individual considering admission, however, it is a reasonable request. Programs may allow family members to tour the facility, depending on the circumstances. Most programs will not allow tours to students or interested onlookers.

When investigating any treatment program, it is reasonable to ask for an evaluation appointment. Sometimes this appointment will be free of charge, but it is worth paying for even if it is not. If you tend to get flustered in this kind of a situation, make out a list of questions ahead of time and take it along. Make notes if you think you might forget something. You are entitled to have your questions answered before you make a decision. Other questions to ask at this point are: Why are you recommending this kind of treatment? and What are the alternatives?

Outpatient Treatment (Therapists and Programs)

Outpatient treatment can allow the eating-disordered person to recover gradually without interrupting day-to-day life. It can be offered through a well-organized, specialized program, but it is most often offered through individual psychotherapists.

Following are some important questions to ask.

What background do you have in treating this specific problem? An interest in the field is of value only when combined with training and expertise. One way therapists develop expertise in this field is through supervision by clinicians with extensive background. This arrangement expands the availability of quality treatment.

Who provides nutritional counseling? Psychotherapists and dietitians have very different kinds of training. Few people have a background in both. A team approach can meet this need, especially for patients who use their preoccupation with food to obscure other issues.

How is weight monitoring handled, if necessary? If a family member is to assume responsibility for monitoring weight it should be a specific part of the family therapy and one that is frequently discussed. Otherwise, it can lead to battles at home over control and independence, just when focus needs to be on improved communication. In any event, weight does need to be monitored somewhere, by someone.

What happens if the patient needs to be hospitalized? Sometimes eating problems and other symptoms such as depression actually get worse in response to talking about difficult issues in therapy. Outpatient therapy can be helpful in dealing with emotional issues but not in addressing the eating behavior. An individual psychotherapist should have some kind of back-up in the event that inpatient treatment is necessary, ideally, access to the inpatient unit chosen.

What other resources are available? It is important to determine if the therapist can provide a referral for family therapy, individual therapy for other family members, and group therapy.

FINDING HELP

The first step in finding treatment often involves making lots of telephone calls. Call your family doctor, the local medical or psychological society, the library, and the mental-health association. Look in the telephone book under such categories as dietitians, hospitals, eating disorders, anorexia, and bulimia for promising listings. Check the facilities listed in the directory section of this book. Try the counseling department at local colleges and high schools. Call women's organizations, parent clubs and physician referral services. Check with the national organizations listed in this book, as well as the psychiatric departments at local hospitals. Ask each of them, "What facilities provide treatment for eating disorders?" Over time you will begin to hear the same names repeated, and that will help you narrow your search. Set aside some time to gather information and take notes. Don't get discouraged because you keep getting referred elsewhere or you get transferred several times on one call. When you find someone who can answer your questions, make a note of the person's name and ask for a direct phone number.

Although major cities have many programs and resources from which to choose, small towns and rural areas will, of course, have fewer. It is important to evaluate options based on both geographic availability and quality of treatment. Driving farther to get better treatment will pay off in the long run. On the other hand, great distances can present obstacles to length of treatment as well as family involvement. Sometimes, particularly when inpatient treatment is needed, a less specialized program close enough to provide aftercare and family therapy will work better than a more specialized program farther away. However, some patients who are very ill or having a hard time getting better may benefit from traveling farther to a better program.

In the last few years, insurance providers have become increasingly involved in making treatment decisions. Most managed care companies limit what treatment is available and who can provide it. When contacting the insurance carrier involved, it is helpful to already have some information about what is needed and what is available in the area. Calls to insurance companies sometimes lead into a maze of voice mail messages, making it important to persevere until finding a human being. If the person you reach cannot answer questions adequately, ask for someone who can. Often a company will assign a "case manager" who then becomes an advocate for the individual in negotiating the red tape.

If you are already working through a family doctor or psychiatrist, there may be an insurance coordinator in the doctor's office who can help, especially with names and phone numbers of specific resource people at the insurance company.

If your insurance provider refuses to cover eating-disorder treatment, check with your state's insurance board to see if the insurance company can legally deny coverage for a specific diagnosis. Sometimes a company will cover treatment

if the eating disorder is a secondary diagnosis, with a primary diagnosis of depression, anxiety, or some other mental disability. If all else fails, contact the human resources department of the employer who provides the insurance. Employers offer health insurance so that their employees and families can get the care they need. If this isn't happening, the employer may wish to know that.

Choosing treatment for an eating disorder is an important decision. The investment in time and energy to evaluate all the options will pay off in, it is hoped, a satisfactory resolution of the problem.

PART 6
Facilities and
Selected Resources

Leigh Cohn, Section Editor

Directory of Facilities and Programs

This directory lists inpatient and residential treatment facilities and programs for which questionnaires have been returned from April to August of 1998. All information has been supplied by personnel from the program or facility. This is not a comprehensive list of all eating-disorder programs, nor is it a list of recommended facilities; rather, it is meant to provide a starting point. Check with a therapist or other local health professional who is knowledgeable about eating disorders for further recommendations; many colleges and universities provide eating-disorders therapy in connection with student health centers. Also check with the national organizations listed in the "Nonprofit Eating Disorders Organizations" in this book, some of which can provide referral lists of programs and professionals.

Abbreviations

BED Binge Eating Disorder
ED Eating Disorders
IOP Intensive Outpatient
NOS Not Otherwise Specified
PTSD Post-Traumatic Stress Disorder

ARIZONA

Prescott

1. Pia's Place
615 Hillside Ave
Prescott, AZ 86301
Contact: Gay Chatfield. 520-445-5081, *fax:* 520-445-0395
Internet: http://piasplace.prescott-az.com/
Date Established: 1994.
Disorders treated: Anorexia nervosa; Bulimia nervosa; Compulsive eating (or BED); Obesity.
Population treated: Women only; Adults.
Programs: Residential or Day-Hospital; Intensive outpatient.
Treatments: Individual therapy; Group therapy; Family therapy; Family groups; Addiction model; Experimental therapy; Medication; Body image; Nutrition counseling; 12-Step.
Treatment setting: Outpatient facility.
Program cost: $2900/mo.
Average length of program: 90 days.
Maximum patients in program: 24.
Average number served per year: 122.

Scottsdale

2. Psychological Pathways
3260 N Hayden Rd, Ste 106
Scottsdale, AZ 85251
Contact: Ray Lemberg, PhD, Dir. (602) 994-9773, *fax:* (602) 994-9785
Date Established: 1983.
Disorders treated: Anorexia nervosa; Bulimia nervosa; Compulsive eating (or BED); Obesity.
Population treated: Adolescents; Young children; Adults.
Programs: Outpatient; Support groups.
Treatments: Individual therapy; Group therapy; Family therapy; Nutrition counseling; Medication.
Average number served per year: 300.
Comments: Multidisciplinary group practice with locations in Scottsdale, Mesa, and Prescott.

3. Willow Creek Eating Disorders Program at Samaritan Behavioral Health Center— Scottsdale
7575 E Earl Dr
Scottsdale, AZ 85251
Contact: Jay L Lewis, PhD. 602-941-7555 *Facility phone:* 602-254-HELP
Date Established: 1990.
Disorders treated: Anorexia nervosa; Bulimia nervosa; Compulsive eating (or BED); Obesity.
Population treated: Women & men; Adolescents.
Programs: Inpatient; Partial hospitalization; Residential or Day-Hospital; Community education programs; Support groups; Follow-up programs.
Treatments: Individual therapy; Group therapy; Family therapy; Family groups; Medication; Body image; Nutrition counseling; Exercise.
Treatment setting: Hospital.
Program cost: $900 inpatient; $300/day for day treatment.
Maximum patients in program: 12.
Follow-up care offered: Followed on outpatient basis by therapists, psychiatrist and nutritionists.

Tucson

4. Life Force LLC

2421 E 6th St
Tucson, AZ 85719
Mailing Address
PO Box 35847
Tucson, AZ 85740-5847
Contact: Cheryl Toner, PhD, CEDS, CPC, ACH. 520-323-3734, *fax:* 520-760-5580, *e-mail:* twofeathers@gci-net.com
Internet: http://jrust@edrecovery.com
Hotline: 800-495-1884
Date Established: 1995.
Disorders treated: Anorexia nervosa; Bulimia nervosa; Compulsive eating (or BED); Obesity; Trauma; Substance abuse.
Population treated: Women & men; Adolescents; College.
Programs: Residential or Day-Hospital; Outpatient; Clinical studies; Community education programs; Intensive outpatient; Support groups; Follow-up programs; Will open 2-wk intensive inpatient lectures and training.
Treatments: Individual therapy; Group therapy; Family therapy; Family groups; Experimental therapy; Body image; Nutrition counseling; Exercise; Biofeedback; Hypnotherapy; Spirituality; Meditation; Guided imagery; Yoga; Tai Chi; Qui Gong; Mandala work.
Treatment setting: Therapist's office.
Average number served per year: 100.
Follow-up care offered: E-mail questionnaires sent.

5. Sierra Tucson

16500 N Lago del Oro Pkwy
Tucson, AZ 85739
Contact: Gail Richtor; Vicki Berkus, MD, PhD. 800-624-9001, *fax:* 520-792-5806, *e-mail:* keppiebog@aol.com
Internet: http://www.sierratucson.com
Date Established: 1988.
Disorders treated: Anorexia nervosa; Bulimia nervosa; Compulsive eating (or BED); Obesity.
Population treated: Adults.
Programs: Inpatient.
Treatments: Individual therapy; Group therapy; Family therapy; Family groups; Addiction model; Experimental therapy; Medication; Body image; Nutrition counseling; 12-Step; Exercise.
Treatment setting: Hospital.
Average length of program: Optimum 30 days.
Maximum patients in program: 62.
Follow-up care offered: 3 mos; 6 mos; 1 yr.

Wickenburg

6. The Meadows

1655 N Tegner
Wickenburg, AZ 85390
Contact: Carole Ryan, RD. 520-684-3926 *Facility phone:* 800-621-4062, *Facility fax:* 520-684-3935
Disorders treated: Anorexia nervosa; Bulimia nervosa; Compulsive eating (or BED); Obesity.
Population treated: Adults.
Programs: Inpatient.

Treatments: Individual therapy; Group therapy; Family therapy; Family groups; Addiction model; Experimental therapy; Medication; Body image; Nutrition counseling; 12-Step; Exercise.
Treatment setting: Hospital.
Program cost: $31,450.
Average length of program: 5 wks open-ended.
Maximum patients in program: 20.
Average number served per year: 380.
Comments: Dual diagnosis facility; addictions, psych eating disorders treated together.

7. Remuda Ranch Programs for Anorexia and Bulimia

One E Apache
Wickenburg, AZ 85390
Contact: Drema Stroud. *Facility phone:* 800-455-1900, *Facility fax:* 520-684-7903, *e-mail:* remuda@good-net.com
Internet: http://www.remuda-ranch.com
Hotline: 800-445-1900
Date Established: 1990.
Disorders treated: Anorexia nervosa; Bulimia nervosa.
Population treated: Women only; Adolescents.
Programs: Inpatient; Partial hospitalization; Residential or Day-Hospital; Outpatient; Community education programs; Intensive outpatient; Support groups; Follow-up programs.
Treatments: Individual therapy; Group therapy; Family therapy; Family groups; Addiction model; Experimental therapy; Medication; Body image; Nutrition counseling; Christian-based; Exercise; Art therapy; Equine therapy.
Treatment setting: Hospital.
Program cost: Sliding scale.
Average length of program: 45 days adult; 60 days adolescent.
Maximum patients in program: 110.
Average number served per year: 681.
Follow-up care offered: 10 days; 30 days; 3, 6, 12, and 24 mos.

8. Rosewood Women's Center for Anorexia, Bulimia, and Related Disorders

36075 S Rincon Rd
Wickenburg, AZ 85390
Contact: Priscilla Bolin. 800-280-1212, *fax:* 423-769-2511 *Facility phone:* 877-4-WOMEN, *Facility fax:* 520-684-9562
Date Established: July 1998.
Disorders treated: Anorexia nervosa; Bulimia nervosa; Compulsive eating (or BED); Substance abuse; PTSD; trauma; panic disorders; anxiety disorders.
Population treated: Women only.
Programs: Inpatient; Community education programs; Female athletes with eating disorders: prevention, intervention, and treatment programs (athlete assistance model).
Treatments: Individual therapy; Group therapy; Family therapy; Family groups; Experimental therapy; Medication; Body image; Nutrition counseling; 12-Step; Exercise; "A Woman's Way through the 12 Steps".
Maximum patients in program: 14.

ARKANSAS
Little Rock
9. Arkansas Children's Hospital, University of Arkansas Medical Sciences
800 Marshall, Ste 512
Little Rock, AR 72202
Contact: Jane A Fitzgerald, PhD. 501-320-4065, *fax:* 501-320-4068
Date Established: 1992.
Disorders treated: Anorexia nervosa; Bulimia nervosa; Compulsive eating (or BED); Obesity.
Population treated: Adolescents; Young children.
Programs: Inpatient; Outpatient; Support groups.
Treatments: Individual therapy; Group therapy; Family therapy; Family groups; Experimental therapy; Medication; Body image; Nutrition counseling.
Treatment setting: Hospital.
Program cost: $600-$800/mo for wkly individual and group therapy.
Maximum patients in program: 25-30.

CALIFORNIA
Greenbrae
10. Anorexia/Bulimia Group of Marin
112 Bretano Way
Greenbrae, CA 94904
Contact: Dr. Lou Rappaport. 415-461-3211, *fax:* 415-561-9156, *e-mail:* CAJAL@aol.com
Date Established: 1983.
Disorders treated: Anorexia nervosa; Bulimia nervosa; Compulsive eating (or BED); Obesity.
Population treated: Women & men; Adolescents; Young children.
Programs: Partial hospitalization; Outpatient; Community education programs; Support groups.
Treatments: Individual therapy; Group therapy; Family therapy; Addiction model; Medication; Body image; Nutrition counseling; Exercise.
Treatment setting: Therapist's office.
Program cost: $120 individual session; group is free.
Maximum patients in program: 20.
Average number served per year: 63.
Follow-up care offered: 3 mo; 6 mo; 2 yrs.

Los Angeles
11. Rader Programs Inc
12099 W Washington Blvd, Ste 204
Los Angeles, CA 90066
Contact: Andrea James. 800-841-1515, *fax:* 310-391-6259, *e-mail:* rader@raderpro.com *Facility phone:* 310-390-9979
Internet: http://www.raderpro.com
Hotline: 800-255-1818
Date Established: 1978.
Disorders treated: Anorexia nervosa; Bulimia nervosa; Compulsive eating (or BED); Obesity; Sexual abuse.
Population treated: Women & men; Adolescents.

Programs: Inpatient; Partial hospitalization; Residential or Day-Hospital; Community education programs; Follow-up programs.
Treatments: Individual therapy; Group therapy; Family therapy; Family groups; Addiction model; Experimental therapy; Medication; Body image; Nutrition counseling; 12-Step; Exercise.
Treatment setting: Hospital.
Maximum patients in program: 16.
Average number served per year: 300.
Follow-up care offered: 6 mos; 1 yr; 2 yrs; 5 yrs.

12. UCLA Neuropsychiatric Hospital Eating Disorders Clinic
UCLA Neuropsychiatric Institute 760 Westwood Plaza
Los Angeles, CA 90024-1759
Contact: Michael Strober. 310-825-5730, *fax:* 310-825-2982, *e-mail:* MStrober@Mednet.ucla.edu
Date Established: 1961.
Disorders treated: Anorexia nervosa; Bulimia nervosa.
Population treated: Women & men; Adults; Adolescents.
Programs: Inpatient; Partial hospitalization; Residential or Day-Hospital; Clinical studies; Intensive outpatient.
Treatments: Individual therapy; Group therapy; Family therapy; Family groups; Experimental therapy; Medication; Nutrition counseling.
Treatment setting: Hospital.
Program cost: $875/day inpatient; $450/day hospital; $220/wk outpatient.
Maximum patients in program: 30.
Average number served per year: 60.
Follow-up care offered: Every 6 mos.

Malibu
13. Monte Nido Residential Treatment Center
27162 Sea Vista Dr
Malibu, CA 90265
Contact: Carolyn Costin. 310-457-9958, *fax:* 310-457-8442, *e-mail:* mntc@idt.net *Facility phone:* 818-222-9534, *Facility fax:* 818-222-3818
Internet: http://www.montenido.com
Date Established: 1996.
Disorders treated: Anorexia nervosa; Bulimia nervosa; Compulsive exercise.
Population treated: Women only; Adults.
Programs: Residential or Day-Hospital; Outpatient; Community education programs; Intensive outpatient; Support groups; Follow-up programs.
Treatments: Individual therapy; Group therapy; Family therapy; Family groups; Experimental therapy; Medication; Body image; Nutrition counseling; Exercise; Cognitive behavioral groups.
Treatment setting: Therapist's office; Residential treatment.
Program cost: $650/day.
Average length of program: 1-6 mos.
Maximum patients in program: 12.
Average number served per year: 39.
Follow-up care offered: With newsletters and alumni group.

Comments: Has a level system which accommodates clients in various stages of treatment; clients start out being served meals or supplements and monitored carefully and gradually out to level four, in which they shop and cook and exercise on their own. Graduates may be approved to continue in program's transitional home.

Northridge

14. The Pathfinder Center

8941 Balvoa Blvd
Northridge, CA 91325
Contact: Jason Scura. 800-785-0883, *fax:* 818-708 9100
Facility phone: 818-885-0883
Date Established: 1993.
Disorders treated: Anorexia nervosa; Bulimia nervosa; Compulsive eating (or BED); Obesity.
Population treated: Adults.
Programs: Inpatient; Partial hospitalization; Residential or Day-Hospital; Outpatient; Intensive outpatient.
Treatments: Individual therapy; Group therapy; Family therapy; Body image; Nutrition counseling; 12-Step; Exercise; Music therapy.
Treatment setting: Inpatient residential.
Program cost: $15,000/mo.
Average length of program: 2-6 mos.
Maximum patients in program: 6-8.
Average number served per year: 50.
Follow-up care offered: Every 3 mos by return visits or telephone.

Palo Alto

15. Packard Children's Hospital at Stanford Eating Disorders Program for Children and Adolescents

750 Welch Rd, Ste 325
Palo Alto, CA 94304
Contact: Seth David Ammerman, MD. 650-725-8293, *fax:* 650-725-8347, *e-mail:* sethamm@sj.bigger.net
Internet: http://www-med.stanford.edu/school/pediatric
Date Established: 1979.
Disorders treated: Anorexia nervosa; Bulimia nervosa; Compulsive eating (or BED); Obesity; Atypical eating disorders.
Population treated: Adolescents; Young children.
Programs: Inpatient; Partial hospitalization; Outpatient.
Treatments: Individual therapy; Group therapy; Family therapy; Medication; Nutrition counseling.
Treatment setting: Hospital.
Maximum patients in program: 12 inpatient; 8 partial.
Average number served per year: Approx 100.
Follow-up care offered: Medical and psychosocial through various research projects and clinical pathways.

San Bernardino

16. Kaiser Permanente

325 W Hospitality Ln
San Bernardino, CA 92408
Contact: May E Moore, PhD. 909-386-5503, *fax:* 909-386-5520
Date Established: 1997.
Disorders treated: Anorexia nervosa; Bulimia nervosa.

Population treated: Women & men; Adolescents.
Programs: Inpatient; Outpatient; Support groups; Individual psychotherpy.
Treatments: Individual therapy; Group therapy; Family therapy; Family groups; Medication; Body image; Nutrition counseling; Exercise.
Treatment setting: Hospital; Therapist's office; Pediatric clinic.
Average length of program: 10-wk educational group.
Follow-up care offered: Wkly or as needed.

San Diego

17. Teen Eating Disorder Solutions

9040 Friars Rd, Ste 400
San Diego, CA 92108
Contact: Trish Stanley, MS, MFCC. 619-455-5557, *fax:* 619-455-6780
Date Established: 1998.
Disorders treated: Anorexia nervosa; Bulimia nervosa; Compulsive eating (or BED); Dual diagnosis; Anxiety and mood disorder.
Population treated: Adolescents.
Programs: Inpatient; Residential or Day-Hospital; Outpatient; Community education programs; Intensive outpatient; Support groups; Follow-up programs.
Comments: Integrated, collaborative, multicomponent nonprofit treatment program, partnered with a free-standing nonprofit psychiatric hospital for inpatient and day hospital.

Stanford

18. Stanford University Medical Center—Eating Disorders Program

Department of Psychaitry and Behavioral Sciences, 401 Quarry Rd
Stanford, CA 94305
Contact: Intake Service. 650-498-9111
Date Established: 1975.
Disorders treated: Anorexia nervosa; Bulimia nervosa; Compulsive eating (or BED); Obesity.
Population treated: Adults; Adolescents.
Programs: Inpatient; Partial hospitalization; Outpatient; Clinical studies.
Treatments: Individual therapy; Group therapy; Medication.
Treatment setting: Hospital; Therapist's office.
Average length of program: Average outpatient 20 wks.
Average number served per year: 150.
Follow-up care offered: Conducted as needed.

COLORADO

Florence

19. Clearview of Colorado

521 West 5th
Florence, CO 81226
Contact: Deb Hadley. 719-784-6337, *fax:* 719-784-6337
Date Established: 1988.
Disorders treated: Anorexia nervosa; Bulimia nervosa; Compulsive eating (or BED).
Population treated: Women only; Adults.

Programs: Inpatient; Residential or Day-Hospital.
Treatments: Individual therapy; Group therapy; Family therapy; Addiction model; Medication; Body image; Nutrition counseling; 12-Step; Christian-based.
Treatment setting: Hospital owned but is a free-standing facility.
Program cost: $205/day.
Average length of program: 60-90 days.
Maximum patients in program: 12.
Average number served per year: 40.
Follow-up care offered: 6 mos; 12 mos; 18 mos.

CONNECTICUT

Greenwich

20. Wilkins Center for Eating Disorders

7 Riverside Rd
Greenwich, CT 06903
Contact: Annita Kahm. 203-968-0860, *fax:* 203-329-0589, *e-mail:* AKahm@aol.com *Facility phone:* 203-531-1909
Date Established: 1973.
Disorders treated: Anorexia nervosa; Bulimia nervosa; Compulsive eating (or BED); Obesity.
Population treated: Women & men; Adolescents; Young children.
Programs: Inpatient; Partial hospitalization; Residential or Day-Hospital; Follow-up programs; Intensive outpatient.
Treatments: Individual therapy; Group therapy; Family therapy; Medication; Nutrition counseling.
Treatment setting: Therapist's office; Medical office.
Program cost: Nutritional counseling $60-$150/hr.
Maximum patients in program: 25.
Average number served per year: 100.
Comments: Multi-modal team approach.

Hartford

21. Institute of Living, Eating Disorders Program

400 Washington St
Hartford, CT 06106
Contact: Margo Maine, PhD or Robert Weinstein, PhD. 860-545-7203, *fax:* 860-545-7253, *e-mail:* MMaine@HARTHOSP.org *Facility phone:* 860-545-7200
Date Established: 1985.
Disorders treated: Anorexia nervosa; Bulimia nervosa; Compulsive eating (or BED).
Population treated: Women & men; Adolescents; Young children.
Programs: Inpatient; Partial hospitalization; Residential or Day-Hospital; Outpatient; Community education programs; Intensive outpatient; Support groups; Follow-up programs.
Treatments: Individual therapy; Group therapy; Family therapy; Family groups; Experimental therapy; Medication; Body image; Nutrition counseling.
Treatment setting: Hospital.
Maximum patients in program: 25.
Average number served per year: 250.

New Canaan

22. Silver Hill Hospital

208 Valley Rd
New Canaan, CT 06840
Contact: Anne Cassidy Dir of Admissions. 203-966-3561, *fax:* 203-966-1075, *e-mail:* info@silverhillhospital.com
Internet: http://www.silverhilllhospital.com
Disorders treated: Anorexia nervosa; Bulimia nervosa.
Population treated: Women & men; Adolescents.
Programs: Inpatient; Partial hospitalization; Residential or Day-Hospital; Outpatient; Community education programs; Intensive outpatient.
Treatments: Individual therapy; Group therapy; Family therapy; Experimental therapy; Medication; Body image; Nutrition counseling; Exercise.
Treatment setting: Hospital.
Maximum patients in program: 30.
Comments: Silver Hill is a nonprofit psychiatric hospital; able to treat patients with dual diagnosis.

DISTRICT OF COLUMBIA

23. Children's National Medical Center

4900 Massachusetts Ave NW
Washington, DC 2
Contact: Darlene M Atkins, PhD. 202-884-2164, *fax:* 202-745-4112
Date Established: 1970.
Disorders treated: Anorexia nervosa; Bulimia nervosa; Compulsive eating (or BED); Obesity.
Population treated: Adolescents; Young children; Ages 10-19.
Programs: Partial hospitalization; Residential or Day-Hospital; Outpatient; Intensive outpatient; Support groups.
Treatments: Individual therapy; Group therapy; Family therapy; Medication; Nutrition counseling; Medical evaluation and treatment by Eating Disorders specialist.
Treatment setting: Hospital; Outpatient satellite office.
Average number served per year: 100+.
Follow-up care offered: Yes.

24. The Donald Delaney Eating Disorders Program of Children's National Medical Center

111 Michigan Ave NW
Washington, DC 20010
Contact: Dr Darlene Atkins or Dr Thomas Siber. 202-884-3066, *fax:* 202-884-3630, *e-mail:* TSilber@cnmc.org
Facility phone: 202-884-2164
Date Established: 1974.
Disorders treated: Anorexia nervosa; Bulimia nervosa.
Population treated: Adolescents; Young children.
Programs: Inpatient; Partial hospitalization; Residential or Day-Hospital; Outpatient; Support groups.
Treatments: Individual therapy; Group therapy; Family therapy; Experimental therapy; Medication; Nutrition counseling.
Treatment setting: Hospital; Therapist's office; Outpatient program.

Average length of program: 1-6 wks inpatient; 1-7 yrs outpatient.
Average number served per year: 96.

FLORIDA

Clearwater

25. Fairwinds Treatment Center

1569 S Ft Harrison
Clearwater, FL 33756
Contact: Sandi Brown. 813-449-0300, *fax:* 813-446-0200
Date Established: 1998.
Disorders treated: Anorexia nervosa; Bulimia nervosa; Obesity.
Population treated: Women & men; Adolescents.
Programs: Inpatient; Outpatient; Community education programs; Support groups.
Treatments: Individual therapy; Group therapy; Family therapy; Family groups; Addiction model; Medication; Body image; Nutrition counseling; 12-Step; Exercise.
Treatment setting: Therapist's office; School.
Maximum patients in program: 30.

26. Windmoor Healthcare of Clearwater

11300 US 19 N
Clearwater, FL 34624
Contact: Beverly Pizzano. 888-834-9246, *fax:* 813-321-0832 *Facility phone:* 813-541-2646, *Facility fax:* 813-541-3163
Hotline: 888-834-2946
Disorders treated: Anorexia nervosa; Bulimia nervosa; Compulsive eating (or BED); Obesity.
Population treated: Women & men; Adults.
Programs: Inpatient; Outpatient; Community education programs; Support groups.
Treatments: Individual therapy; Group therapy; Family groups; Addiction model; Medication; Body image; 12-Step.
Treatment setting: Hospital.
Maximum patients in program: 163 beds in hospital; 10 women's program.
Average number served per year: 823.
Comments: In the process of developing specific education unit. Currently have women's program, dual diagnosis, crisis stabilization, and elder unit.

Coconut Creek

27. The Renfrew Center

7700 Renfrew Ln
Coconut Creek, FL 33073
Contact: Donna Vitz. 800-332-8415, *fax:* 954-698-9007, *e-mail:* inquiries@renfrew.org
Internet: http://www.renfrew.org
Date Established: 1990.
Disorders treated: Anorexia nervosa; Bulimia nervosa; Compulsive eating (or BED).
Population treated: Females 14 years old and up.
Programs: Inpatient; Partial hospitalization; Residential or Day-Hospital; Outpatient; Clinical studies; Community education programs; Intensive outpatient; Support groups; Follow-up programs.

Treatments: Individual therapy; Group therapy; Family therapy; Family groups; Experimental therapy; Medication; Body image; Nutrition counseling; Exercise.
Maximum patients in program: Inpatient 42.
Average number served per year: 275.
Follow-up care offered: Conducted via research surveys.

Fort Myers

28. Columbia Gulf Coast Hospital/No More Diets

13681 Doctor's Way
Fort Myers, FL 33905
Contact: Laurel Savoy, MS, RD, LD. 941-768-8441
Date Established: 1996.
Disorders treated: Anorexia nervosa; Bulimia nervosa; Compulsive eating (or BED); Obesity.
Population treated: Women & men; Adolescents; Young children.
Programs: Inpatient; Outpatient; Community education programs; Support groups.
Treatments: Individual therapy; Family therapy; Family groups; Body image; 12-Step; Exercise.
Treatment setting: Hospital; Therapist's office.
Program cost: Classes $10-15/session; Individual $54 initial, $27 followup, 1-4 visits.
Average length of program: 10-15 sessions.
Maximum patients in program: 30.
Average number served per year: 40.

Naples

29. The Willough at Naples

9001 Tamiami Trail E
Naples, FL 33413
Contact: Margaret Allen. 941-775-4500, *fax:* 941-775-6488, *e-mail:* willough1@aol.com
Date Established: 1983.
Disorders treated: Anorexia nervosa; Bulimia nervosa; Compulsive eating (or BED); Obesity; Addictions.
Population treated: Women & men; Adults.
Programs: Inpatient; Partial hospitalization; Residential or Day-Hospital; Outpatient; Community education programs; Intensive outpatient; Support groups; Follow-up programs.
Treatments: Individual therapy; Group therapy; Family therapy; Family groups; Addiction model; Experimental therapy; Medication; Body image; Nutrition counseling; 12-Step; Christian-based; Exercise.
Treatment setting: Hospital.
Average number served per year: 830.
Follow-up care offered: Through contact with Dr. Walter Kay.

North Miami

30. American Family Counseling Tract III

19501 NE 10th Ave, Ste 305
North Miami, FL 33179
Contact: Deborah Saland, PsyD, CCSW. 305-653-1716, *fax:* 305-653-7040 *Facility phone:* 954-653-9842
Hotline: 954-772-9842
Date Established: 1997.

Disorders treated: Anorexia nervosa; Bulimia nervosa; Compulsive eating (or BED); Obesity.
Population treated: Women & men; Adults; Adolescents.
Programs: Partial hospitalization; Residential or Day-Hospital; Outpatient; Intensive outpatient; Support groups; Follow-up programs.
Treatments: Individual therapy; Group therapy; Family therapy; Family groups; Experimental therapy; Medication; Body image; Nutrition counseling; 12-Step; Blending of addiction model with psychodynamic.
Treatment setting: Therapist's office; Clinic.
Program cost: $2550/wk.
Maximum patients in program: 30.
Average number served per year: 50.
Follow-up care offered: Aftercare group 1 x/wk with individual therapy as needed.

North Miami Beach
31. Institute for Human Potential
19501 NE 10th Ave, Ste 305
North Miami Beach, FL 33179
Contact: Dr. Deborah Saland. 305-653-1716, *fax:* 305-653-7040
Date Established: 1997.
Disorders treated: Anorexia nervosa; Bulimia nervosa; Compulsive eating (or BED); Obesity; Trauma.
Population treated: Women & men; Adults.
Programs: Inpatient; Partial hospitalization; Residential or Day-Hospital; Outpatient; Intensive outpatient; Support groups; Follow-up programs.
Treatments: Individual therapy; Group therapy; Family therapy; Addiction model; Experimental therapy; Medication; Body image; Nutrition counseling.
Treatment setting: Hospital; Therapist's office.
Program cost: $1500/week.
Maximum patients in program: 25.
Average number served per year: 60.
Follow-up care offered: Survey.

Tallahassee
32. Canopy Cove Residential Day Treatment
2300 Killearn Center Blvd
Tallahassee, FL 32308
Contact: Lisa McLoughlin, EdS, MS. 800-236-7524, *fax:* 850-893-6994, *e-mail:* labrogdon@nettally.com
Internet: http://www.canopycove.com
Hotline: 800-236-7524
Date Established: 1992.
Disorders treated: Anorexia nervosa; Bulimia nervosa; Compulsive eating (or BED); Obesity; Eating disorders with diabetes.
Population treated: Women & men; Adolescents; Young children; College.
Programs: Residential or Day-Hospital; Outpatient; Community education programs; Intensive outpatient; Support groups; Follow-up programs; Meal groups.
Treatments: Individual therapy; Group therapy; Family therapy; Experimental therapy; Medication; Body image; Nutrition counseling; Recovery model.
Treatment setting: Therapist's office; Treatment center.
Program cost: $8600 day treatment; $1410 residential.

Average length of program: Minimum 4 wk stay.
Maximum patients in program: 10.
Average number served per year: 75.
Follow-up care offered: Phone contact, questionnaire at 3, 6, 9, 12 mos.

Tampa
33. Hyde Park Counseling Center
207 Verne St
Tampa, FL 33606
Contact: Fred Hill. 813-258-4605, *fax:* 813-258-4705, *e-mail:* HYDEPARK@aol.com
Hotline: 888-869-4367
Date Established: 1996.
Disorders treated: Anorexia nervosa; Bulimia nervosa.
Population treated: Women only.
Programs: Inpatient; Partial hospitalization; Residential or Day-Hospital; Outpatient; Intensive outpatient; Support groups; Male population on outpatient only.
Treatments: Individual therapy; Group therapy; Family therapy; Family groups; Addiction model; Experimental therapy; Body image; Nutrition counseling; 12-Step; Exercise.
Program cost: $4,260 1st mo, phase I (30 days); $3,000 each additional mo; cost includes therapy, food, and lodging.
Maximum patients in program: 17.
Average number served per year: 54.

34. Turning Point of Tampa Florida
5439 Beaumont Center Blvd Ste 1010
Tampa, FL 33634
Contact: Robin Piper and Dr. Daisy DeGamuza. 813-882-3003, *fax:* 813-885-6974, *e-mail:* tpotampa@aol.com *Facility phone:* 800-397-3006
Date Established: 1987.
Disorders treated: Anorexia nervosa; Bulimia nervosa; Compulsive eating (or BED); Obesity.
Population treated: Women & men; Adults.
Programs: Residential or Day-Hospital; Intensive outpatient; Support groups; Follow-up programs; Drug and alcohol addictions.
Treatments: Group therapy; Family therapy; Family groups; Addiction model; Experimental therapy; Medication; Body image; Nutrition counseling; 12-Step; Exercise; AA, NA, Codep, and OA meetings; Individual therapy.
Treatment setting: Therapist's office; Residential treatment center; Halfway house.
Average length of program: 30 days; 60 days; 90 days.
Maximum patients in program: 8-12 ED; 30-40 combined CD and ED.
Average number served per year: Approx 45 ED and 250 combined CD and ED.

35. University of South Florida Eating Disorders Program
3515 E Fletcher Ave
Tampa, FL 33613
Contact: Sherry McKnight. (813) 974-2926, *fax:* (813) 974-3223, *e-mail:* SMcKnigh@com1.med.usf.edu

Facility phone: (813) 974-8900
Date Established: 1978.
Disorders treated: Anorexia nervosa; Bulimia nervosa; Compulsive eating (or BED); Obesity.
Population treated: Women & men; Adolescents; Young children.
Programs: Inpatient; Residential or Day-Hospital; Outpatient.
Treatments: Individual therapy; Group therapy; Family therapy; Medication; Body image; Nutrition counseling.
Treatment setting: Hospital; Therapist's office.
Maximum patients in program: 50.
Average number served per year: 100.
Follow-up care offered: Conducted either by phone or in person.

GEORGIA

Atlanta

36. Atlanta Center for Eating Disorders

2300 Peachford Rd, Ste 2010
Atlanta, GA 30338
Contact: Dr. Linda Buchanan or Dr. Rick Kilmer. 770-458-8711, *fax:* 770-458-8640
Date Established: 1994.
Disorders treated: Anorexia nervosa; Bulimia nervosa; Compulsive eating (or BED); Obesity; Anxiety disorders.
Population treated: Women & men; Adolescents; Young children.
Programs: Outpatient; Partial hospitalization; Clinical studies; Community education programs; Intensive outpatient; Support groups; Follow-up programs.
Treatments: Individual therapy; Group therapy; Family therapy; Family groups; Experimental therapy; Body image; Nutrition counseling.
Treatment setting: Center.
Program cost: PHP $250/day; IOP and individual $180/day.
Average length of program: Up to 8hrs/day.
Maximum patients in program: 30.
Average number served per year: 100.
Follow-up care offered: Conducted at discharge only.

Smyrna

37. Ridgeview Institute—Women's Center

3995 S Cobb Dr
Smyrna, GA 30080
Contact: Sandie Clarck, LCSW. 770-431-8200, *fax:* 770-434-5136 *Facility phone:* 770-434-4567
Date Established: 1986.
Disorders treated: Anorexia nervosa; Bulimia nervosa; Compulsive eating (or BED); Obesity.
Population treated: Women only; Adolescents.
Programs: Inpatient; Partial hospitalization; Residential or Day-Hospital; Outpatient; Community education programs; Intensive outpatient; Support groups.
Treatments: Individual therapy; Group therapy; Family therapy; Family groups; Medication; Body image; Nutrition counseling.
Treatment setting: Hospital; Therapist's office.
Follow-up care offered: 3 and 6 mos.

HAWAII

Aiea

38. Kali Mohala Specialty Hospital

Aiea, HI 96701
Contact: Kristen Linsey-Dudley RD, MPH. 808-671-8511
Facility phone: 800-999-8899
Date Established: 1987.
Disorders treated: Anorexia nervosa; Bulimia nervosa; Compulsive eating (or BED); Obesity.
Population treated: Women & men; Adolescents; Young children.
Programs: Inpatient; Partial hospitalization; Residential or Day-Hospital; Support groups; Follow-up programs.
Treatments: Individual therapy; Group therapy; Family therapy; Family groups; Medication; Body image; Nutrition counseling; Exercise.
Treatment setting: Hospital.
Average length of program: 1 wk inpatient; 3 wks partial.
Maximum patients in program: 10.
Average number served per year: 50.
Comments: Focus is short-term hospitalization to partial hospital, then intensive outpatient. Works in conjunction with eating-disorders clinic with the same approach and overlapping staff.

Honolulu

39. Kapiolani Counseling Center, Eating Disorders Program

1319 Punahou St, 6th Floor
Honolulu, HI 96826
Contact: Neal Anzai, MD, Kristen Lindsey-Dudley, RD, MPH. 808-983-8368, *fax:* 808-983-8629
Date Established: 1986.
Disorders treated: Anorexia nervosa; Bulimia nervosa; Compulsive eating (or BED).
Population treated: Women & men; Adults; Adolescents; Young children; College.
Programs: Inpatient; Outpatient; Community education programs; Intensive outpatient; Support groups; Follow-up programs; Intensive nutrition services (individual & group) package.
Treatments: Individual therapy; Group therapy; Family therapy; Family groups; Experimental therapy; Medication; Body image; Nutrition counseling; Nutrition groups; Psycho-educational groups for patient & family.
Treatment setting: Hospital; Therapist's office.
Average length of program: 6 mos-5 yrs outpatient treatment.
Maximum patients in program: 200.
Average number served per year: 200+.
Follow-up care offered: Follow-ups after completion of program on case-by-case basis.

ILLINOIS

Centralia

40. St. Mary's Hospital

400 N Pleasant Ave
Centralia, IL 62801

Contact: Dr Natalie Alsop. 618-532-6731 ext 5665, *fax:* 618-532-6739
Date Established: 1997.
Disorders treated: Anorexia nervosa; Bulimia nervosa; Obesity.
Population treated: Women & men; Adolescents; Young children.
Programs: Partial hospitalization; Outpatient; Community education programs; Support groups.
Treatments: Individual therapy; Group therapy; Family therapy; Family groups; Medication; Body image; Nutrition counseling.
Treatment setting: Hospital; Therapist's office.
Average length of program: 8-wk structured group therapy; individual and family therapy duration as needed.

Chicago

41. Rush—Presbyterian—St. Luke's Eating Disorder Program

1653 W Congress Pkwy
Chicago, IL 60612
Contact: Dr John Mead or Dr Gary Strokosch. 312-942-6656, *fax:* 312-733-0263, *e-mail:* gstrokosch@aol.com
Hotline: 312-942-3034 (answering service)
Date Established: 1987.
Disorders treated: Anorexia nervosa; Bulimia nervosa.
Population treated: Women & men; Adults; Adolescents; Young children; College.
Programs: Inpatient; Outpatient; Clinical studies; Community education programs; Follow-up programs.
Treatments: Individual therapy; Family therapy; Experimental therapy; Medication; Body image; Nutrition counseling; Exercise.
Treatment setting: Hospital; Therapist's office.
Average number served per year: 100.
Follow-up care offered: Outpatient therapy/phone follow-up.

Elk Grove Village

42. Alexian Brothers Medical Center

800 Biesterfield
Elk Grove Village, IL 60007
Contact: John L Levitt, PhD. 847-437-5500 ext 4017, *fax:* 847-228-5566, *e-mail:* JLevitt334@aol.com
Internet: http://www.alexian.org/
Hotline: 800-432-5005
Date Established: 1992.
Disorders treated: Anorexia nervosa; Bulimia nervosa; Compulsive eating (or BED); Obesity; Traumatic disorders; Self-injury; Dual diagnosis.
Population treated: Women & men; Adolescents; Young children.
Programs: Inpatient; Partial hospitalization; Residential or Day-Hospital; Outpatient; Community education programs; Intensive outpatient; Support groups; Follow-up programs; Clinical studies.
Treatments: Individual therapy; Group therapy; Family therapy; Family groups; Medication; Body image; Nutrition counseling; Christian-based; Exercise.
Treatment setting: Hospital; Therapist's office.

Average length of program: 2-6 wks overall with progressive step-down over time.
Average number served per year: 150.
Follow-up care offered: Inpatients contacted by phone at 6 mos.
Comments: Adults, adolescents treated together and apart throughout the day; children treated separately from others.

Highland Park

43. Eating Disorders Unit, Highland Park Hospital

718 Glenview Ave
Highland Park, IL 60035
Contact: Ann Willits and Robert Pero. 847-480-3720, *fax:* 847-480-3797 *Facility phone:* 847-432-8000 ext 2617, *Facility fax:* 847-480-2647
Hotline: 847-480-3720
Date Established: 1985.
Disorders treated: Anorexia nervosa; Bulimia nervosa; Compulsive eating (or BED).
Population treated: Women & men; Ages 13 and up.
Programs: Partial hospitalization; Outpatient; Community education programs; Intensive outpatient; Support groups.
Treatments: Individual therapy; Group therapy; Family therapy; Family groups; Experimental therapy; Medication; Body image; Nutrition counseling; Cognitive-behavioral; Psychodrama.
Maximum patients in program: 15.
Average number served per year: 150.
Follow-up care offered: Ongoing.

Lake Forest

44. Rush Behavioral Health

800 Westmoreland Ste 800
Lake Forest, IL 60045
Contact: Steve Ruohomaki, LCSW. 847-735-3300, *fax:* 847-735-6400
Date Established: 1995.
Disorders treated: Anorexia nervosa; Bulimia nervosa; Compulsive eating (or BED); Obesity.
Population treated: Adults.
Programs: Partial hospitalization; Outpatient; Intensive outpatient; Support groups; Follow-up programs; Residential or Day-Hospital.
Treatments: Individual therapy; Group therapy; Family groups; Addiction model; Experimental therapy; Medication; Nutrition counseling; 12-Step.
Treatment setting: Hospital; Clinic.
Program cost: $125-$359/treatment episode.
Maximum patients in program: 20.
Follow-up care offered: Annually.

Naperville

45. Linden Oaks Hospital

852 West St
Naperville, IL 60540
Contact: Dr Santucci/Dr Prinz. 630-305-5500, *fax:* 630-305-5083

Date Established: 1991.
Disorders treated: Anorexia nervosa; Bulimia nervosa; Compulsive eating (or BED).
Population treated: Women & men; Adolescents; Young children.
Programs: Inpatient; Partial hospitalization; Residential or Day-Hospital; Outpatient; Community education programs; Intensive outpatient; Support groups; Follow-up programs.
Treatments: Individual therapy; Group therapy; Family therapy; Family groups; Addiction model; Experimental therapy; Medication; Body image; 12-Step; Exercise.
Treatment setting: Hospital; Therapist's office; School.
Maximum patients in program: 20.
Average number served per year: 170.

Park Ridge

46. Lutheran General Hospital/Eating Disorders Program

1775 W Dempster St
Park Ridge, IL 60068
Contact: Dr Kathleen Traub. 847-723-8151, *fax:* 847-723-7481, *e-mail:* Kathy.Traub@advocatehealth.com
Date Established: 1988.
Disorders treated: Anorexia nervosa; Bulimia nervosa; Compulsive eating (or BED); Obesity; Comorbid diagnoses.
Population treated: Women & men; Adolescents; Young children.
Programs: Residential or Day-Hospital; Outpatient; Community education programs; Intensive outpatient; Support groups; Follow-up programs; Inpatient.
Treatments: Individual therapy; Group therapy; Family therapy; Family groups; Experimental therapy; Medication; Body image; Nutrition counseling; Exercise.
Treatment setting: Hospital.
Program cost: $384/day (8 am-6 pm, includes 3 meals and snacks).
Average length of program: Partial hospitalization 4-6 wks.
Maximum patients in program: 10-15.
Average number served per year: 26.
Comments: Inpatient hospitalization is available if needed.

Peoria

47. OSF Saint Francis Medical Center Eating Disorders Program

530 NE Glen Oak Ave
Peoria, IL 61637
Contact: Gail Koch, LRD, MA, LCPC. 309-655-2738, *fax:* 309-655-7138
Date Established: 1983.
Disorders treated: Anorexia nervosa; Bulimia nervosa.
Population treated: Women & men; Adolescents.
Programs: Partial hospitalization; Outpatient; Support groups.
Treatments: Individual therapy; Group therapy; Family therapy; Family groups; Experimental therapy; Medication; Body image; Nutrition counseling; Exercise.
Treatment setting: Hospital.

Program cost: Partial Hospitalization $335/day; Weekend $190/day; Outpatient $2.50/hr.
Average length of program: 4-8 wks.
Average number served per year: 120.
Follow-up care offered: Discharge evaluations only.

INDIANA

Bloomington

48. Bloomington Hospital Eating Disorders Program

PO Box 1149, Dept 638
Bloomington, IN 47402
Contact: Jane Taylor, MSW. 812-336-9219, *fax:* 812-336-9219 *Facility phone:* 800-222-9589
Date Established: 1986.
Disorders treated: Anorexia nervosa; Bulimia nervosa.
Population treated: Women & men.
Programs: Outpatient; Intensive outpatient; Support groups.
Treatments: Individual therapy; Group therapy; Family therapy; Family groups; Medication; Body image; Nutrition counseling.
Treatment setting: Hospital; Therapist's office.
Program cost: Approx $3,600.
Average length of program: 8 wks.
Maximum patients in program: 8.
Average number served per year: 46.

Evansville

49. Life Balance Program—Mulberry Center

420 Mulberry St
Evansville, IN 47713-1231
Contact: Marvel Harrison, PhD; Janie Chapell. 505-662-9200, *fax:* 505-662-4044, *e-mail:* marvel@trail.com *Facility phone:* 800-788-6541
Internet: http://www.liferesources.com
Hotline: 800-788-6541
Date Established: 1993.
Disorders treated: Anorexia nervosa; Bulimia nervosa; Compulsive eating (or BED); Obesity; Body image; Chronic dieting.
Population treated: Women & men; Adults; Adolescents.
Programs: Inpatient; Partial hospitalization; Residential or Day-Hospital; Outpatient; Community education programs; Intensive outpatient; Support groups; Follow-up programs.
Treatments: Individual therapy; Group therapy; Family therapy; Family groups; Addiction model; Experimental therapy; Medication; Body image; Nutrition counseling; 12-Step; Exercise.
Treatment setting: Hospital; Therapist's office.
Program cost: 11-day residential treatment program approx $3000.
Average length of program: 11-day intensive program; Individual therapy designed by client.
Maximum patients in program: 8/process group; 2-3 groups/clinic.
Average number served per year: 75.
Follow-up care offered: 1 yr with questionnaires.
Comments: Program to assist people in finding resolution to disordered eating & body image problems; inte-

grates group therapy with focused action therapy, imagery, self-reflection, journaling, physical activity, psycho-education, and movement therapy.

50. Mother & Baby Care of Southern Indiana, Inc—E.A.T.S. Program

4900 Shamrock Dr Ste 105
Evansville, IN 47715-7325
Contact: Sue Keith, RN, Program Director. 812-477-2568, *fax:* 812-477-2994, *e-mail:* sekeith@evansville.net
Date Established: 1997.
Disorders treated: Anorexia nervosa; Bulimia nervosa; Compulsive eating (or BED); Obesity.
Population treated: Women & men; Adolescents; Young children.
Programs: Outpatient; Community education programs; Intensive outpatient; Support groups; Follow-up programs.
Treatments: Individual therapy; Group therapy; Family therapy; Family groups; Experimental therapy; Body image; Nutrition counseling; 12-Step; Christian-based; Exercise.
Treatment setting: Therapist's office; Agency.
Program cost: $75/session or sliding fee scale.
Average length of program: 6-8 wks.
Maximum patients in program: 8-10.
Average number served per year: 25.
Follow-up care offered: 3 mos; 6 mos; 9 mos, 1 yr.
Comments: Services not denied to anyone for lack of ability to pay.

Fort Wayne

51. Medical Nutritional Therapists Inc

310 E DuPont Rd
Fort Wayne, IN 46825
Contact: James A. Holb RD, LD. 219-489-9009, *fax:* 219-484-4396
Date Established: 1985.
Disorders treated: Anorexia nervosa; Bulimia nervosa; Compulsive eating (or BED); Obesity.
Population treated: Women & men; Adolescents; Young children.
Programs: Outpatient.

Indianapolis

52. Eating Disorders Center of Indiana

3945 Eagle Creek Pkwy, Ste C
Indianapolis, IN 46254
Contact: Tony Shantz, MA. 317-329-7071, *fax:* 317-329-2721, *e-mail:* ECPC@aol.com
Date Established: 1997.
Disorders treated: Anorexia nervosa; Bulimia nervosa; Eating disorders not otherwise specified.
Population treated: Women & men; Adolescents; Young children.
Programs: Inpatient; Outpatient; Community education programs; Intensive outpatient; Support groups; Follow-up programs.
Treatments: Individual therapy; Group therapy; Family therapy; Family groups; Experimental therapy; Medication; Body image; Nutrition counseling.

Treatment setting: Clinic.
Average length of program: 10-wk intensive outpatient.
Maximum patients in program: 8-10.
Average number served per year: Approx 100.
Follow-up care offered: At end of intensive outpatient, then at 3 mos and 1 yr.
Comments: Multidisciplinary staff including 3 PhD psychologists, 1 LCSW 1 MS, RD and 2 MDs, specialize in children and adolescents. Adults are also treated.

South Bend

53. Memorial Hospital HOPE Program (Healthy Options for Problem Eaters)

707 N Michigan St
South Bend, IN 46601
Contact: Valerie Staples. 219-284-3153, *fax:* 219-284-3609
Hotline: 219-284-3000
Date Established: 1985.
Disorders treated: Anorexia nervosa; Bulimia nervosa; Compulsive eating (or BED).
Population treated: Women & men; Adolescents.
Programs: Inpatient; Partial hospitalization; Outpatient; Intensive outpatient; Support groups; Follow-up programs; Community education programs.
Treatments: Individual therapy; Group therapy; Family therapy; Family groups; Experimental therapy; Medication; Body image; Nutrition counseling.
Treatment setting: Hospital; Therapist's office.
Program cost: Approx $1200 for BED 1x/wk group for 16 wks; $3500-$4000 for 8-10 wks of inpatient 3x/wk; $98/hr for individual; $150/3 hr group.
Average length of program: 8-10 wks.
Maximum patients in program: 8/group.

IOWA

Cedar Rapids

54. Mercy Women's Center Eating Disorders Program

701 10th St, SE
Cedar Rapids, IA 52403
Contact: Marcey Scholtfelt, RN, MSN. 319-398-6774, *fax:* 319-369-4495 *Facility phone:* 319-398-6821
Date Established: 1981.
Disorders treated: Anorexia nervosa; Bulimia nervosa; Compulsive eating (or BED).
Population treated: Adults; Young children.
Programs: Outpatient; Community education programs; Support groups; Inpatient available on general psychiatric unit; Also offer info and referral via phone.
Treatments: Individual therapy; Group therapy; Family therapy; Body image; Nutrition counseling; Exercise.
Treatment setting: Hospital; Therapist's office.
Program cost: Individual $80/hr; Groups vary.
Average length of program: 6 mos to 2 yrs average.
Maximum patients in program: 20-30.
Average number served per year: 60.
Follow-up care offered: Annually.
Comments: Also offer information and referral by phone (30-50 calls/mo).

Des Moines

55. Iowa Lutheran Hospital Eating Disorder Program

700 E University
Des Moines, IA 50316
Contact: Wanda Wray or Eating Disorder Staff. 515-263-5672, *fax:* 515-263-5637 *Facility phone:* 515-263-5276
Hotline: 800-562-4944
Date Established: 1985.
Disorders treated: Anorexia nervosa; Bulimia nervosa.
Population treated: Women & men; Adolescents.
Programs: Partial hospitalization; Outpatient; Community education programs; Intensive outpatient; Support groups; Follow-up programs.
Treatments: Individual therapy; Group therapy; Family therapy; Family groups; Medication; Body image; Nutrition counseling; Exercise.
Treatment setting: Hospital.
Program cost: $38.74/hr.
Average length of program: 3-4 wks, 3 days/wk.
Maximum patients in program: 8-10.
Average number served per year: 52.
Follow-up care offered: Phone or face-to-face in support group. 3-4 wks; 6 mos.

Iowa City

56. University of Iowa Hospitals and Clinics Eating Disorders Program

The University of Iowa Department of Psychiatry, 200 Hawkins Dr, Ste 2880 JPP
Iowa City, IA 52242-1057
Contact: Arnold E. Anderson and Kay Evans. AEA: 319-356-1354, *fax:* 319-356-2587, *e-mail:* arnold-anderson@uiowa.edu *Facility phone:* 319-353-6952
Internet: http://www.uihc.uiowa.edu/pubinfo/eatdis/eatdis.htm
Date Established: 1991.
Disorders treated: Anorexia nervosa; Bulimia nervosa; Compulsive eating (or BED).
Population treated: All ages over 11, including males.
Programs: Inpatient; Partial hospitalization; Residential or Day-Hospital; Outpatient; Clinical studies; Community education programs; Intensive outpatient; Support groups; Follow-up programs; Education and consultation.
Treatments: Individual therapy; Group therapy; Family therapy; Family groups; Addiction model; Experimental therapy; Medication; Body image; Nutrition counseling; Exercise; Cognitive-behavioral therapy.
Treatment setting: Hospital.
Maximum patients in program: 14 inpatients; 25 partial hospital; over 100 outpatients (including individual, group, and/or family group).
Average number served per year: Approx 200.
Follow-up care offered: Follow-up by phone with patient, referral therapist, and occasionally for ongoing research.

Waterloo

57. Covenant Medical Center—Choices Eating Disorders Program

3421 W 9th St
Waterloo, IA 50702
Contact: Barb Knipp. 319-272-8031, *fax:* 319-272-8597
Date Established: 1988.
Disorders treated: Anorexia nervosa; Bulimia nervosa; Compulsive eating (or BED).
Population treated: Women & men; Adolescents.
Programs: Inpatient; Partial hospitalization; Outpatient; Intensive outpatient; Support groups.
Treatments: Individual therapy; Group therapy; Family therapy; Medication; Body image; Nutrition counseling.
Treatment setting: Hospital.
Comments: Has an assessment clinic that operates twice/mo. Assessments include physical by an M.D., food history by dietician, and interviews by counselor. Recommendations follow review by treatment team.

KANSAS

Salina

58. Salina Regional Health Center

400 S Santa Fe
Salina, KS 67410
Contact: Rose M. Anderson. 785-452-6070, *fax:* 785-452-6106 *Facility phone:* 785-452-7000
Date Established: 1998.
Disorders treated: Anorexia nervosa; Bulimia nervosa; Compulsive eating (or BED); Obesity.
Population treated: Adults.
Programs: Partial hospitalization; Outpatient.
Treatments: Individual therapy; Group therapy; Family therapy; Nutrition counseling.
Treatment setting: Hospital.
Maximum patients in program: 10.
Follow-up care offered: Weekly for 6 wks.

Topeka

59. Menninger Eating Disorders Program

PO Box 829
Topeka, KS 66606
Contact: Nikki Donaldson. 800-351-9058 ext 5676, *fax:* 785-273-0379, *e-mail:* donaldnn@menninger.edu
Internet: http://www.menniger.edu
Date Established: 1983.
Disorders treated: Anorexia nervosa; Bulimia nervosa; Compulsive eating (or BED); Obesity; Activity disorder.
Population treated: Women & men; Adolescents; Young children.
Programs: Inpatient; Partial hospitalization; Residential or Day-Hospital; Outpatient; Clinical studies; Community education programs; Intensive outpatient; Support groups; Follow-up programs.
Treatments: Individual therapy; Group therapy; Family therapy; Family groups; Body image; Nutrition counseling; Exercise.
Treatment setting: Hospital; Therapist's office; School.
Average length of program: 2-4 wks.
Maximum patients in program: 12.

Follow-up care offered: Once/wk.

LOUISIANA

Baton Rouge

60. Our Lady of the Lake Eating Disorders Program

8080 Margaret Ann Dr
Baton Rouge, LA 70809
Contact: Dr. Renee Bruno. 504-765-6033, *fax:* 504-765-6315
Disorders treated: Anorexia nervosa; Bulimia nervosa.
Population treated: Women & men; All ages.
Programs: Inpatient; Partial hospitalization; Residential or Day-Hospital; Clinical studies; Community education programs; Intensive outpatient; Support groups; Follow-up programs.
Treatments: Individual therapy; Group therapy; Family therapy; Family groups; Experimental therapy; Medication; Body image; Nutrition counseling; Exercise.
Treatment setting: Hospital; Therapist's office.
Program cost: Inpatient: approximately $675/day; partial $360/day.
Average length of program: Average inpatient 2 wks; average partial 2-4 wks.
Maximum patients in program: 12.
Average number served per year: 200-300.
Follow-up care offered: Monthly.
Comments: Outpatient clinic appointments available so same social worker, psychiatrist, and dietician can follow patient throughout full continuum of care.

New Orleans

61. Eating Disorders Recovery Center, River Oaks Hospital

1525 River Oaks Rd W
New Orleans, LA 70123
Contact: Paula Ga, PhD. 504-734-1740, *fax:* 504-733-7020
Internet: http://www.riveroakshospital.com
Hotline: 800-366-1740
Date Established: 1997.
Disorders treated: Anorexia nervosa; Bulimia nervosa; Compulsive eating (or BED); Obesity.
Population treated: Women & men; Adolescents.
Programs: Inpatient; Partial hospitalization; Outpatient.
Treatments: Individual therapy; Group therapy; Family therapy; Experimental therapy; Medication; Body image; Nutrition counseling.
Treatment setting: Hospital.
Average length of program: 2-4 wks.
Maximum patients in program: 10.

62. Tulane Behavioral Health Center Eating Disorders Clinic

1040 Calhoun St
New Orleans, LA 70118
Contact: Susan Willard, MSW. 800-548-4183, *fax:* 504-894-7295
Date Established: 1982.

Disorders treated: Anorexia nervosa; Bulimia nervosa; Compulsive eating (or BED); Obesity.
Population treated: Women & men; Adolescents; Young children.
Programs: Inpatient; Partial hospitalization; Residential or Day-Hospital; Outpatient; Community education programs; Intensive outpatient; Support groups; Follow-up programs.
Treatments: Individual therapy; Group therapy; Family therapy; Family groups; Experimental therapy; Medication; Body image; Nutrition counseling; Exercise.
Treatment setting: Hospital; Therapist's office.
Maximum patients in program: 9 beds.

MAINE

Bangor

63. The Acadia Hospital

PO Box 422, 268 Stillwater Ave
Bangor, ME 04402-0422
Contact: Annette Adams. 207-973-6064, *fax:* 207-973-6109, *e-mail:* aadams@emh.org *Facility phone:* 207-973-6100
Date Established: 1992.
Disorders treated: Anorexia nervosa; Bulimia nervosa.
Population treated: Women & men; Adolescents; Young children.
Programs: Inpatient; Outpatient; Community education programs; Intensive outpatient; Support groups.
Treatments: Individual therapy; Group therapy; Family groups; Medication.
Treatment setting: Hospital; School.
Maximum patients in program: 100.
Average number served per year: 49 inpatients.

Westbrook

64. Eating Disorder Program at Westbrook Hospital

40 Park Rd
Westbrook, ME 04092
Contact: Carol Crosby, LCSW, DCSW, Prog Dir; Jean Douba, Admin Coord. 207-854-8464, *fax:* 207-839-8711, *e-mail:* ppuchalski@Westbrook.Hospital.org, *Facility fax:* 207-856-2590
Date Established: 1986.
Disorders treated: Anorexia nervosa; Bulimia nervosa; Compulsive eating (or BED); Eating disorders nonspecified.
Population treated: Women & men; Adolescents; Ages 13 and up.
Programs: Inpatient; Partial hospitalization; Outpatient; Community education programs; Support groups.
Treatments: Individual therapy; Group therapy; Family therapy; Family groups; Experimental therapy; Medication; Body image; Nutrition counseling; Exercise.
Treatment setting: Hospital.
Program cost: $800-$900/day inpatient; $600-$800 5-day/wk partial hospital 12-hr program daily.
Average length of program: 10-14 inpatient; 2-3 wks partial hospital program.
Maximum patients in program: 8-12.

Average number served per year: 140.
Follow-up care offered: 1 mo; 6 mos; 1 yr.
Comments: Small community-based hospital with separate eating disorders wing; full medical facility; non-locked unit; overtly suicidal clients not appropriate until stablized; some managed care contracts apply.

MARYLAND
Baltimore

65. Johns Hopkins Eating Disorders Program

Johns Hopkins Hospital, Meyer 101, Wolfe St
Baltimore, MD 21287
Contact: Linda Ryan or Janis Walker. 410-955-3863, *e-mail:* LRYAN@Welchlink.welch.jhu.edu
Internet: http://www.med.jhu.edu/jhhpsychiatry/ed1.
htm#about
Date Established: 1976.
Disorders treated: Anorexia nervosa; Bulimia nervosa; Compulsive eating (or BED); Co-morbid affective disorders and OCO.
Population treated: Women & men; Adolescents.
Programs: Inpatient; Partial hospitalization; Residential or Day-Hospital; Outpatient.
Treatments: Individual therapy; Group therapy; Family therapy; Family groups; Medication; Body image; Nutrition counseling; Exercise; Cognitive-behavioral therapy.
Treatment setting: Hospital; Therapist's office.
Program cost: Approx $1000/day inpatient; approx $500/day partial hospitalization; outpatient consultation $355; outpatient follow-up $90-$150.
Average length of program: Average inpatient 14 days; day hospital 21 days.
Maximum patients in program: 20.
Average number served per year: Approx 150 inpatient and day hospital; initial consultations 84; day hospital visits 1704.
Follow-up care offered: Outpatient clinic provides follow-up at patients request, usually on a weekly basis. Outcomes monitoring phone call follow-ups of all patients are conducted 1 and 12 mos after discharge.

Towson

66. Center for Eating Disorders PA

7620 York Rd, Jordan Ctr, 4th Fl
Towson, MD 21204
Contact: Harry A Brandt, MD, Dir. 410-427-1200, *fax:* 410-427-2001, *e-mail:* hbrandt@eating-disorders.com
Internet: http://www.eating-disorders.com
Disorders treated: Anorexia nervosa; Bulimia nervosa; Compulsive eating (or BED); Obesity.
Population treated: Women & men; Adolescents.
Programs: Inpatient; Partial hospitalization; Outpatient; Clinical studies; Community education programs; Intensive outpatient; Support groups; Follow-up programs.
Treatments: Individual therapy; Group therapy; Family therapy; Family groups; Medication; Body image; Nutrition counseling.
Treatment setting: Hospital; Therapist's office.
Average number served per year: 400 inpatient/day.
Follow-up care offered: Follow-up evaluations conducted.

MASSACHUSETTS
Boston

67. Children's Hospital—Boston Bader Inpatient Psychiatric Unit

300 Longwood Ave
Boston, MA 02215
Contact: Susan E. Frates, MS, RD. 617-355-7600
Disorders treated: Anorexia nervosa; Bulimia nervosa; Compulsive eating (or BED); Obesity.
Population treated: Adolescents; Young children.
Programs: Inpatient.
Treatments: Individual therapy; Group therapy; Family therapy; Family groups; Medication; Body image; Nutrition counseling.
Treatment setting: Hospital.
Maximum patients in program: Approximately 20.
Comments: Eating-disordered patients are placed on either the Anorexia Protocol, Bulima Protocol, or a specialized eating-disorder NOS Protocol.

Greenfield

68. Franklin Partial Hospitalization Eating Disorder Program

164 High St
Greenfield, MA 01301
Contact: James Gardner, LICSW; Denise Green, PhD.
413-773-2546, *fax:* 413-773-2374
Date Established: 1996.
Disorders treated: Anorexia nervosa; Bulimia nervosa.
Population treated: Women only; 16 yrs and older.
Programs: Partial hospitalization; Outpatient; Intensive outpatient.
Treatments: Group therapy; Body image; Nutrition counseling.
Treatment setting: Hospital.
Program cost: $150 for 3-hr program.
Average length of program: 3-hr program, once/wk, for 5 mos.
Maximum patients in program: 10.
Average number served per year: 21.

Waltham

69. Deaconess Waltham Hospital Eating Disorder Services

5 Hope Ave
Waltham, MA 02254-9116
Contact: Dennis Czajkowski, PHD. 781-647-6700
Date Established: 1994.
Disorders treated: Anorexia nervosa; Bulimia nervosa; Compulsive eating (or BED); Eating disorders and diabetes.
Population treated: Women & men; Adults; Adolescents.
Programs: Inpatient; Partial hospitalization; Residential or Day-Hospital; Community education programs; Intensive outpatient; Support groups; Evening treatment.
Treatments: Individual therapy; Group therapy; Family therapy; Family groups; Medication; Body image; Nutrition counseling; Cognitive behavioral.
Treatment setting: Hospital.

Maximum patients in program: 12-14.
Average number served per year: 80-100.

Westwood

70. Westwood Lodge Hospital, Eating Disorders Program

45 Clapboardtree St
Westwood, MA 02090
Contact: Laura J Weisberg, PhD, Director. 781-762-7764 ext 480, *fax:* 781-762-0550, *e-mail:* weiswant@datablost.net
Hotline: 800-222-2237
Date Established: 1989.
Disorders treated: Anorexia nervosa; Bulimia nervosa; Compulsive eating (or BED); Chemical dependency; Trauma; General psychiatry.
Population treated: Women & men; Adolescents.
Programs: Inpatient; Partial hospitalization; Residential or Day-Hospital; Outpatient; Community education programs; Intensive outpatient.
Treatments: Individual therapy; Group therapy; Family therapy; Family groups; Medication; Body image; Nutrition counseling; psychodynamic, cognitive and dialectical behavorial and expressive therapies, as well as nutrional counseling and psychopharmacology.
Treatment setting: Hospital; Therapist's office.
Program cost: Inpatient approximately $1000/day; partial hospital/day treatment approximately $300/day.
Maximum patients in program: 20 inpatient/partial hospital.
Average number served per year: Approx 200.

MICHIGAN

Flint

71. McLaren Regional Medical Center Weight Management Center

4448 Oak Bridge Dr
Flint, MI 48532
Contact: Ruth Clements, RD. 810-733-3278, *fax:* 810-733-7549
Date Established: 1990.
Disorders treated: Anorexia nervosa; Bulimia nervosa; Compulsive eating (or BED); Obesity.
Population treated: Women & men; Adolescents; Young children.
Programs: Inpatient; Outpatient; Intensive outpatient; Support groups; Follow-up programs.
Treatments: Individual therapy; Group therapy; Family therapy; Family groups; Medication; Nutrition counseling; 12-Step; Christian-based; Exercise.
Treatment setting: Hospital.
Program cost: $48-$3,000 depending on treatment required.
Average length of program: wkly for 26 wks.
Maximum patients in program: 150.
Average number served per year: 650.
Follow-up care offered: One hour consults 1 or 2 times/wk.

Grand Rapids

72. Forest View Mental Health Services Center for the Treatment of Eating Disorders

1055 Medical Park Dr, SE
Grand Rapids, MI 49546
Contact: Pamela Beane. 616-942-9610, *fax:* 616-954-3131
Internet: http://www.forrestview.com
Hotline: 800-949-8439
Date Established: 1984.
Disorders treated: Anorexia nervosa; Bulimia nervosa; Compulsive eating (or BED).
Population treated: Women & men; Adolescents; Young children.
Programs: Inpatient; Partial hospitalization; Outpatient; Community education programs; Intensive outpatient; Support groups; Follow-up programs.
Treatments: Individual therapy; Group therapy; Family therapy; Family groups; Experimental therapy; Medication; Body image; Nutrition counseling; 12-Step.
Treatment setting: Hospital.

73. Pine Rest Christian Mental Health Services

300 68th St SE
Grand Rapids, MI 49501-0165
Contact: Betsy Buist. 616-455-5000, *fax:* 616-455-5370
Disorders treated: Anorexia nervosa; Bulimia nervosa; Compulsive eating (or BED); Obesity; Trauma.
Population treated: Women & men; Adolescents; Young children.
Programs: Inpatient; Partial hospitalization; Outpatient; Intensive outpatient.
Treatments: Individual therapy; Group therapy; Family therapy; Body image; Nutrition counseling; Christian-based; Exercise.
Treatment setting: Hospital.
Average length of program: 3-21 days.
Maximum patients in program: 6.

MINNESOTA

Minneapolis

74. Fairview—University Medical Center Eating Disorders Program

2450 Riverside Ave
Minneapolis, MN 55406
Contact: Alexis Houck. 612-672-2953, *fax:* 612-672-7520
Hotline: 612-672-2952
Date Established: 1979.
Disorders treated: Anorexia nervosa; Bulimia nervosa; MDD; Obsessive compulsive disorder; Anxiety disorders.
Population treated: Women & men; Adolescents.
Programs: Inpatient; Partial hospitalization; Community education programs; Intensive outpatient.
Treatments: Individual therapy; Group therapy; Family therapy; Experimental therapy; Medication; Body image; Nutrition counseling; relapse prevention, family education.
Treatment setting: Hospital.

Average length of program: 4 wks.

75. University of Minnesota Eating Disorder Program

PO Box 393, Rays Bldg, University of Minnesota Hospital
Minneapolis, MN 55455
Contact: Dr Elke Eckert. 612-626-6871, *fax:* 612-626-5591
Date Established: 1974.
Disorders treated: Anorexia nervosa; Bulimia nervosa; Compulsive eating (or BED).
Population treated: Women & men; Adolescents; Young children.
Programs: Inpatient; Partial hospitalization; Residential or Day-Hospital; Outpatient; Clinical studies; Community education programs; Intensive outpatient; Support groups; Follow-up programs.
Treatments: Individual therapy; Group therapy; Family therapy; Medication; Body image; Nutrition counseling.
Treatment setting: Clinic; Hospital.
Average length of program: Hospital 10 days-3 wks; partial hospital program 2-4 wks.
Average number served per year: 100.

Pine City

76. Pine Shores

PO Box 139
Pine City, MN 55063
Contact: Lynette Kuzel. 612-444-4500, *fax:* 612-444-6965
Disorders treated: Anorexia nervosa; Compulsive eating (or BED); Obesity.
Population treated: Women & men; Adults.
Programs: Inpatient.
Treatments: Individual therapy; Group therapy; Nutrition counseling; 12-Step; Exercise.
Treatment setting: Inpatient treatment.
Average length of program: 21 days; 28 days; 60 days.
Maximum patients in program: 38.
Follow-up care offered: Aftercare.

Rochester

77. Mayo Clinic Eating Disorders Program

200 First St SW
Rochester, MN 55905
Contact: Donald E McAlpine, MD. 507-284-0877, *fax:* 507-284-5370, *e-mail:* mcalpine.donald@mayo.edu
Date Established: 1986.
Disorders treated: Anorexia nervosa; Bulimia nervosa.
Population treated: Women & men; Adolescents.
Programs: Inpatient; Partial hospitalization; Residential or Day-Hospital; Outpatient; Clinical studies; Intensive outpatient; Support groups; Follow-up programs.
Treatments: Individual therapy; Group therapy; Family therapy; Body image; Nutrition counseling.
Treatment setting: Hospital.
Average number served per year: 100.
Follow-up care offered: Weekly to monthly.
Comments: Full range of outpatient, intermediate (day hospital) and inpatient programs. Serve both the local community and worldwide referrals.

Saint Louis Park

78. The Eating Disorders Institute, Methodist Hospital Health System Minnesota

6490 Excelsior Blvd, Ste 315E
Saint Louis Park, MN 55426
Contact: Rhond Whetstine, Tammy Van Huen. 612-993-6200, *fax:* 612-993-6742
Internet: http://www.healthsystem.minnesota.com
Date Established: 1986.
Disorders treated: Anorexia nervosa; Bulimia nervosa.
Population treated: Women & men; Adolescents.
Programs: Inpatient; Partial hospitalization; Outpatient; Community education programs; Intensive outpatient; Support groups; Follow-up programs.
Treatments: Individual therapy; Group therapy; Family therapy; Family groups; Experimental therapy; Medication; Body image; Nutrition counseling; Exercise.
Treatment setting: Hospital; Therapist's office; Outpatient clinic.
Average length of program: 2-4 wks, inpatient; 2-4 partial; 6 mos-1 yr, outpatient.
Maximum patients in program: 10 beds in patient unit.
Average number served per year: 157 outpatients; 115 inpatients.

MISSOURI

Kansas City

79. Baptist Medical Center, Eating Disorder Unit

6601 Rockhill Rd
Kansas City, MO 64131
Contact: Ann Gabrick, MSW, LSCSW. 816-276-7819, *fax:* 816-926-2253 *Facility phone:* 816-276-7818
Hotline: 816-276-7818
Date Established: 1992.
Disorders treated: Anorexia nervosa; Bulimia nervosa; Compulsive eating (or BED); Eating disorders not otherwise specified; Medically related proglems (reflux, etc.).
Population treated: Women & men; Adults; Adolescents.
Programs: Inpatient; Partial hospitalization; Residential or Day-Hospital; Outpatient; Community education programs; Support groups; Free assessment to diagnose and refer.
Treatments: Individual therapy; Group therapy; Family therapy; Family groups; Experimental therapy; Medication; Body image; Nutrition counseling; Exercise; Spirituality component; Pastoral counselor.
Treatment setting: Hospital; Therapist's office.
Average length of program: 2 wks-3 mos.
Maximum patients in program: 8 Inpatient; 4 day treatment.
Average number served per year: Approx 1200.
Follow-up care offered: Aftercare or contact with referring therapist; initially on monthly basis.

Saint Louis

80. Anorexia Bulimia Treatment and Education Center, Saint John's Mercy Medical Center

615 S New Ballas Rd
Saint Louis, MO 63141

Contact: Joshua Calhoun, MD. 314-569-6898, *fax:* 314-995-4197, *e-mail:* calhjw.stlo.sonhs.com
Date Established: 1984.
Disorders treated: Anorexia nervosa; Bulimia nervosa.
Population treated: Women & men; Adolescents; Young children.
Programs: Inpatient; Partial hospitalization; Residential or Day-Hospital; Outpatient; Community education programs; Intensive outpatient; Support groups.
Treatments: Individual therapy; Group therapy; Family therapy; Medication; Body image; Nutrition counseling.
Treatment setting: Hospital.
Average number served per year: 40+.
Follow-up care offered: Yes.

81. BJC Behavioral Health Center

605 Old Ballas Rd, Ste 250
Saint Louis, MO 63141
Contact: Lynn Stark, RN MSN. 314-569-7161, *fax:* 314-569-9434 *Facility phone:* 800-597-2793
Date Established: 1997.
Disorders treated: Anorexia nervosa; Bulimia nervosa.
Population treated: Women & men; Adolescents; Young children.
Programs: Partial hospitalization; Intensive outpatient.
Treatments: Individual therapy; Group therapy; Family therapy; Family groups; Medication; Body image; Nutrition counseling; Exercise.
Treatment setting: Outpatient center.
Program cost: $400 partial day treatment.
Maximum patients in program: 13.

NEBRASKA

Omaha

82. Nebraska Health Systems Eating Disorders Program

600 S 42nd St
Omaha, NE 68198-5600
Contact: Mary Legino, PhD. 402-559-5524, *fax:* 402-559-9218, *e-mail:* MLegino@edu.com
Internet: http://www.unmc.edu/edp/edp.htm
Date Established: 1990.
Disorders treated: Anorexia nervosa; Bulimia nervosa; Compulsive eating (or BED); Obesity; Concomitatant psychopathology.
Population treated: Women & men; Adolescents; Young children.
Programs: Inpatient; Partial hospitalization; Intensive outpatient.
Treatments: Individual therapy; Group therapy; Family therapy; Family groups; Experimental therapy; Medication; Body image; Nutrition counseling; Exercise; cognitive behavioral treatment model.
Treatment setting: Hospital.
Average length of program: 3-4 wks combined inpatient/partial hospital days.
Maximum patients in program: 20.
Follow-up care offered: 6, 18, 24, 36, 48 mos.
Comments: Comprehensive outpatient treatment program as well as inpatient and partial programs.

NEVADA

Reno

83. ABC Nutrition Services

457 Court St
Reno, NV 89523
Contact: Barbara Cox, RD. 702-324-1900, *fax:* 702-746-8396, *e-mail:* Dietpro@aol.com
Date Established: 1991.
Disorders treated: Anorexia nervosa; Bulimia nervosa; Compulsive eating (or BED); Obesity; Nutrition related medical problems (i.e., hypoglycemia, diabetes mellitus, cholecystitis).
Population treated: Women only; Men only; Women & men; Adults; Adolescents; Young children.
Programs: Outpatient; Follow-up programs.
Treatments: Nutrition counseling.
Treatment setting: Therapist's office.
Program cost: $80/hr every 2 wks in conjunction with therapist appointments.
Average length of program: 3 mos and up.
Maximum patients in program: 50-60.
Average number served per year: Approx 400.
Follow-up care offered: Every 2 wks until patient terminates treatment.

NEW HAMPSHIRE

Hampstead

84. Hampstead Hospital Eating Disorders Treatment Center

218 East Road
Hampstead, NH 03841
Contact: Michelle Wilson. 603-329-5311 ext 3252, *fax:* 602-329-4746
Internet: http://www.hampsteadhospital.com
Date Established: 1998.
Disorders treated: Anorexia nervosa; Bulimia nervosa; Compulsive eating (or BED).
Population treated: Women & men; Adolescents 15 and over.
Programs: Inpatient; Partial hospitalization; Support groups.
Treatments: Individual therapy; Group therapy; Family therapy; Family groups; Experimental therapy; Medication; Body image; Nutrition counseling; Exercise.
Treatment setting: Hospital.
Comments: Center's philosophy is based on a relational and solution-focused model which provides treatment that is nuturing and goal oriented. Goal is to assist patients in developing healthy eating patterns while identifying internal conflicts and underlying feelings; staff members help patients discover internal strengths and develop alternate, healthy coping strategies while challenging distorted and negative thinking that perpetuates symptoms.

Lebanon

85. Children's Hospital at Dartmouth Adolescent Eating Disorders Program

1 Medical Center Dr
Lebanon, NH 03756
Contact: Carole A. Stashwick, MD. 603-650-5473, *fax:* 603-650-5458, *e-mail:* Carole.A.Stashwick@dartmouth. edu
Internet: http://www.hitchcock.org/pages/CHaD/CHaD. htmlhttp://www.hitchcock.org/pages/CHaD
Date Established: 1998.
Disorders treated: Anorexia nervosa; Bulimia nervosa.
Population treated: Adolescents; Young children.
Programs: Inpatient; Partial hospitalization; Residential or Day-Hospital; Outpatient; Intensive outpatient; Support groups.
Treatments: Individual therapy; Group therapy; Family therapy; Medication; Body image; Nutrition counseling; Exercise.
Treatment setting: Hospital.
Maximum patients in program: 4 in partial program; unlimited in outpatient program.
Average number served per year: 25-30.

NEW JERSEY
Princeton

86. The Medical Center at Princeton Eating Disorders Program

253 Witherspoon St
Princeton, NJ 08540
Contact: Robin Boudette, PhD. 609-497-4490, *fax:* 609-497-4412
Date Established: 1996.
Disorders treated: Anorexia nervosa; Bulimia nervosa; Compulsive eating (or BED); Obesity; Trauma.
Population treated: Women & men; Young children.
Programs: Inpatient; Partial hospitalization; Community education programs; Intensive outpatient; Support groups.
Treatments: Individual therapy; Group therapy; Family therapy; Family groups; Experimental therapy; Medication; Body image; Nutrition counseling.
Treatment setting: Hospital.
Maximum patients in program: 14 inpatients; 30 outpatients.
Average number served per year: 125.
Follow-up care offered: Referred to outpatient treatment providers.

Skillman

87. Princeton Eating Disorders Center

154 Tammarack Cir
Skillman, NJ 08558
Contact: Ayman Ramay, MD. 609-924-5250, *fax:* 609-924-8113
Disorders treated: Anorexia nervosa; Bulimia nervosa; Compulsive eating (or BED); Obesity.
Population treated: Women & men; Adolescents.
Programs: Inpatient; Partial hospitalization; Outpatient; Intensive outpatient; Support groups.

Treatments: Individual therapy; Group therapy; Family therapy; Nutrition counseling.
Treatment setting: Hospital; Therapist's office.
Maximum patients in program: 8/group.
Average number served per year: 32.
Follow-up care offered: Annually.

Somerville

88. Somerset Medical Center Eating Disorders Program

110 Rehill Ave
Somerville, NJ 08876-2598
Contact: Vernetter Clarke, Unit secretary. 908-685-2847, *fax:* 908-685-2458
Date Established: 1985.
Disorders treated: Anorexia nervosa; Bulimia nervosa.
Population treated: Women & men; Adolescents.
Programs: Inpatient; Partial hospitalization; Intensive outpatient; Support groups.
Treatments: Individual therapy; Group therapy; Family therapy; Family groups; Experimental therapy; Medication; Body image; Nutrition counseling; Exercise.
Treatment setting: Hospital.
Average length of program: 14-21 days inpatient.
Maximum patients in program: 26.
Average number served per year: 250.
Follow-up care offered: After discharge from each level of care.

Tinton Falls

89. Monmouth Psychological Associates Eating Disorders Program

620 Shrewsbury Ave
Tinton Falls, NJ 07701
Contact: Donald E. Erwin, PhD. 732-530-9029, *fax:* 732-530-0387
Hotline: 800-870-9029
Date Established: 1982.
Disorders treated: Anorexia nervosa; Bulimia nervosa.
Population treated: Women & men; Adolescents.
Programs: Inpatient; Partial hospitalization; Outpatient; Community education programs; Intensive outpatient; Support groups; Follow-up programs; Nutritional analysis and education.
Treatments: Individual therapy; Group therapy; Family therapy; Experimental therapy; Body image; Nutrition counseling.
Program cost: Approximately $240/wk.
Average length of program: 4-6 mos.
Comments: Multimodal, multidisciplinary outpatient practice. Patients also evaluated for residential, inpatient care at Somerset Medical Center. Free, biweekly discussion groups.

NEW YORK
Bayside

90. Holliswood Hospital

38-24 213th St
Bayside, NY 11361
Contact: Robin Korngold. 718-776-8181 ext 359

Disorders treated: Anorexia nervosa; Bulimia nervosa; Compulsive eating (or BED).
Population treated: Women & men; Adolescents; Young children.
Programs: Inpatient; Outpatient.
Treatments: Individual therapy; Group therapy; Family therapy; Body image; 12-Step.
Treatment setting: Hospital; Therapist's office.
Program cost: Individual $75-$100; Group $25-$30.
Maximum patients in program: 6-8 for groups.
Comments: 2 groups: adolescents who are anorexic and bulimic; compulsive overeaters between 34-55.

Brooklyn

91. Helping To End Eating Disorders—Brookdale Hospital and Medical Center

9620 Church Ave
Brooklyn, NY 11212
Contact: Ira M Sacker, MD. 718-240-6451, *fax:* 718-240-6420, *e-mail:* Sacker MD @aol.com
Internet: http://www.eatingdis.com
Date Established: 1987.
Disorders treated: Anorexia nervosa; Bulimia nervosa; Compulsive eating (or BED); Obesity; All forms of addictive behaviors.
Population treated: Women & men; Adolescents; Young children.
Programs: Inpatient; Outpatient; Clinical studies; Community education programs; Intensive outpatient; Support groups; Follow-up programs.
Treatments: Individual therapy; Group therapy; Family therapy; Family groups; Experimental therapy; Medication; Body image; Nutrition counseling; Exercise.
Treatment setting: Hospital; Therapist's office; School; Groups.
Maximum patients in program: 100.
Average number served per year: 200.
Follow-up care offered: Monthly by telephone.
Comments: H.E.E.D. presently involved in prevention model to this program; going into schools beginning with kindergarteners to do lessons on self-esteem and body image with follow-up materials for teachers.

Manhasset

92. North Shore University Hospital

400 Community Dr
Manhasset, NY 11030
Contact: Marcie Schneider, MD or Martin Fisher MD. 516-622-5075, *fax:* 516-622-5074 *Facility phone:* 516-869-6831, *Facility fax:* 516-869-6834
Date Established: Inpatient since 1980; day program since 1995.
Disorders treated: Anorexia nervosa; Bulimia nervosa; Obesity; Compulsive eating (or BED).
Population treated: Adults; Adolescents; Young children; Young children up through age 40.
Programs: Inpatient; Partial hospitalization; Outpatient; Clinical studies; Intensive outpatient; Follow-up programs.
Treatments: Individual therapy; Group therapy; Family therapy; Family groups; Experimental therapy; Medica-

tion; Body image; Nutrition counseling; Exercise; Medical treatment and management.
Treatment setting: Hospital; Outpatient office; Day Program.
Maximum patients in program: Inpatient 7; day program 10; outpatient unlimited.
Average number served per year: 100.
Comments: Day treatment program meets 5 days/wk. Daily activities include group, individual, and family psychotherapy, psychopharmacology, physical therapy, art and recreational therapy, nutritionally balanced meals, and ongoing medical care.

New Hyde Park

93. Schneider Children's Hospital Eating Disorders Center

269-01 76th Ave
New Hyde Park, NY 11040
Contact: Neville H Golden, MD. 718-470-3275, *fax:* 718-347-2315, *e-mail:* golden@lij.edu
Date Established: 1975.
Disorders treated: Anorexia nervosa; Bulimia nervosa.
Population treated: Adolescents; Young children.
Programs: Inpatient; Partial hospitalization; Outpatient; Clinical studies; Community education programs; Support groups.
Treatments: Individual therapy; Group therapy; Family therapy; Experimental therapy; Medication; Nutrition counseling; Exercise; medical monitoring.
Treatment setting: Hospital.
Average length of program: Inpatient 3-4 wks; Partial hospital further 3-5 wks.
Maximum patients in program: Inpatient 15.
Average number served per year: 190.
Follow-up care offered: Weekly 4-6 wks; then every 7 wks.

New York

94. (NYSPI) New York State Psychiatric Institute

722 W 168th St, Unit 98
New York, NY 10032
Contact: Claire Barrett, anorexia; Christina Grey, bulimia; Dara Lucks, binge eating. 212-543-5316 (AN); 543-5739 (BN/BED), *fax:* 212-543-5607, *e-mail:* EDRU@nyspimail.cpmc.columbia.edu
Internet: http://www.nyspi.cpmc.columbia.edu/nyspi/depts/psypharm/eating~1/index.htm
Date Established: 1979.
Disorders treated: Anorexia nervosa; Bulimia nervosa; Compulsive eating (or BED).
Population treated: Women only (AN; BN); Women and men (BED).
Programs: Inpatient; Outpatient; Clinical studies; Follow-up programs.
Treatments: Individual therapy; Group therapy; Medication; Nutrition counseling; Cognitive behavioral therapy.
Treatment setting: Hospital.
Program cost: Free of charge in exchange for participation in research.

Average length of program: BN inpatient, 6-8 wks; BN outpatient 5 mos; AN inpatient 3-4 wks; AN outpatient 1 yr.
Average number served per year: Approximately 60.
Follow-up care offered: Every 3-4 mos up to 1 yr after discharge.

95. The Renfrew Center

15 E 36th St, Ste 1D
New York, NY 10016
Contact: Lori Lynn Bauer, CSW. 212-947-7111, *fax:* 212-947-2633 *Facility phone:* 1-800-736-3739
Date Established: 1985.
Disorders treated: Anorexia nervosa; Bulimia nervosa; Obesity.
Population treated: Women & men; Women only in programs and groups; Men and women in individual treatment.
Programs: Inpatient; Partial hospitalization; Residential or Day-Hospital; Outpatient; Clinical studies; Community education programs; Intensive outpatient; Support groups; Inpatient in Philadelphia & Florida locations.
Treatments: Individual therapy; Group therapy; Family therapy; Experimental therapy; Body image; Nutrition counseling.
Treatment setting: Therapist's office; Meeting room.
Average length of program: Day Treatment: 5 days/wk, 9am-3pm; Intensive outpatient: 3 eves/wk, 5:30-9:30 pm.
Maximum patients in program: 10.

New York City

96. Program for Managing Eating Disorders

420 E 76th St
New York City, NY 10021
Contact: Charlie Murkofsky MD. 212-580-1530, *fax:* 212-875-0530, *e-mail:* cpw247ed@aol.com *Facility phone:* 212-434-5584, *Facility fax:* 212-434-5513
Date Established: 1993.
Disorders treated: Anorexia nervosa; Bulimia nervosa; Compulsive eating (or BED).
Population treated: Women & men; Adolescents.
Programs: Partial hospitalization; Residential or Day-Hospital; Outpatient; Community education programs; Intensive outpatient; Support groups; Follow-up programs.
Treatments: Individual therapy; Group therapy; Family therapy; Family groups; Medication; Body image; Nutrition counseling; Multi-family group.
Treatment setting: Hospital; Therapist's office.
Program cost: $375 full day; $200 half day.
Maximum patients in program: 25.
Average number served per year: 130.
Follow-up care offered: Periodic as-needed aftercare group.
Comments: Program is only facility licensed IOP/partial program in New York City. Provides access to care for Medicaid/Medicare patients along with traditional.

Rochester

97. Adolescent Eating Disorders Program

601 Elmwood Ave
Rochester, NY 14642
Contact: Teri Litteer, RN, PNP. 716-275-2964, *fax:* 716-242-9733
Date Established: 1985.
Disorders treated: Anorexia nervosa; Bulimia nervosa; Compulsive eating (or BED); Obesity; Adolescent medicine.
Population treated: Adolescents; Young children.
Programs: Inpatient; Partial hospitalization; Residential or Day-Hospital; Outpatient; Clinical studies; Community education programs; Intensive outpatient; Support groups; Follow-up programs.
Treatments: Individual therapy; Group therapy; Family therapy; Family groups; Medication; Body image; Nutrition counseling; Cognitive behavioral.
Treatment setting: Hospital.
Maximum patients in program: 70.
Average number served per year: 150.
Follow-up care offered: Survey every 4 yrs to determine long-term outcome.
Comments: Developmentally based assessment and treatment program based in the department of pediatrics with close link to department of psychiatry at the University of Rochester.

98. Strong Behavioral Health; University of Rochester, Medical Center—Eating Disorder Treatment Service

300 Crittenden Blvd, University of Rochester Medical Center
Rochester, NY 14642
Contact: Mary Tantillo, PhD RNC's, Dept of Psychiatry. 716-275-0324, *fax:* 716-273-1093, *e-mail:* mtantillophd@worldnet.att.net *Facility phone:* 716-275-4202 (to schedule appointment)
Date Established: 1990.
Disorders treated: Anorexia nervosa; Bulimia nervosa; Compulsive eating (or BED).
Population treated: Women & men; Adults; Adolescents.
Programs: Inpatient; Partial hospitalization; Outpatient; Support groups.
Treatments: Individual therapy; Group therapy; Family therapy; Family groups; Medication; Body image; Nutrition counseling; Relational therapy (Stone Center approach) interview with cognitive behavioral approach throughout continuum.
Treatment setting: Hospital.
Maximum patients in program: 75-100.
Average number served per year: 79.
Follow-up care offered: 6 mos and 12 mos last 3 yrs of aftercare.

Syracuse

99. Benjamine Rush Center—Adult Services—Eating Disorders Track

650 Salina St
Syracuse, NY 13202
Contact: Sherie Ramsgard, RD, MSD. 315-476-2176 ext 233, *fax:* 315-476-0127
Hotline: 800-647-6479
Disorders treated: Anorexia nervosa; Bulimia nervosa.
Population treated: Women & men; Adolescents.
Programs: Inpatient.

Treatments: Individual therapy; Group therapy; Family therapy; Family groups; Medication; Body image; Nutrition counseling; Exercise.
Treatment setting: Hospital.
Average length of program: 2 wks.
Maximum patients in program: 10.
Follow-up care offered: Upon discharge ensure adequate outpatient treatment.

White Plains

100. Cornell Eating Disorders Program

New York Hospital—Cornell Medical Center, 21 Bloomingdale Rd
White Plains, NY 10605
Contact: Katherine Halmi, MD, Director. 914-997-5875, *fax:* 914-997-5781, *e-mail:* khalmi%westnyh@nyh.med.cornell.edu
Date Established: 1979.
Disorders treated: Anorexia nervosa; Bulimia nervosa; Compulsive eating (or BED); Obesity.
Population treated: Adolescents; Young children; Adults.
Programs: Inpatient; Partial hospitalization; Residential or Day-Hospital; Outpatient; Clinical studies; Community education programs; Intensive outpatient; Follow-up programs.
Treatments: Individual therapy; Group therapy; Family therapy; Family groups; Medication; Body image; Nutrition counseling; Cognitive Behavior Therapy.
Treatment setting: Hospital; Therapist's office; PHP.
Maximum patients in program: 300-400.
Average number served per year: 500-600.
Follow-up care offered: 2 mos; 6 mos; 12 mos; 18 mos; 2-5 yrs.

NORTH CAROLINA

Durham

101. Duke University Diet and Fitness Center

804 W Trinity Ave
Durham, NC 27701
Contact: Ronette L Kolotkin, PhD. 919-684-6331 ext 239, *fax:* 919-682-8869
Date Established: 1972.
Disorders treated: Compulsive eating (or BED); Obesity.
Population treated: Adults; Elderly.
Programs: Residential or Day-Hospital; Intensive outpatient; Follow-up programs.
Treatments: Individual therapy; Group therapy; Experimental therapy; Body image; Nutrition counseling; Exercise; Lifestyle modification.
Treatment setting: Hospital.
Program cost: 1 wk $2,495; 2 wks $4,495; 4 wks $5,595.
Maximum patients in program: 120.
Average number served per year: 1200.

102. Structure House

3017 Pickett Rd
Durham, NC 27705
Contact: Lee Kern, MSW. 919-313-3124 *Facility phone:* 919-493-4205, *Facility fax:* 919-490-0191, *e-mail:* info@structurehouse.com

Internet: http://www.structurehouse.com
Date Established: 1977.
Disorders treated: Compulsive eating (or BED); Obesity.
Population treated: Women & men; Adults.
Programs: Residential or Day-Hospital.
Treatments: Individual therapy; Group therapy; Body image; Nutrition counseling; Exercise; psychoeducational classes, workshops, intensive groups.
Treatment setting: Residential setting.
Program cost: $1,196/wk for 4 wks.
Average length of program: 4 wks.
Maximum patients in program: 110.
Average number served per year: 600.
Follow-up care offered: 3 mos; 18 mos.
Comments: Treatment team comprises psychotherapists, exercise staff, a nutritionist, and a nurse.

Fletcher

103. Hope Program, Park Ridge Hospital, Fletcher

PO Box 1569
Fletcher, NC 28732
Contact: Jane Lawson. 828-681-2726, *fax:* 828-681-2742, *e-mail:* jlawson@buncombe.main.nc.us
Internet: http://main.nc.us/HOPE/
Hotline: 800-954-4673
Date Established: 1986.
Disorders treated: Anorexia nervosa; Bulimia nervosa; Compulsive eating (or BED).
Population treated: Women only; Adolescents; Young children; Will take adolescent males.
Programs: Inpatient; Partial hospitalization; Intensive outpatient; Support groups.
Treatments: Individual therapy; Group therapy; Family groups; Family therapy; Addiction model; Experimental therapy; Medication; Body image; Nutrition counseling; 12-Step; Christian-based.
Treatment setting: Hospital; Therapist's office.
Maximum patients in program: 26.
Average number served per year: 200.

Hendersonville

104. Hope Program, Park Ridge Hospital, Hendersonville

136 Homestead Farms Cir
Hendersonville, NC 28792
Contact: Kelly Brown. 828-684-1115, *fax:* 828-687-6064
Disorders treated: Anorexia nervosa; Bulimia nervosa; Compulsive eating (or BED); Obesity; Post-traumatic stress disorder; Depression.
Population treated: Women only; Adolescents; Geriatric.
Programs: Inpatient; Partial hospitalization; Outpatient; Intensive outpatient.
Treatments: Individual therapy; Group therapy; Family therapy; Addiction model; Experimental therapy; Medication; Body image; Nutrition counseling; 12-Step; Christian-based.
Treatment setting: Hospital; Therapist's office.
Maximum patients in program: 12-15.

NORTH DAKOTA

Grand Forks

105. Altru Hospital—Psychiatry/Chemical Dependency

PO Box 6002
Grand Forks, ND 58206-6002
Contact: Mike Dewald. 701-780-5950, *fax:* 701-780-3477, *e-mail:* mdewald@medpark.grand-forks.nd.us
Hotline: 701-780-5900
Date Established: 1980.
Disorders treated: Anorexia nervosa; Bulimia nervosa.
Population treated: Women & men; Adolescents.
Programs: Inpatient; Partial hospitalization; Outpatient.
Treatments: Individual therapy; Group therapy; Family therapy; Family groups; Body image; Nutrition counseling; 12-Step; Exercise.
Treatment setting: Hospital.
Average number served per year: 730.
Follow-up care offered: By referral evaluation or by staff post-discharge.

OHIO

Akron

106. Eating Disorders Program; Children's Hospital

1 Perkins Square
Akron, OH 44308
Contact: Holly Berchin, RN, MNS, CS. 330-379-8493, *fax:* 330-258-3856, *e-mail:* BMURPHY@chmca.org *Facility phone:* 330-379-8590
Date Established: 1988.
Disorders treated: Anorexia nervosa; Bulimia nervosa; Compulsive eating (or BED); Obesity; Depression; Obsessive-compulsive disorder.
Population treated: Adolescents; Young children.
Programs: Inpatient; Partial hospitalization; Residential or Day-Hospital; Outpatient; Support groups.
Treatments: Individual therapy; Group therapy; Family therapy; Medication; Nutrition counseling.
Treatment setting: Hospital; Therapist's office.
Program cost: Therapy $114/hr.
Average length of program: 6-12 mos.
Average number served per year: 80-100.
Comments: Family therapy a requirement. Team approach used. Includes therapists, RD, psychiatrists, and primary care pediatricians.

Cleveland

107. Cleveland Clinic Foundation—Eating Disorder Intensive Outpatient Program

9500 Euclid Ave
Cleveland, OH 44195
Contact: Mary Kenney; John Glazer, MD; Eating Disorder Evaluation Center Ellen Rome, MD, MPH. 216-444-6148, *fax:* 216-445-5749, *e-mail:* kenneym@cesmtp.ccf.org; romee@cesmtp.ccf.org *Facility phone:* 216-444-6142
Date Established: 1996.

Disorders treated: Anorexia nervosa; Bulimia nervosa; Compulsive eating (or BED).
Population treated: Women & men; Adolescents; Adults.
Programs: Partial hospitalization (children and adolescents only, 7-17 yrs); Intensive outpatient (adolescents and young adults, 13-40 yrs).
Treatments: Group therapy; Family groups; Experimental therapy; Medication; Body image; Nutrition counseling.
Treatment setting: Hospital.
Program cost: Intensive outpatient $3500.
Average length of program: Intensive outpatient 6 wks, 9 hrs of group therapy/wk.
Maximum patients in program: 8.

Columbus

108. Center for the Treament of Eating Disorders (CTED)

445 E. Dublin Granville Rd
Columbus, OH 43229
Contact: Laura Hill, PhD. 614-785-7450, *fax:* 614-785-7471 *Facility phone:* 614-846-2833
Date Established: 1983.
Disorders treated: Anorexia nervosa; Bulimia nervosa; Compulsive eating (or BED); Obesity.
Population treated: Women & men; Adolescents; Young children.
Programs: Partial hospitalization; Residential or Day-Hospital; Outpatient; Community education programs; Intensive outpatient; Support groups.
Treatments: Individual therapy; Group therapy; Family therapy; Family groups; Medication; Nutrition counseling; Marital therapy.
Treatment setting: Hospital; Therapist's office.
Program cost: $145 initial visit.
Average length of program: 6 mos-2 yrs.
Comments: During course of treatment patients meet in individual and/or group therapy sessions, see psychiatrist if needed, work with staff dietician and personal physician. If inpatient treatment is needed, CTED works with patient's insurance company to provide referrals. In addition to weekly therapy session, patients are encouraged to attend the eating disorder support groups. Three groups meet simultaneously for persons with bulimia nervosa, anorexia nervosa, binge eating disorder, and one group for family and friends.

Dayton

109. Children's Medical Center

One Children's Plaza
Dayton, OH 45404
Contact: Dr. David Rube. 937-226-8300 ext 8042, *fax:* 937-463-5076
Date Established: 1993.
Disorders treated: Anorexia nervosa; Bulimia nervosa; Compulsive eating (or BED).
Population treated: Women & men; Adolescents; Young children.
Programs: Inpatient; Outpatient; Support groups; Follow-up programs.

Treatments: Individual therapy; Group therapy; Family therapy; Family groups; Medication; Nutrition counseling.
Treatment setting: Hospital; Therapist's office.
Maximum patients in program: 30.
Average number served per year: 15.

Toledo

110. Toledo Center for Eating Disorders

7261 W Central Ave
Toledo, OH 43617
Contact: David M Garner, PhD. 419-843-2000, *fax:* 419-843-1336, *e-mail:* garnerdm@aol.com
Date Established: 1994.
Disorders treated: Anorexia nervosa; Bulimia nervosa; Compulsive eating (or BED); Obesity.
Population treated: Women & men; Adolescents.
Programs: Residential or Day-Hospital; Outpatient; Clinical studies; Community education programs; Intensive outpatient.
Treatments: Individual therapy; Group therapy; Family therapy; Family groups; Medication; Body image; Nutrition counseling.
Treatment setting: Treatment center.
Maximum patients in program: 60.
Average number served per year: 150.
Follow-up care offered: By phone or in person. Patients complete standardized self-report.

OKLAHOMA

Oklahoma City

111. Professional Help for Eating Disorders at St Anthony

1000 N Lee
Oklahoma City, OK 73101
Contact: Jodi Dodson. 405-272-6216, *fax:* 405-272-8346
Hotline: 405-272-6216
Date Established: 1997.
Disorders treated: Anorexia nervosa; Bulimia nervosa; Compulsive eating (or BED); Obesity.
Population treated: Women & men; Adolescents.
Programs: Inpatient; Outpatient; Community education programs; Support groups.
Treatments: Individual therapy; Group therapy; Family therapy; Family groups; Addiction model; Experimental therapy; Medication; Body image; Nutrition counseling; Christian-based.
Treatment setting: Hospital; Therapist's office; Clinic.
Program cost: Intensive outpatient approx $4,000.
Average length of program: 8 wks.
Maximum patients in program: 8.
Average number served per year: 40.
Follow-up care offered: By appointment.

Tulsa

112. Laureate Psychiatric Clinic and Hospital

6655 S Yale Ave
Tulsa, OK 74136
Contact: Craig Johnson, PhD. *Facility phone:* 918-491-3702, *Facility fax:* 918-481-4065

Internet: http://www.laureate.com
Hotline: 918-491-5600
Date Established: 1990.
Disorders treated: Anorexia nervosa; Bulimia nervosa.
Population treated: Women only; Adolescents; Young children.
Programs: Inpatient; Partial hospitalization; Residential or Day-Hospital; Outpatient; Clinical studies; Community education programs; Intensive outpatient; Follow-up programs.
Treatments: Individual therapy; Group therapy; Family therapy; Family groups; Experimental therapy; Medication; Body image; Nutrition counseling; 12-Step; Exercise.
Treatment setting: Hospital.
Average length of program: 30 days-2 yrs.
Maximum patients in program: 15 bed acute care, 16-20 bed partial hospital additional intensive outpaient.
Follow-up care offered: 6 and 12 mos; questionnaires via mail and telephone.
Comments: Nationally based program. 95% of patients are from out of state. Apartment-like setting in transitional living allows patients to stay on campus for an extended period.

OREGON

Portland

113. Kartini Clinic for Disordered Eating

2800 N Vancouver, Ste 121
Portland, OR 97227
Contact: Julie O'Toole, MD, MPH. 503-249-8851, *fax:* 503-282-3409, *e-mail:* kartiniore@aol.com
Date Established: 1998.
Disorders treated: Anorexia nervosa; Bulimia nervosa; Compulsive eating (or BED); Obesity.
Population treated: Adolescents; Young children; Up to age 16; no lower age limit.
Programs: Inpatient; Intensive outpatient.
Treatments: Group therapy; Nutrition counseling; Medical model.
Treatment setting: Hospital; MD's office.
Comments: Was established as an intensive outpatient program to serve children and adolescents through age 16 who have conditions of disordered eating. Such children may be hospitalized for inpatient medical stabilization at Emanuel Children's hospital in Portland. Day treatment program with hospital being developed.

114. Providence/St. Vincent Medical Center

9206 SW Barnes Rd, 5th floor
Portland, OR 97225
Contact: Barbara Oyler. 503-216-7080, *fax:* 503-216-2485
Hotline: 503-216-7080
Date Established: 1983.
Disorders treated: Anorexia nervosa; Bulimia nervosa.
Population treated: Women & men; Adolescents; Selected dual diagnosis with alcohol and chemical dependency.
Programs: Inpatient; Residential or Day-Hospital; Intensive day-treatment program 8am to 7pm M-F with week-

end medical monitoring for some; inpatient available for short-term medical and psychiatric stabilization.
Treatments: Individual therapy; Group therapy; Family therapy; Family groups; Medication; Body image; 12-Step.
Treatment setting: Hospital.
Program cost: Daily average $550. Inpatient $900-$1,000.
Average length of program: 4-8 wks on a tapered schedule.
Maximum patients in program: 25-30.
Average number served per year: 254.
Follow-up care offered: Outpatient and medications available weekly.

PENNSYLVANIA

Hershey

115. Adolescent Eating Disorders Program

Milton S. Hershey Medical Center
Hershey, PA 17033
Contact: Dr Richard Levine. 717-531-8006, *fax:* 717-531-8985, *e-mail:* RLL@psu.edu
Date Established: 1996.
Disorders treated: Anorexia nervosa; Bulimia nervosa.
Population treated: Adolescents.
Programs: Inpatient; Outpatient; Support groups.
Treatments: Individual therapy; Group therapy; Family therapy; Medication; Nutrition counseling.
Treatment setting: Hospital.
Average number served per year: 100.

116. Penn State Geisenger Health System— Penn State Children's Hospital

PO Box 850, 500 University Dr
Hershey, PA 17033
Contact: John Horn. 717-531-6771
Date Established: 1996.
Disorders treated: Anorexia nervosa; Bulimia nervosa; Compulsive eating (or BED).
Population treated: Adolescents; Young children.
Programs: Inpatient; Outpatient; Support groups.
Treatments: Individual therapy; Group therapy; Family therapy; Body image; Nutrition counseling.
Treatment setting: Hospital; Clinic.
Program cost: $200/90-min visit.
Average length of program: 90-min visit, 30-min each medical/psychology/nutrition.
Average number served per year: 75-80.

Mt. Gretna

117. Philhaven, Women's Day Hospital Program and Mt. Gretua Intensive Outpatient Program

283 S Butler Rd, PO Box 550
Mt. Gretna, PA 17064
Contact: Dr Rosa Cabezas. 717-270-2421, *fax:* 717-270-2455, *e-mail:* rac@philhaven.com *Facility phone:* 717-273-8871
Internet: http://www.philhaven.com
Date Established: 1993.

Disorders treated: Anorexia nervosa; Bulimia nervosa; Compulsive eating (or BED); Body-image; Women's issues.
Population treated: Women only.
Programs: Partial hospitalization; Intensive outpatient.
Treatments: Individual therapy; Group therapy; Family therapy; Experimental therapy; Medication; Body image; Nutrition counseling.
Treatment setting: Psychiatric facility.
Program cost: Day Program $240-$300/day; IOP-$150/day.
Average length of program: Day program 8-10 days; IOP 9 3-hr days.
Maximum patients in program: 15-20.
Average number served per year: Day program 112; IOP 13.

Orfeild

118. Kids Peace National Centers for Kids in Crisis; National Hospital for Kids in Crisis; Athlete Center; Acute/Intensive Residential Program

5300 Kids Peace Dr
Orfeild, PA 10869
Contact: Admissions. 610-799-8586 *Facility phone:* 610-799-8800, *Facility fax:* 610-799-8801
Hotline: 800 FOR A KID
Date Established: 1994.
Disorders treated: Anorexia nervosa; Bulimia nervosa; Compulsive eating (or BED); Self-injurious behaviors.
Population treated: Adolescents; Young children.
Programs: Inpatient; Residential or Day-Hospital.
Treatments: Individual therapy; Group therapy; Family therapy; Addiction model; Experimental therapy; Medication; Body image; Nutrition counseling; Exercise; Wilderness training experience.
Treatment setting: Hospital; School; Residential treatment center.
Average length of program: Residential treatment up to 2 yrs.
Maximum patients in program: 50 hospital; 50 residential.
Average number served per year: Approx 75.
Follow-up care offered: 3 mos; 6 mos.

Philadelphia

119. Belmont Center for Comprehensive Treatment Eating Disorders Program

4200 Monument Rd
Philadelphia, PA 19131
Contact: Susan Ice, MD. 215-581-3842, *fax:* 215-879-2443 *Facility phone:* 215-877-2000
Date Established: 1985.
Disorders treated: Anorexia nervosa; Bulimia nervosa; Compulsive eating (or BED).
Population treated: Women only; Adolescent girls.
Programs: Inpatient; Partial hospitalization; Residential or Day-Hospital; Outpatient; Support groups; Halfway house.

Treatments: Individual therapy; Group therapy; Family therapy; Family groups; Experimental therapy; Medication; Body image; Nutrition counseling; Exercise.
Treatment setting: Hospital; Therapist's office.
Maximum patients in program: 20.
Average number served per year: 250.

120. The Renfrew Center

475 Spring Ln
Philadelphia, PA 19127
Contact: Judi Goldstein, MSS, LSW, Vice President for Professional Relations & Education. 800-736-3739, *fax:* 215-482-7390, *e-mail:* inquiry@renfrew.org
Internet: http://www.renfrew.org
Hotline: 800-736-3739
Date Established: 1985.
Disorders treated: Anorexia nervosa; Bulimia nervosa; Compulsive eating (or BED); Obesity; Women's mental health.
Population treated: Women & men; Adolescents; Young children.
Programs: Inpatient; Partial hospitalization; Residential or Day-Hospital; Outpatient; Community education programs; Intensive outpatient; Support groups; Follow-up programs; Multifamily group/National professional network for clients who may be unable to access Renfrew's services.
Treatments: Individual therapy; Group therapy; Family therapy; Family groups; Experimental therapy; Medication; Body image; Nutrition counseling; 12-Step; Exercise; Feminist therapy; Cognitive behavioral therapy.
Treatment setting: Therapist's office.
Average number served per year: 2,100.
Follow-up care offered: At discharge; 3 mos post-discharge; 1 yr post-discharge through self-report questionnaire.
Comments: Outpatient treatment offices at Coconut Creek, FL; Allendale, NJ; Jericho, NY; New York, NY; Philadelphia, PA.

Pittsburgh

121. St. Francis Medical Center/Eating Disorder Services

400 45th St
Pittsburgh, PA 15201
Contact: Jerry E Smith, PhD. 412-622-4545 ext 320, *fax:* 412-622-7183
Date Established: 1984.
Disorders treated: Anorexia nervosa; Bulimia nervosa; Compulsive eating (or BED); Obesity; Affective disorders.
Population treated: Women & men; Adolescents.
Programs: Inpatient; Partial hospitalization; Outpatient; Residential or Day-Hospital; Community education programs; Intensive outpatient; Support groups.
Treatments: Individual therapy; Group therapy; Family therapy; Family groups; Addiction model; Medication; Nutrition counseling; 12-Step.
Treatment setting: Hospital.
Program cost: $1,200/day inpatient; $165 intensive partial; $95/outpatient session.

Average length of program: Inpatient 7 days; intensive 21 days; outpatient 3 mos.
Average number served per year: 400.

Scranton

122. Behavioral Healthcare Center

1016 Pittston Ave, Ste 201
Scranton, PA 18505
Contact: Richard Sibert, MD. 717-961-8803, *fax:* 717-961-8879
Date Established: 1994.
Disorders treated: Anorexia nervosa; Bulimia nervosa; Compulsive eating (or BED).
Population treated: Women & men; Adolescents; Young children.
Programs: Inpatient; Residential or Day-Hospital; Outpatient; Community education programs; Intensive outpatient; Follow-up programs.
Treatments: Individual therapy; Group therapy; Family therapy; Addiction model; Experimental therapy; Medication; Body image; Nutrition counseling; 12-Step; Exercise; Dietitian.
Treatment setting: Hospital; Therapist's office.
Maximum patients in program: 10/group.
Average number served per year: 15.
Follow-up care offered: Monthly consultations with psychiatrists and team members.
Comments: Participated in National Eating Disorders Awareness week in office and schools locally. Group therapy offered as demand occurs. Work with local hospitals (Mercy and Moses Taylor) developing referral network known as the Comprehensive Eating Disorders Coalition affiliated with EDAP.

RHODE ISLAND

Providence

123. Hasbro Partial Hospitalization Program

593 Eddy St
Providence, RI 02903
Contact: Suzanne Riggs, MD, or Thomas Roesler, MD. 401-444-8638, *fax:* 401-444-7018
Date Established: 1998.
Disorders treated: Anorexia nervosa; Bulimia nervosa.
Population treated: Adolescents; Young children.
Programs: Inpatient; Partial hospitalization.
Treatments: Individual therapy; Group therapy; Family therapy; Medication; Nutrition counseling.
Treatment setting: Hospital.
Program cost: $600/day.
Maximum patients in program: 6.
Comments: This unit treats children and adolescents with a variety of medical conditions including eating disorders. The unit is a collaboration between the Department of Pediatrics and a university medical school affiliated children's hospital.

SOUTH CAROLINA

Charleston

124. Medical University of South Carolina Institute of Psychiatry, Eating Disorders Program

171 Ashley Ave
Charleston, SC 29425
Contact: Timothy Brewerton, MD. 843-792-9888, *fax:* 843-792-5503, *e-mail:* psynews@musc.edu
Internet: http://www.musc.edu/psychiatry
Date Established: 1987.
Disorders treated: Anorexia nervosa; Bulimia nervosa; Compulsive eating (or BED); Obesity.
Population treated: Women & men; Adolescents; Young children.
Programs: Inpatient; Partial hospitalization; Residential or Day-Hospital; Outpatient; Clinical studies; Community education programs; Intensive outpatient; Support groups; Follow-up programs; Apartment program available.
Treatments: Individual therapy; Group therapy; Family therapy; Family groups; Medication; Body image; Nutrition counseling; Exercise; Cognitive behavioral therapy.
Treatment setting: Hospital.
Average length of program: Min 3 wks in day treatment.
Maximum patients in program: Day treatment 10.
Average number served per year: 150.

Greenville

125. Behavioral Health Services/Marshall I Pickens Hospital

701 Grove Rd
Greenville, SC 29605-5601
Contact: Jo Powell. 864-455-8988, *fax:* 864-455-4540
Date Established: 1994.
Disorders treated: Anorexia nervosa; Bulimia nervosa; Compulsive eating (or BED); OCD; Anxiety.
Population treated: Women & men; Adolescents; Young children.
Programs: Inpatient; Partial hospitalization; Residential or Day-Hospital; Outpatient; Community education programs; Intensive outpatient.
Treatments: Individual therapy; Group therapy; Family therapy; Family groups; Experimental therapy; Medication; Nutrition counseling; 12-Step.
Treatment setting: Hospital; Therapist's office.

SOUTH DAKOTA

Yankton

126. Human Services Center—Adolescent Psychologic Program

PO Box 76, 3515 Broadway Avenue
Yankton, SD 57078
Contact: Jody M Smith, MA. 605-668-3331, *fax:* 605-668-3193, *e-mail:* jodys@hsc-dhs.state.sd.us
Date Established: 1992.
Disorders treated: Anorexia nervosa; Bulimia nervosa.
Population treated: Adolescents; Age 13-17.
Programs: Inpatient; Community education programs.

Treatments: Individual therapy; Group therapy; Family therapy; Medication; Nutrition counseling; Exercise.
Treatment setting: Hospital.
Program cost: Sliding scale.
Average length of program: 3 wks.
Average number served per year: 10.
Comments: State facility only for residents of South Palch will continue as long as necessary regardless of ability to pay.

TEXAS

Buffalo Gap

127. Shades of Hope Treatment Center

PO Box 639
Buffalo Gap, TX 79508
Contact: Cindy Henson. 915-572-3843, *fax:* 915-572-3405
Date Established: 1988.
Disorders treated: Anorexia nervosa; Bulimia nervosa; Compulsive eating (or BED); Obesity.
Population treated: Women & men; Adolescents.
Programs: Inpatient; Residential or Day-Hospital; Outpatient; Community education programs; Intensive outpatient; Support groups; Follow-up programs.
Treatments: Individual therapy; Group therapy; Family therapy; Family groups; Addiction model; Experimental therapy; Medication; Body image; Nutrition counseling; 12-Step; Christian-based; Exercise.
Treatment setting: Residential treatment center.
Program cost: $350/day inpatient.
Average length of program: 42 days.
Maximum patients in program: 20.
Follow-up care offered: Aftercare 1 mo and 1 yr. Aftercare group once weekly for 1 yr.

Dallas

128. Presbyterian Hospital Dallas Eating Disorders Program

8200 Walnut Hill Ln
Dallas, TX 75231
Contact: R Lynn Markle, MD, Clinical Director. 214-369-5797, *fax:* 214-369-6356 *Facility phone:* 214-345-5500,
Facility fax: 214-345-8618
Internet: http://pbsnet.phs.care.org
Date Established: 1995.
Disorders treated: Anorexia nervosa; Bulimia nervosa; Compulsive eating (or BED); Atypical eating disorders.
Population treated: Women & men; Adults.
Programs: Inpatient; Residential or Day-Hospital; Support groups; Outpatient education group therapy plus aftercare.
Treatments: Individual therapy; Group therapy; Family groups; Medication; Body image; Nutrition counseling; Art therapy; Recreation Therapy.
Treatment setting: Hospital; Therapist's office.
Program cost: Inpatient $435; day hospital $232 (includes 3 meals).
Maximum patients in program: 12.
Average number served per year: 95.
Comments: In the process of gathering information on patient population re echocardiograph & bone densitometry.

129. UT Southwestern—Children's Medical Center of Dallas

5323 Harry Hines Blvd
Dallas, TX 75235-9070
Contact: David A Waller, MD. 214-648-3898, *fax:* 214-648-7980, *e-mail:* dwalle@mednet.swmed.edu
Date Established: 1983.
Disorders treated: Anorexia nervosa; Bulimia nervosa; Other psychiatric eating disorders.
Population treated: Adolescents; Young children.
Programs: Inpatient; Partial hospitalization; Residential or Day-Hospital; Outpatient; Clinical studies; Intensive outpatient; Support groups; Follow-up programs.
Treatments: Individual therapy; Group therapy; Family therapy; Family groups; Experimental therapy; Medication; Body image; Nutrition counseling.
Treatment setting: Hospital.
Maximum patients in program: 20.
Average number served per year: 50.
Follow-up care offered: As needed.

Richardson

130. Paul Meier New Life Day Hospital

2071 N Collins Blvd
Richardson, TX 75080
Contact: Jacquelyn Jeffrey. 972-437-4698, *fax:* 972-690-9309
Date Established: 1988.
Disorders treated: Anorexia nervosa; Bulimia nervosa; Compulsive eating (or BED); Obesity.
Population treated: Adults; Outpatient—all ages.
Programs: Partial hospitalization; Outpatient; Intensive outpatient.
Treatments: Individual therapy; Group therapy; Family therapy; Family groups; Addiction model; Experimental therapy; Medication; Body image; Nutrition counseling; 12-Step; Christian-based.
Treatment setting: Day hospital and outpatient facility.
Program cost: Day hospital $355/day; sliding scale available.
Average length of program: Average 2 wks.
Maximum patients in program: Day hospital 20.
Average number served per year: Day hospital 1800; outpatient 7000.
Follow-up care offered: Yes.

UTAH

Orem

131. Center for Change

1790 N State St
Orem, UT 84057
Contact: Lisa VonColln or Denise Stewart. 801-224-8255, *fax:* 801-224-8301, *e-mail:* mail@cfchange.com
Internet: http://www.cfchange.com
Date Established: 1995.
Disorders treated: Anorexia nervosa; Bulimia nervosa; Compulsive eating (or BED); Obesity; Posttraumatic stress disorder; Abuse; Depression.
Population treated: Women only; Adolescents.

Programs: Inpatient; Partial hospitalization; Residential or Day-Hospital; Outpatient; Clinical studies; Community education programs; Intensive outpatient; Support groups; Follow-up programs.
Treatments: Individual therapy; Group therapy; Family therapy; Family groups; Addiction model; Experimental therapy; Medication; Body image; Nutrition counseling; 12-Step; Christian-based; Exercise.
Treatment setting: Hospital.
Program cost: $750/day.
Average length of program: 60-90 days.
Maximum patients in program: 16.
Average number served per year: 78.
Follow-up care offered: On discharge; in 6 mos; then annually.

VERMONT

Brattleboro

132. Brattleboro Retreat Eating Disorder Services

Box 803
Brattleboro, VT 05302
Contact: Sandra Campbell PsyD. 802-345-5550, *fax:* 802-258-3788 *Facility phone:* 802-258-3707
Internet: http://www.bratretreat.org
Date Established: 1985.
Disorders treated: Anorexia nervosa; Bulimia nervosa; Compulsive eating (or BED); Obesity.
Population treated: Women & men; Adolescents.
Programs: Inpatient; Partial hospitalization; Outpatient; Intensive outpatient.
Treatments: Individual therapy; Group therapy; Family therapy; Medication; Nutrition counseling.
Treatment setting: Hospital; Therapist's office.
Average number served per year: 100+.

Essex Junction

133. Family Therapy Associates: Continuum

15 Pinecrest Dr
Essex Junction, VT 05452
Contact: Jodie Bisson, MA. 802-878-4399, *fax:* 802-878-0633
Disorders treated: Anorexia nervosa; Bulimia nervosa; Compulsive eating (or BED).
Population treated: Women only; Adolescents.
Programs: Partial hospitalization; Community education programs; Intensive outpatient; Follow-up programs.
Treatments: Individual therapy; Group therapy; Family therapy; Family groups; Experimental therapy; Medication; Body image; Nutrition counseling; Dialectical behavior skill training; Case management; Emergency on-call services.
Treatment setting: Clinic.
Program cost: $300/day partial hospital all inclusive; $175/day intensive outpatient all inclusive.
Average length of program: 5-6 hrs/day partial hospital—LOS 20-25 days; 3-4 hours/day intensive outpatient—LOS 17 days.
Maximum patients in program: 10.
Average number served per year: 127.

Follow-up care offered: 30 day follow-up interviews conducted either face-to-face or over the phone.
Comments: After-care consists of DBT skill training/supportive counseling group once/wk for 90 min.

Ludlow

134. Green Mountain at Fox Run

Fox Ln Box 164
Ludlow, VT 05149
Contact: Elena M Ramerez, PhD. 802-228-8885, *fax:* 802-228-8887, *e-mail:* eramerez@wctv.com *Facility phone:* 800-448-8106, *e-mail:* greenmountain@foxrun.com
Internet: http://fitwoman.com
Date Established: 1973.
Disorders treated: Anorexia nervosa; Bulimia nervosa; Compulsive eating (or BED); Obesity.
Population treated: Women only; Adults.
Programs: Residential or Day-Hospital.
Treatments: Individual therapy; Group therapy; Body image; Nutrition counseling; Exercise; Lectures; Workshops.
Treatment setting: Therapist's office; Residential program.
Average length of program: Minimum 1 wk; recommended full program 4 wks.
Maximum patients in program: 40.
Average number served per year: 350.
Follow-up care offered: Feedback given on progress, 3 mos, 6 mos, 1 yr.

VIRGINIA

New Kent

135. Cumberland Hospital for Children and Adolescents

9407 Cumberland Rd
New Kent, VA 23125
Contact: Marianne Henley. 800-368-3472, *fax:* 804-966-5639
Date Established: 1983.
Disorders treated: Anorexia nervosa; Bulimia nervosa; Compulsive eating (or BED); Obesity; Organic eating disorders; Disordered diabetic eating.
Population treated: Women & men; Adolescents; Young children.
Programs: Inpatient.
Treatments: Individual therapy; Group therapy; Family therapy; Family groups; Experimental therapy; Medication; Body image; Nutrition counseling; Exercise.
Treatment setting: Hospital.
Program cost: Approx $1,000/day.
Average length of program: average 60-90 days.
Maximum patients in program: 52.
Average number served per year: 25.
Follow-up care offered: At 3 and 12 mos via telephone.
Comments: Specializes in treating diabetics with eating disorders.

WASHINGTON

Edmons

136. The Center for Counseling and Health Resources, Inc.

547 Dayton
Edmons, WA 98020
Contact: Gregg Jantz, PhD. 425-771-5166, *fax:* 425-670-2807, *e-mail:* DRJANTZ@AOL.COM, *e-mail:* THECENTERINC@MSN.COM
Internet: http://www.aplaceofhope.com
Date Established: 1984.
Disorders treated: Anorexia nervosa; Bulimia nervosa; Compulsive eating (or BED); Obesity; Post-traumatic stress disorder; Depression.
Population treated: Women & men; Adolescents; Young children.
Programs: Partial hospitalization; Support groups; Community education programs; Follow-up programs.
Treatments: Individual therapy; Group therapy; Family therapy; Family groups; Addiction model; Medication; Body image; Nutrition counseling; 12-Step; Christian-based; Exercise.
Treatment setting: Clinic.
Program cost: Sliding scale; approx $3,200 total.
Average length of program: 2 yrs.
Maximum patients in program: 1,000.
Average number served per year: 1,500.
Follow-up care offered: Once a year.
Comments: Serve greater Seattle and Washington state and have options for out-of-state. All services state licensed also for chemical dependency.

Richland

137. Lourdes Counseling Center

1175 Carondelet Dr
Richland, WA 99352
Contact: Nadine Houtrouw, RD, CD, CDE. 509-943-9104 ext 350, *fax:* 509-943-7241
Disorders treated: Anorexia nervosa; Bulimia nervosa; Compulsive eating (or BED); Obesity.
Population treated: Women & men; Adolescents; Young children.
Programs: Inpatient; Outpatient.
Treatments: Individual therapy; Nutrition counseling; Christian-based.
Treatment setting: Hospital; Therapist's office.
Program cost: $990/day included in normal hospitalization for other mental illness.
Maximum patients in program: 35.
Follow-up care offered: Conducted through outpatient services as needed.
Comments: Treatment for eating disorders conducted in conjunction with dietitian, physician, and mental-health counselors.

Seattle

138. Swedish Medical Center Eating Disorders Program

PO Box 70707
Seattle, WA 98107

Contact: Linda Zobrist. 206-781-6345, *fax:* 206-781-6186
Internet: http://www.swedish.org
Date Established: 1986.
Disorders treated: Anorexia nervosa; Bulimia nervosa; Compulsive eating (or BED).
Population treated: Women & men; Adolescents.
Programs: Inpatient; Partial hospitalization; Outpatient; Community education programs; Intensive outpatient; Support groups.
Treatments: Individual therapy; Group therapy; Family therapy; Family groups; Experimental therapy; Medication; Body image; Nutrition counseling; Exercise; Art therapy.
Treatment setting: Hospital.
Average length of program: Intensive outpatient 8 wks; inpatient varies; individual average is 2-3 wks.
Maximum patients in program: 10 inpatient; 10 outpatient.
Average number served per year: 300.
Follow-up care offered: Yes.

WEST VIRGINIA

Morgantown

139. Chestnut Ridge Hospital, Eating Disorder Outpatient

22 Alderman Dr
Morgantown, WV 26505
Contact: Ceia A Collins. 304-594-0752
Date Established: 1991.
Disorders treated: Anorexia nervosa; Bulimia nervosa; Compulsive eating (or BED).
Population treated: Women & men; Adults; Adolescents.
Programs: Inpatient; Partial hospitalization; Outpatient; Community education programs; Intensive outpatient; Support groups.
Treatments: Individual therapy; Group therapy; Family therapy; Body image; Nutrition counseling; Exercise.
Treatment setting: Hospital; Therapist's office.
Follow-up care offered: Yes, as needed.

WISCONSIN

Brown Deer

140. Charter Behavioral Health System of Wisconsin

4600 W Schroeder Drive
Brown Deer, WI 53223
Contact: Dr Susan Kachler. 414-362-1228, *fax:* 414-355-6726 *Facility phone:* 414-355-2273
Internet: http://www.charterbehavioral.com
Hotline: 800-789-1988
Disorders treated: Anorexia nervosa; Bulimia nervosa; Compulsive eating (or BED).
Population treated: Women & men.
Programs: Inpatient; Partial hospitalization; Outpatient; Intensive outpatient.
Treatments: Individual therapy; Group therapy; Family therapy; Family groups; Experimental therapy; Medication; Body image; Nutrition counseling.
Treatment setting: Hospital; Therapist's office.

Program cost: Outpatient $100/session.

La Crosse

141. Gunderson Lutheran Eating Disorders Program

1910 South Ave
La Crosse, WI 54601
Contact: Sarah Stinson. 608-791-4707, *fax:* 608-791-4732 *Facility phone:* 800-362-9567 ext 4707
Internet: http://www.gundluth.org
Date Established: 1990.
Disorders treated: Anorexia nervosa; Bulimia nervosa; Compulsive eating (or BED); Obesity; Eating disorder not otherwise specified (NOS).
Population treated: Women & men; Adolescents; Young children.
Programs: Outpatient; Community education programs.
Treatments: Individual therapy; Group therapy; Family therapy; Family groups; Body image; Nutrition counseling.
Treatment setting: Hospital; Therapist's office.
Average number served per year: 125.
Comments: The program currently is restructuring the intake/assessment process to be more comprehensive and begin family education.

Oconomowac

142. Residential Eating Disorders Center—Rogers Memorial Hospital

37400 Valley Rd
Oconomowac, WI 53018
Contact: Paul Mueller. 920-496-5878, *fax:* 920-496-0809
Facility phone: 414-646-4411, *Facility fax:* 414-646-7802
Internet: http://www.rogershosp.org
Date Established: 1995.
Disorders treated: Anorexia nervosa; Bulimia nervosa; Compulsive eating (or BED).
Population treated: Women & men; Adults; Adolescents; 12- to 18-year-old males separate unit.
Programs: Inpatient; Residential or Day-Hospital; Community education programs; Support groups.
Treatments: Individual therapy; Group therapy; Family therapy; Family groups; Experimental therapy; Medication; Body image; Nutrition counseling; 12-Step; Dance movement, art, music therapies and ropes challenge course.
Treatment setting: Hospital.
Program cost: $14,100/30 days.
Average length of program: 30-60 days.
Maximum patients in program: 30.
Average number served per year: 181.
Comments: Intensive residential treatment program treating voluntary patients with a motivation to change. Care limited to 3 hr/wk. Non-locked facility.

Waukesha

143. Center for Behavioral Health, Waukesha Hospital System, Eating Disorders Treatment and Education Program

725 American Ave
Waukesha, WI 53188
Contact: Mary Leiske. 414-544-2484, *fax:* 414-544-1213, *e-mail:* mary.leiske@whs.org *Facility phone:* 800-326-2011 ext 4036, *Facility fax:* 414-544-1213
Hotline: 800-326-2011 ext 4036
Date Established: 1991.
Disorders treated: Anorexia nervosa; Bulimia nervosa; Compulsive eating (or BED).
Population treated: Women & men; Adolescents; Young children.
Programs: Inpatient; Partial hospitalization; Outpatient; Community education programs; Intensive outpatient; Support groups.
Treatments: Individual therapy; Group therapy; Family therapy; Family groups; Experimental therapy; Medication; Body image; Nutrition counseling; Biopsychosocial model.
Treatment setting: Hospital; Therapist's office.
Maximum patients in program: 50.
Average number served per year: 215.

Wauwatosa

144. Milwaukee Psychiatric Hospital Eating Disorders Program

1220 Dewey Ave
Wauwatosa, WI 53213
Contact: Anthony T Machi, MD. 414-454-6619, *fax:* 414-454-6039 *Facility phone:* 414-454-6600, *Facility fax:* 414-454-6737
Date Established: 1982.
Disorders treated: Anorexia nervosa; Bulimia nervosa; Compulsive eating (or BED); Obesity.
Population treated: Women & men; Adolescents; Young children.
Programs: Inpatient; Partial hospitalization; Residential or Day-Hospital; Outpatient; Support groups; Follow-up programs.
Treatments: Individual therapy; Group therapy; Family therapy; Family groups; Experimental therapy; Medication; Body image; Nutrition counseling; 12-Step.
Treatment setting: Hospital; Therapist's office; School.
Maximum patients in program: 200-400.
Average number served per year: 200.
Follow-up care offered: Only provided if patient reconnects with the agency.

List of Facilities

Note: Numbers refer to entry numbers.

Books on Eating Disorders

This comprehensive bibliography of books on eating disorders and related topics contains most titles that have been published since the late 1980s, and a few older, classic texts. Eating-disorders literature was rather obscure until the mid-1980s; in fact, prior to 1984 there were fewer than 40 books in print. Around that time awareness about "bulimia" became generally widespread in the form of numerous newspaper, magazine, and television feature stories. The 1990s has seen an even greater number of books on these topics, with 20–40 new titles published each year compared to seven in 1982 or even 13 in 1987. This trend is likely to continue as more and more recovered individuals want to tell their stories, therapists share treatment insights, and more books are written for educational purposes.

To make this list more manageable, books are divided into the following subject areas, though many titles might be suited to more than one category:

I.   General Information on Eating Disorders
II.   General Self-Help
III.   Anorexia Nervosa and Bulimia
IV.   Compulsive Eating, Binge Eating and Obesity
V.   Body Image and Size Acceptance
VI.   Educational
VII.   For Young People
VIII. For Parents and Loved Ones
IX.   Personal Stories, Biography, and Fiction
X.   Professional Texts
XI.   Sociocultural and Historical Perspectives

I. GENERAL INFORMATION ON EATING DISORDERS

Arenson, G. *Substance Called Food*. New York: McGraw-Hill, 1989.

Bennett, W. & Gurin, J. *Dieter's Dilemma: Eating Less and Weighing More*. New York: Basic Books, 1982.

Berg, F. *Health Risks of Weight Loss*. Hettinger, ND: Healthy Weight Journal, 1992.

Bruch, H. *Eating Disorders: Obesity, Anorexia Nervosa and the Person Within*. New York: Basic Books, 1973.

Claude-Pierre, P. *Secret Language of Eating Disorders*. New York: Random House, Inc., 1997.

Costin, C. *Eating Disorder Sourcebook*. Los Angeles, CA: Lowell House, 1996.

Friedman, S. *When Girls Feel Fat*. Vancouver, BC: Salal Books, 1997.

Frissell, S. & Harney, P. *Eating Disorders and Weight Control*. Springfield, NJ: Enslow Publishers, 1998.

Hesse-Biber, S. *Am I Thin Enough Yet?* Cary, NC: Oxford University Press, Inc., 1996.

Lemberg, R. (Ed.). *Eating Disorders: A Reference Sourcebook*. Phoenix, AZ: The Oryx Press, 1999.

Moe, B. *Coping with Eating Disorders*. New York: Rosen Publishing Group, 1995.

O'Halloran, M.S. *Focus on Eating Disorders: A Reference Handbook*. Santa Barbara, CA: ABC-CLIO, 1993.

Woodman, M. *Addiction to Perfection*. Toronto: Inner City Books, 1982.

Woodman, M. *The Owl Was a Baker's Daughter: Obesity, Anorexia Nervosa and the Repressed Feminine*. Toronto: Inner City Books, 1980.

Zerbe, K. *Body Betrayed: A Deeper Understanding of Women, Eating Disorders and Treatment*. Carlsbad, CA: Gürze Books, 1993.

II. GENERAL SELF-HELP

Abraham, S. & Llewellyn-Jones, D. *Eating Disorders: The Facts—Fourth Edition*. Oxford: Oxford University Press, 1997.

Abramson, E. *Emotional Eating: A Practical Guide to Taking Control*. New York: Lexington Books, 1993.

Asada, C. & Haase, J. *Conscious Eating: How to Stop Eating in Response to Everything!* Seattle, WA: Peanut Butter Publishing, 1997.

Barnhill, J. & Taylor, N. *If You Think You Have an Eating Disorder*. New York: Dell Publishing, 1998.

Billigmeier, S. *Inner Eating*. Nashville, TN: Thomas Nelson, 1991.

Bray-Garretson, H. & Cook, K. *Chaotic Eating: A Guide to Recovery*. Grand Rapids, MI: Zondervan Publishing House, 1992.

Champion, V. *Change Your Relationship with Food: Soar Above the Battlefield*. Tempe, AZ: Feeding the Heart, 1997.

Cohen, M.A. *French Toast for Breakfast: Declaring Peace with Emotional Eating*. Carlsbad, CA: Gürze Books, 1995.

David, M. *Nourishing Wisdom: A Mind/Body Approach to Nutrition and Well-Being*. New York: Random House, Inc., 1991.

Elisabeth, L. *Inner Harvest: Daily Meditations for Recovery from Eating Disorders.* Center City, MN: Hazelden, 1990.

Garrison, T. & Levitsky, D. *Fed Up! A Woman's Guide to Freedom from the Diet/Weight Prison.* New York: Carroll & Graf Publishers, 1993.

Greeson, J. *It's Not What You're Eating, It's What's Eating You.* New York: Simon & Schuster, 1991.

Hirschmann, J. & Munter, C. *When Women Stop Hating Their Bodies.* New York: Random House, Inc., 1995.

Hollis, J. *Fat is a Family Affair.* New York: HarperCollins Publishers, 1985.

Kano, S. *Making Peace with Food.* New York: HarperCollins Publishers, 1989.

Katrina, K., King, N. & Hayes, D. *Moving Away From Diets.* Lake Dallas, TX: Helm Seminars, Publishing, 1996.

Lefever, R. *How to Combat Anorexia, Bulimia and Compulsive Overeating.* London: Promise Publishing Limited, 1988.

Levine, M. *I Wish I Were Thin. . . I Wish I Were Fat: The Real Reasons We Overeat and What We Can Do About It.* Huntington Station, NY: Vanderbilt Press, 1997.

Mallord, L. *No More Black Days: Complete Freedom from Depression, Eating Disorders and Compulsive Behaviors.* Venice, CA: White Stone Publishers, 1992.

Marx, R. *It's Not Your Fault: Overcoming Anorexia and Bulimia through Biopsychiatry.* New York: Penguin, 1991.

McFarland, B. *Shame and Body Image.* Deerfield Beach, FL: Health Communications, 1990.

Meltsner, S. *Body & Soul: A Guide to Lasting Recovery from Compulsive Eating and Bulimia.* Center City, MN: Hazelden, 1993.

Minirth, F., Meier, P., Hemfelt, R., Sneed, S. & Hawkins, D. *Love Hunger: Recovery from Food Addiction.* Nashville, TN: Thomas Nelson, 1990.

Normandi, C. & Roark, L. *It's Not About Food: Healing from the Obsession with Food and Weight.* New York, NY: Putnam Publishing Group, 1998.

Omichinski, L. *You Count, Calories Don't—Third Edition.* Winnipeg: Tamos Books, Inc., 1993.

Price, D. *Healing the Hungry Self: The Diet-Free Solution to Lifelong Weight Management.* New York: Plume, 1998.

Radcliffe, R. *Enlightened Eating.* Minneapolis, MN: EASE, 1996.

Rodin, J. *Body Traps.* New York: William Morrow, 1992.

Rose, L. *Life Isn't Weighed on the Bathroom Scale.* Waco, TX: WRS Group, 1994.

Roth, G. *Feeding the Hungry Heart.* Bergenfield, NJ: Penguin, 1983.

Schroeder, C. *Fat Is Not a Four-Letter Word.* Minneapolis, MN: DCI Publishing/Chronomid, 1992.

Sheppard, K. *Food Addiction: The Body Knows.* Deerfield Beach, FL: Health Communications, 1993.

Smith, P. *Food Trap.* Lake Mary, FL: Creation House, 1991.

Sward, S. *You Are More Than What You Weigh.* Denver, CO: Wholesome Publishing, 1995.

Virtue, D. *Constant Craving: What Your Food Cravings Mean and How to Overcome Them.* Carlsbad, CA: Hay House, 1995.

Worth, J. *Toad Within: How to Control Eating Choices.* Dubuque, IA: Islewest Publishing, 1995.

Zimbelman, L. *Stop Eating Your Feelings: Workbook & Guide.* Rancho Palos Verdes, CA: Women and Their Families in Recovery, 1997.

III. ANOREXIA NERVOSA & BULIMIA

Boskind-White, M. & White, W. *Bulimiarexia: The Binge-Purge Cycle.* New York: W. W. Norton & Co., Inc., 1983.

Bruch, H. *Golden Cage: The Enigma of Anorexia Nevosa.* New York: Random House, Inc., 1978.

Buckroyd, J. *Anorexia & Bulimia: Your Questions Answered.* Rockport, MA: Element Books, 1996.

Cooper, P. *Bulimia Nervosa & Binge-Eating: A Guide to Recovery.* London: Robinson Publishing, 1995.

Crisp, A. *Anorexia Nervosa: Let Me Be.* London: Academic Press, 1980.

Crisp, A., Joughin, N., Halek, C. & Bowyer, C. *Anorexia Nervosa: The Wish to Change.* East Sussex, UK: Psychology Press, 1996.

Fodor, V. *Desperately Seeking Self: An Inner Guidebook for People with Eating Problems.* Carlsbad, CA: Gürze Books, 1997.

Hall, L. & Cohn, L. *Bulimia: A Guide to Recovery—Fifth Edition.* Carlsbad, CA: Gürze Books, 1998.

Hall, L. & Ostroff, M. *Anorexia Nervosa: A Guide to Recovery.* Carlsbad, CA: Gürze Books, 1998.

Jantz, G. *Hope, Help, & Healing for Eating Disorders.* Wheaton, IL: Harold Shaw Publishers, 1995.

Kolodny, N. *When Food's a Foe: How You Can Confront and Conquer Your Eating Disorder.* Boston, MA: Little, Brown and Company, 1992.

Levenkron, S. *Treating & Overcoming Anorexia Nervosa.* New York: Warner Books, Inc., 1982.

MacLeod, S. *The Art of Starvation.* New York: Schocken Books, 1981.

O'Neill, C. *Starving for Attention.* New York: Continuum, 1982.

Orbach, S. *Hunger Strike: The Anorectic's Struggle as a Metaphor for Our Age.* New York: W. W. Norton & Co., Inc., 1986.

Remuda Ranch. *Beyond The Looking Glass: Daily Devotions.* Wickenburg, AZ: Remuda Ranch, 1992.

Rumney, A. *Dying to Please: Anorexia Nervosa and Its Cure.* Jefferson, NC: McFarland, 1983.

Sandbek, T. *Deadly Diet: Recovering from Anorexia and Bulimia—Second Edition.* Oakland, CA: New Harbinger Publications, 1993.

Schmidt, U. & Treasure, J. *Getting Better Bit(e) by Bit(e).* East Sussex, UK: Lawrence Erlbaum Associates, 1993.

Siegel, M., Brisman, J. & Weinshel, M. *Surviving an Eating Disorder—Revised Edition.* New York: Harper & Row, 1997.

Treasure, J. *Anorexia Nervosa: A Survival Guide for Families, Friends and Sufferers.* East Sussex, UK: Psychology Press, 1997.

Vredevelt, P., Newman, D. & Harry, B. (Eds.). *Thin Disguise: Overcoming and Understanding Anorexia and Bulimia.* Nashville, TN: Thomas Nelson, 1996.

Way, E. *Anorexia Nervosa and Recovery.* Binghamton, NY: The Haworth Press, 1993.

Weiss, L., Katzman, M. & Wolchik, S. *You Can't Have Your Cake & Eat It Too: A Program for Controlling Bulimia.* Phoenix, AZ: Golden Psych Press, 1986.

IV. COMPULSIVE EATING, BINGE EATING & OBESITY

"A.", Jim. *Recovery from Compulsive Eating: A Complete Guide to the Twelve Step Program.* Center City, MN: Hazelden, 1994.

Alpert, J. *I Always Start My Diet on Monday: A Unique Approach to Permanently Conquer Emotional Overeating.* Northfield, IL: Pearl Publishing, 1997.

Anonymous. *Twelve Steps & Twelve Traditions.* Rio Rancho, NM: Overeaters Anonymous, 1995.

Bruno, B. *Worth Your Weight.* Bethel, CT: Rutledge Books, Inc., 1996.

Fairburn, C. *Overcoming Binge Eating.* New York: Guilford Press, 1995.

Foreyt, J. & Goodrick, K. Living *Without Dieting.* New York: Warner Books, Inc., 1992.

Gaesser, G. *Big Fat Lies: The Truth about Your Weight and Your Health.* New York: Fawcett Columbine, 1996.

Hirschmann, J. & Munter, C. *Overcoming Overeating.* New York: Random House, Inc., 1988.

Johnston, A. *Eating in the Light of the Moon.* Secaucus, NJ: Carol Publishing Group, 1996.

Katherine, A. *Anatomy of a Food Addiction.* Carlsbad, CA: Gürze Books, 1991.

"L," Elisabeth, & Jennings, J. *Twelve Steps for Overeaters: An Interpretation of the Twelve Steps of Overeaters Anonymous.* Center City, MN: Hazelden, 1996.

Levine, M. *I Wish I Were Thin—I Wish I Were Fat.* Huntington Station, NY: Vanderbilt Press, 1997.

Miller, P. *If I'm So Smart Why Do I Eat Like This?* New York: Warner Books, 1988.

Newman, L. *Eating Our Hearts Out.* Freedom, CA: Crossing Press, 1993.

Roth, G. *Breaking Free from Compulsive Eating.* Bergenfield, NJ: Penguin, 1984.

Roth, G. *Why Weight: A Guide to Ending Compulsive Eating.* Bergenfield, NJ: Penguin, 1989.

Simpson, C. *Coping with Compulsive Eating.* New York: Rosen Publishing Group, 1997.

Ward, S. *Beyond Feast or Famine: Daily Affirmations for Compulsive Eaters.* Deerfield Beach, FL: Health Communications, 1990.

V. BODY IMAGE AND SIZE ACCEPTANCE

Brannon-Quan, T. & Licavoli, L. *Love Your Body: A Guide to Transforming Body Image.* Kearney, NE: Morris Publishing, 1996.

Cash, T. *Body Image Workbook.* Oakland, CA: New Harbinger Publications, 1997.

Dixon, M. *Love the Body You Were Born With.* New York: Berkley Putnam Group, 1994.

Emme & Paisner, D. *True Beauty: Positive Attitudes and Practical Tips from the World's Leading Plus-Size Model.* New York: G.P. Putnam's Sons, 1996.

Erdman, C. *Nothing to Lose: A Guide to Sane Living in a Larger Body.* New York: HarperCollins Publishers, 1995.

Freedman, R. *Bodylove: Learning to Like Ourselves and Our Looks.* New York: HarperCollins Publishers, 1988.

Hillman, C. *Love Your Looks: How to Stop Criticizing and Start Appreciating Your Appearance.* New York: Fireside, 1996.

Hutchinson, M. *Transforming Body Image.* Freedom, CA: Crossing Press, 1985.

Johnson, C. *Self Esteem Comes in All Sizes.* New York: Bantam/Doubleday/Dell, 1995.

Johnston, J. *Appearance Obsession.* Deerfield Beach, FL: Health Communications, 1994.

Mayer, K. *Real Women Don't Diet.* Silver Spring, MD: Bartleby Press, 1993.

Naidus, B. *One Size Does Not Fit All.* Littleton, CO: Aigis Publications, 1993.

Newman, L. *SomeBody to Love: A Guide to Loving the Body You Have.* Chicago, IL: Third Side Press, 1992.

Thone, R. *Fat: A Fate Worse than Death?* New York: Harrington Park Press, 1997.

Wiley, C. *Journeys to Self-Acceptance: Fat Women Speak.* Freedom, CA: Crossing Press, 1994.

VI. EDUCATIONAL

Alexander-Mott, L. & Lumsden, B. *Understanding Eating Disorders: Anorexia Nervosa, Bulimia Nervosa and Obesity.* Bristol, PA: Taylor & Francis, 1994.

Friedman, S. *Girls in the 90's.* Vancouver: Salal Books, 1994.

Levine, M. & Hill, L. *Five-Day Lesson Plan on Eating Disorders (Grades 7-12).* Tulsa, OK: National Eating Disorders Organization, 1991.

Shiltz, T. *Eating Concerns Support Group Curriculum, Grades 7-12.* Greenfield, WI: Community Recovery Press, 1997.

Whitaker, L. & Davis W. (Eds.). *Bulimic College Student.* Binghamton, NY: The Haworth Press, 1989.

VII. FOR YOUNG PEOPLE

Bode, J. *Food Fight: A Guide to Eating Disorders for Preteens and their Parents.* New York: Simon & Schuster, 1997.

Cooke, K. *Real Gorgeous: The Truth about Body and Beauty.* New York: W. W. Norton & Co., Inc., 1996.

Folkers, G. & Engelmann, J. *Taking Charge of My Mind & Body.* Minneapolis, MN: Free Spirit Publishing, Inc., 1997.

Hall, L.F. *Perk! The Story of a Teenager with Bulimia.* Carlsbad, CA: Gürze Books, 1997.

Ikeda, J. & Naworski, P. *Am I Fat?* Santa Cruz, CA: ETR Associates, 1992.

Kubersky, R. *Everything You Need to Know About Eating Disorders.* New York: The Rosen Publishing Group, 1992.

Pipher, M. *Hunger Pains: From Fad Diets to Eating Disorders.* Holbrook, MA: Adams Media Group, 1995.

Ward, C. *Compulsive Eating: The Struggle to Feed the Hunger Inside.* New York: Rosen Publishing Group, 1998.

VIII. FOR PARENTS AND LOVED ONES

Berg, F. *Afraid to Eat: Children & Teens in Weight Crisis.* Hettinger, ND: Healthy Weight Journal, 1997.

Costin, C. *Your Dieting Daughter...Is She Dying for Attention?* New York: Brunner/Mazel, 1997.

Goodman, L. *Is Your Child Dying to be Thin?* Pittsburgh, PA: Dorrance Publishing Co. Inc., 1992.

Hirschmann, J. & Zaphiropoulos, L. *Preventing Childhood Eating Problems.* Carlsbad, CA: Gürze Books, 1993.

Jablow, M. *Parent's Guide to Eating Disorders and Obesity.* New York: Dell Publishing, 1992.

Maine, M. *Father Hunger: Fathers, Daughters & Food.* Carlsbad, CA: Gürze Books, 1991.

Riebel, L. & Kaplan, J. *Someone You Love is Obsessed with Food: What You Need to Know about Eating Disorders.* Center City, MN: Hazelden, 1989.

Sherman, R. & Thompson, R. *Bulimia: A Guide for Family & Friends.* Lexington, MA: Lexington Books, 1990.

Waterhouse, D. *Like Mother, Like Daughter.* New York: Warner Books, Inc., 1997.

IX. PERSONAL STORIES, BIOGRAPHY & FICTION

Bitter, C. *Good Enough.* Penfield, NY: HopeLines, 1998.

Bruch, J. *Unlocking the Golden Cage: An Intimate Biography of Hilde Bruch, M.D.* Carlsbad, CA: Gürze Books, 1996.

Fontana, C. *Stick Figure: A Personal Journey through Anorexia and Bulimia.* Melbourne: Hill of Content, 1996.

Foster, P. (Ed.). *Minding the Body: Women Writers on Body and Soul.* New York: Bantam/Doubleday/Dell, 1994.

Grant, S. *Passion of Alice.* Boston, MA: Houghton Mifflin Company, 1995.

Hall, L. *Full Lives: Women Who Have Freed Themselves from Food and Weight Obsession.* Carlsbad, CA: Gürze Books, 1993.

Hanauer, C. *My Sister's Bones.* New York: Bantam/Doubleday/Dell, 1996.

Hornbacher, M. *Wasted: A Memoir of Anorexia & Bulimia.* New York: HarperCollins Publishers, 1998.

Hulan, L. *Pain Behind the Smile: My Battle with Bulimia.* Nashville, TN: Eggman Publishing, 1995.

Kragnow, M. *My Life as a Male Anorexic.* New York: Harrington Park Press, 1996.

Latimer, J. *Beyond the Food Game.* Denver, CO: LivingQuest, 1993.

Levenkron, S. *Best Little Girl in the World.* New York: Warner Books, Inc., 1978.

Medoff, J. *Hunger Point.* New York: HarperCollins Publishers, 1997.

Miller, C. *My Name is Caroline.* Carlsbad, CA: Gürze Books, 1991.

Newman, L. *Fat Chance.* New York: G.P. Putnam's Sons, 1994.

Newman, L. *Good Enough to Eat.* Ithaca, NY: Firebrand Books, 1986.

Rosen, J. *Eve's Apple.* New York: Random House, 1997.

Roth, G. *Appetites.* Bergenfield, NJ: Penguin, 1996.

Roth, G. *When Food is Love.* Bergenfield, NJ: Penguin, 1991.

Rowland, C. *Monster Within: Overcoming Bulimia.* Grand Rapids, MI: Baker Book House, 1984.

Shelley, R. *Anorexics on Anorexia.* Bristol, PA: Taylor and Francis, 1997.

Shute, J. *Life Size.* Boston, MA: Houghton Mifflin Company, 1992.

Smith, C. & Runyon, B. *Diary of an Eating Disorder: A Mother and Daughter Share Their Healing Journey.* Dallas, TX: Taylor Publishing, 1998.

Thayne, E. & Markosian, B. *Hope and Recovery: A Mother-Daughter Story about Anorexia Nervosa, Bulimia, and Manic Depression.* New York: Franklin Watts, 1992.

X.   PROFESSIONAL TEXTS

Agras, W. *Eating Disorders: Management of Obesity, Bulimia and Anorexia Nervosa.* Oxford: Pergamon Press, 1987.

Allison, D. (Eds.). *Handbook of Assessment Methods for Eating Behaviors and Weight Related Problems.* Thousand Oaks, CA: Sage Publications, 1995.

Allison, D. & Pi-Sunyer, F. (Eds.). *Obesity Treatment: Establishing Goals, Improving Outcomes, and Reviewing the Research Agenda.* New York: Plenum Publishing Group, 1995.

American Psychiatric Association. *Practice Guideline for Eating Disorders.* Washington, D.C.: American Psychiatric Association, 1993.

Andersen, A. *Practical Comprehensive Treatment of Anorexia Nervosa and Bulimia.* Baltimore, MD: John Hopkins Press, 1985.

Andersen, A. (Ed.). *Males with Eating Disorders.* New York: Brunner/Mazel, 1990.

Bemporad, J. & Herzog, D. (Eds.). *Psychoanalysis and Eating Disorders.* New York: Guilford Press, 1989.

Brownell, K. & Fairburn, C. (Eds.). *Eating Disorders and Obesity: A Comprehenisve Handbook.* New York: Guilford Press, 1995.

Brownell, K. & Foreyt, J. (Eds.). *Handbook of Eating Disorders.* New York: Basic Books, 1986.

Brownell, K., Rodin, J. & Wilmore, J. (Eds.). *Eating, Body Weight, and Performance in Athletes: Disorders of Modern Society.* Malvern, PA: Lea & Febiger, 1992.

Button, E. *Eating Disorders: Personal Construct Therapy and Change.* Chichester, UK: Wiley, 1993.

Capaldi, E. (Ed.). *Why We Eat What We Eat: The Psychology of Eating.* Washington, DC: American Psychological Assoc., 1996.

Cash, T. & Pruzinsky, T. (Eds.). *Body Image: Develop, Deviance and Changes.* New York: Guilford Press, 1990.

Ciliska, D. *Beyond Dieting.* New York: Brunner/Mazel, 1990.

Cooper, P.J. & Stein, A. (Eds.). *Feeding Problems and Eating Disorders in Children and Adolescents.* Philadelphia, PA: Harwood Academic Publ., 1992.

Crisp, A. & McClelland, L. *Anorexia Nervosa: Guidelines for Assessment and Treatment in Primary and Secondary Care—Second Edition.* East Sussex, UK: Psychology Press, 1996.

Crowther, J., Tennenbaum, D., Hobfoll, S. & Stephens, M. *Etiology of Bulimia Nervosa: The Individual and Familial Context.* Washington, DC: Hemisphere Publishing Corporation, 1992.

Dokter, D. (Ed.). *Arts Therapies & Clients with Eating Disorders.* Bristol, PA: Taylor & Francis, 1995.

Emmett, S. (Ed.). *Theory and Treatment of Anorexia Nervosa and Bulimia: Biomedical, Sociocultural and Psychological Perspectives.* New York: Brunner/Mazel, 1985.

Epling, W.F. & Pierce, W.D. *Activity Anorexia: Theory, Research, and Treatment.* Mahwah, NJ: Lawrence Erlbaum Associates, 1996.

Fairburn, C. & Wilson, T. (Eds.). *Binge Eating: Nature, Assessment and Treatment.* New York: Guilford Press, 1993.

Fallon, P., Katzman, M. & Wooley, S. (Eds.). *Feminist Perspectives on Eating Disorders.* New York: Guilford Press, 1994.

Ferrari, E., Brambilla, F. & Solerte, S. (Eds.). *Primary and Secondary Eating Disorders: A Psychoneuroendocrine and Metabolic Approach.* New York: Pergamon Press, 1994.

Garfinkel, P. & Garner, D. *Anorexia Nervosa: A Multidimensional Perspective.* New York: Brunner/Mazel, 1982.

Garner, D. & Garfinkel, D. (Eds.). *Diagnostic Issues in Anorexia Nervosa and Bulimia.* New York: Brunner/Mazel, 1988.

Garner, D. & Garfinkel, P. (Eds.). *Handbook of Treatment for Eating Disorders.* New York: Guilford Press, 1997.

Halmi, K. *Psychobiology & Treatment of Anorexia Nervosa and Bulimia.* Washington, DC: American Psychiatric Press, 1993.

Hardoff, D. & Chigier, E. (Eds.). *Eating Disorders in Adolescents and Young Adults.* London: Freund Publ., 1988.

Harper-Giuffre, H. & MacKenzie, K. (Eds.). *Group Psychotherapy for Eating Disorders.* Washington, DC: American Psychiatric Press, 1992.

Herzog, W., Deter, H.C., Vandereycken, W. (Eds.). *Course of Eating Disorders: Long-Term Follow-*

up Studies of Anorexia and Bulimia Nervosa. Berlin: Springer-Verlag, 1992.

Hoek, H., Treasure, J. & Katzman, M. (Eds.). *Neurobiology in the Treatment of Eating Disorders.* New York: John Wiley & Sons, 1998.

Hornyak, L. & Baker, E. (Eds.). *Experiential Therapies for Eating Disorders.* New York: Guilford Press, 1989.

Hsu, G. *Eating Disorders.* New York: Guilford Press, 1990.

Hudson, J. & Pope, H. (Eds.). *Psychobiology of Bulimia.* Washington, DC: American Psychiatric Press, 1987.

Johnson, C. (Eds.). *Psychodynamic Treatment of Anorexia Nervosa and Bulimia.* New York: Guilford Press, 1991.

Johnson, C. & Connors, M. *Etiology & Treatment of Bulimia Nervosa.* New York: Basic Books, 1987.

Kaplan, A. & Garfinkel, P. (Ed.). *Medical Issues and Eating Disorders.* New York: Brunner/Mazel, 1993.

Kinoy, B. (Eds.). *Eating Disorders: New Directions in Treatment & Recovery.* Irvington, NY: Columbia University Press, 1994.

Krueger, D. *Body Self: Psychological Self.* New York: Brunner/Mazel, 1989.

Lask, B. & Bryant-Waugh, R. (Eds.). *Childhood Onset: Anorexia Nervosa and Related Eating Disorders.* East Sussex, UK: Lawrence Erlbaum Associates, 1993.

Levens, M. *Eating Disorders and Magical Control of the Body: Treatment through Art Therapy.* London: Routledge, 1995.

McFarland, B. *Brief Therapy and Eating Disorders.* San Francisco, CA: Jossey-Bass, Inc., 1995.

Mitchell, J. *Bulimia Nervosa.* Minneapolis, MN: University of Minnesota Press, 1990.

Mitchell, J. (Ed.). *Anorexia Nervosa and Bulimia: Diagnosis and Treatment.* Minneapolis, MN: University of Minnesota Press, 1985.

Piran, N. & Kaplan, A. (Eds.). *Day Hospital Group Treatment Program for Anorexia Nervosa and Bulimia Nervosa.* New York: Brunner/Mazel, 1990.

Pirke, K.M., Vandereycken, W. & Ploog, D. (Eds.). *The Psychobiology of Bulimia Nervosa.* New York: Springer-Verlag, 1988.

Reiff, D. & Lampson-Reiff, K. *Eating Disorders: Nutrition Therapy in the Recovery Process.* Gaithersburg, MD: Aspen Publishers, 1992.

Schmidt, U. & Treasure, J. *Clinician's Guide to Getting Better Bit(e) by Bit(e).* London: Psychology Press, 1997.

Schneider, L., Cooper, S. & Halmi, K. (Eds.). *Psychobiology of Human Eating Disorders: Preclinical and Clinical Perspectives.* New York: New York Academy of Medicine, 1989.

Schwartz, H. (Ed.). *Bulimia: Psychoanalytic Treatment and Theory—Second Edition.* Madison, CT: International Universities Press, 1990.

Schwartz, M. & Cohn, L. (Eds.). *Sexual Abuse and Eating Disorders.* New York: Brunner/Mazel, 1996.

Smolak, L., Levine, M. & Striegel-Moore, R. (Eds.). *Developmental Psychopathology of Eating Disorders.* Mahwah, NJ: Lawrence Erlbaum Associates, 1996.

Steinhausen, H. (Ed.). *Eating Disorders in Adolescence: Anorexia and Bulimia Nervosa.* Hawthorne, NY: Walter De Gruyter, 1996.

Stierlin, H. & Weber, G. *Unlocking the Family Door: A Systematic Approach to the Understanding and Treatment of Anorexia Nervosa.* New York: Brunner/Mazel, 1989.

Stunkard, A. & Stellar, E. (Eds.). *Eating and Its Disorders.* Philadelphia, PA: Lippincott-Raven Publishers, 1984.

Szmuckler, G., Dare, C. & Treasure, J. *Handbook of Eating Disorders Theory, Treatment, and Research.* New York: John Wiley & Sons, 1996.

Thompson, J. K. (Eds.). *Body Image, Eating Disorders and Obesity.* Washington, DC: American Psychological, 1996.

Thompson, R. & Sherman, R. *Helping Athletes With Eating Disorders.* Champaign, IL: Human Kinetics Publishers, Inc., 1993.

Van Den Broucke, S., Vandereycken, W. & Norre, J. *Eating Disorders and Marital Relations.* London: Routledge, 1997.

Vandereycken, W., Kog, E. & Vanderlinden, J. (Eds.). *Family Approach to Eating Disorders.* Dana Point, CA: PMA Publishing, 1989.

Vanderlinden, J. *Dissociative Experiences, Trauma and Hypnosis: Research Findings & Clinical Applications in Eating Disorders.* Delft, The Netherlands: Uitgeverij Eburon, 1993.

Vanderlinden, J., Norre, J. & Vandereycken, W. *Practical Guide to Treatment of Bulimia Nervosa.* New York: Brunner/Mazel, 1989.

Vanderlinden, J. & Vandereycken, W. *Trauma, Dissociation and Impulse Dyscontrol in Eating Disorders.* New York: Brunner/Mazel, 1997.

Wadden, T. & VanItallie, T. (Eds.). *Treatment of the Seriously Obese Patient.* New York: Guilford Press, 1992.

Walsh, B.T. *Eating Behavior in Eating Disorders.* Washington, DC: American Psychiatric Press, 1988.

Werne, J. (Eds.). *Treating Eating Disorders.* San Francisco, CA: Jossey-Bass, Inc., 1996.

Weston, L.A. & Savage, L.M. (Eds.). *Obesity: Advances in Understanding and Treatment.* Southborough, MA: IBC Biomedical Library, 1996.

Williamson, D. *Assessment of Eating Disorders: Obesity, Anorexia, and Bulimia Nervosa.* Needham Heights, MA: Alyn & Bacon, 1992.

Wilson, C.P., Hogan, C. & Mintz, I. (Eds.). *Psychodynamic Technique in the Treatment of Eating Disorders.* Northvale, NJ: Jason Aronson, Inc., 1992.

Woodside, B., Shekter-Wolfson, L., Brandes, J. & Lackstrom, J. *Eating Disorders & Marriage.* New York: Brunner/Mazel, 1993.

Woodside, D. B. & Shekter-Wolfson, L. (Eds.). *Family Approaches in Treatment of Eating Disorders.* Washington, DC: American Psychiatric Press, 1991.

Yager, J. (Ed.). *Eating Disorders* (Psychiatric Clinics of North America). Philadelphia, PA: WB Saunders, 1996.

Yager, J., Gwirtsman, H. & Edelstein, C. (Eds.). *Special Problems in Managing Eating Disorders.* Washington, DC: American Psychiatric Press, 1992.

Yates, A. *Compulsive Exercise & Eating Disorders.* New York: Brunner/Mazel, 1991.

XI. SOCIOCULTURAL AND HISTORICAL PERSPECTIVES

Bloom, C. & Gitter, A., Gutwill, S., Kogel, L. & Zaphiropoulos, L. *Eating Problems: A Feminist Psychoanalytic Treatment Model.* New York: Basic Books, 1994.

Bordo, S. *Unbearable Weight: Feminism, Western Culture, and the Body.* Berkeley, CA: University of California Press, 1993.

Brown, C. & Jasper, K. *Consuming Passions.* Toronto: Second Story Press, 1993.

Brown, L. & Rothblum, E. *Overcoming Fear of Fat.* Binghamton, NY: The Haworth Press, 1989.

Brumberg, J. *Body Project: An Intimate History of American Girls.* New York: Random House, Inc., 1997.

Brumberg, J. *Fasting Girls: A History of Anorexia Nervosa.* Bergenfield, NJ: Penguin, 1989.

Chernin, K. *Hungry Self: Women, Eating and Identity.* New York: HarperCollins Publishers, 1985.

Chernin, K. *Obsession.* New York: HarperCollins Publishers, 1981.

Chernin, K. *Reinventing Eve.* New York: HarperCollins Publishers, 1989.

Dolan, B. & Gitzinger, I. (Eds.). *Why Women? Gender Issues and Eating Disorders.* Atlantic Highland, NJ: Humanities Press, 1994.

Fraser, L. *Losing It: False Hopes and Fat Profits in the Diet Industry.* New York: Penguin, 1997.

Gaesser, G. *Big Fat Lies.* New York: Random House, Inc., 1996.

Goodman, W.C. *Invisible Woman: Confronting Weight Prejudice in America.* Carlsbad, CA: Gürze Books, 1995.

Gordon, R. *Anorexia & Bulimia: Anatomy of a Social Epidemic.* Williston, VT: Blackwell Publishers, 1990.

Hancock, E. *Girl Within.* New York: Random House, Inc., 1989.

Harris, M. *Down from the Pedestal: Moving Beyond Idealized Images of Womanhood.* New York: Anchor Books, 1994.

Heywood, L. *Dedication to Hunger: The Anorexic Aesthetic in Modern Culture.* Berkeley, CA: University of California Press, 1996.

Jackson, E. *Food and Transformation: Imagery and Symbolism of Eating.* Toronto: Inner City Books, 1996.

Klein, R. *Eat Fat.* New York: Pantheon Books, 1996.

MacSween, M. *Anorexic Bodies: A Feminist and Sociological Perspective on Anorexia Nervosa.* London: Routledge, 1996.

Malson, H. *Thin Woman: Feminism, Post-Structuralism, and the Social Psychology of Anorexia Nervosa.* London: Routledge, 1998.

Meadow, R. & Weiss, L. *Good Girls Don't Eat Dessert: Women's Conflicts about Eating and Sexuality.* Binghamton, NY: The Haworth Press, 1992.

Millman, M. *Such a Pretty Face: Being Fat in America.* New York: W. W. Norton & Co., Inc., 1980.

Nasser, M. *Culture and Weight Consciousness.* New York: Routledge, 1997.

Orbach, S. *Fat Is a Feminist Issue.* New York: Putnam Berkley Group, 1978.

Orenstein, P. *SchoolGirls: Young Women, Self-Esteem and the Confidence Gap.* New York: Bantam/Doubleday/Dell, 1994.

Pipher, M. *Reviving Ophelia: Saving the Selves of Adolescent Girls.* New York: Random House, Inc., 1994.

Ryan, J. *Little Girls in Pretty Boxes: The Making and Breaking of Elite Gymnasts and Figure Skaters.* New York: Doubleday Dell Publishing, 1995.

Thompson, B. *Hunger So Wide and So Deep.* Minneapolis, MN: University of Minnesota Press, 1994.

Vandereycken, W. & van Deth, R. *From Fasting Saints to Anorexic Girls: The History of Self-Starvation.* New York: New York University Press, 1994.

Williams, G. *Internal Landscapes and Foreign Bodies: Eating Disorders and Other Pathologies.* London: Routledge, 1998.

Winkler, M. & Cole, L. (Eds). *Good Body: Asceticism in Contemporary Culture.* New Haven, CT: Yale University Press, 1994.

Wolf, N. *Beauty Myth.* New York: William Morrow, 1991.

Periodicals on Eating Disorders

The following publications are the primary journals and newsletters used in the eating-disorders field. Additionally, several nonprofit organizations (see "Nonprofit Eating Disorders Organizations") publish newsletters that are available to their members.

PERIODICALS

Eating Awareness & Self Enhancement. EASE, PO Box 8032, Minneapolis, MN 55408, 612-226-5640. Bimonthly, self-help newsletter.

Eating Disorders: The Journal of Treatment and Prevention. Taylor & Francis, 1900 Frost Road, Ste 101, Bristol, PA 19007-1598, 800-821-8312. Quarterly, peer-reviewed journal.

Eating Disorders Review. Gürze Books, PO Box 2238, Carlsbad, CA 92018, 760- 434-7533. Bimonthly, clinical newsletter.

Healthy Weight Journal. Decker Inc., 4 Hughson St. S., PO Box 620, Hamilton, ON L8N 3K7 Canada, 800-568-7281. Bimonthly journal with reports on weight issues.

International Journal of Eating Disorders. John Wiley & Sons, 605 Third Ave., New York, NY 10158, 212-850-6000. Bimonthly, peer-reviewed journal.

International Journal of Obesity. Macmillan Press, Ltd., Brunel Rd., Basingstoke, Hants, RG21 2XS, UK. Monthly peer reviewed journal.

Obesity Research. North American Association for the Study of Obesity, 6400 Perkins Rd., Baton Rouge, LA 70808, 504-763-0934. Bimonthly, peer-reviewed journal.

BIBLIOGRAPHIES OF JOURNAL ARTICLES

In addition to print indexes to journal articles, such as *Index Medicus* or *Psychological Abstracts,* there are two bibliographical sources dedicated to eating disorders:

Celeste Morrow's Home Page
http://www.cmorrow.net/biblio.htm
Updated regularly, includes bibliographies on eating disorders and on perfectionism, body image, and dance.

NEDO: National Eating Disorders Organization, 6655 S. Yale Ave., Tulsa, OK 74136, 918-481-4044. Publishes a semiannual bibliography of most recent journal articles on eating disorders for NEDO members; back issues may be requested.

ADDITIONAL RESOURCES

Eating Disorder Resource Catalogue. Gürze Books, PO Box 2238, Carlsbad, CA 92018, 800-756-7533. Free resource that includes more than 125 books on eating disorders, lists of eating disorders nonprofit associations and treatment facilities, and basic facts about eating disorders. Catalogue is also available online at http://www.bulimia.com.

Nonprofit Eating Disorders Organizations

The following, comprehensive list of U.S. organizations are all primarily devoted to eating-disorders education, treatment, and prevention. Additionally, some organizations are concerned with size-acceptance and wellness, and two membership associations for eating-disorders professionals (AED and IAEDP) are included.

AED: Academy for Eating Disorders Degnon Associates, Inc.
6728 Old McLean Village Dr.
McLean, VA 22101-3906
703-556-9222
http://www.acadeatdis.org
For eating-disorders professionals: promotes effective treatment, develops prevention initiatives, stimulates research, and sponsors an international conference and an Internet chat line for members.

AABA: American Anorexia/Bulimia Association
165 W. 46th St., #1108
New York, NY 10036
212-575-6200
http://www.members.aol.com/AmanBu
A source of public information, support groups, referrals, speakers, educational programs, and professional training. Quarterly newsletter.

ANAD: National Association of Anorexia Nervosa & Associated Disorders
P.O. Box 7
Highland Park, IL 60035
847-831-3438
http://www.healthtouch.com/level1/leaflets/anad/anad001.htm
Distributes listings of therapists, hospitals, and informative materials; and sponsors support groups, conferences, advocacy campaigns, research, and a crisis hotline.

Anorexia and Bulimia Association of Rhode Island
94 Waterman St
Providence, RI 02906
401-861-2335
Provides support groups and other services for adults with anorexia nervosa, bulimia nervosa, and binge eating disorder.

ANRED: Anorexia Nervosa and Related Eating Disorders, Inc.
(*see also* NEDO)
6655 S. Yale Ave.
Tulsa, OK 74136
918-481-4044
http://www.anred.com
Provides free and low-cost information on eating disorders and compulsive exercise. Publishes booklets, brochures, fact sheets, and a monthly newsletter. Recently merged with NEDO.

CRAED: Capital Region Association for Eating Disorders
1653 Central Ave
Albany, NY 12205
518-464-9043
Provides support groups and refers to doctors, nutritionists, and counselors; furnishes speakers to the community including schools.

EDAP: Eating Disorders Awareness & Prevention
603 Stewart St., Ste 803
Seattle, WA 98101
206-382-3587
http://members.aol.com/edapinc/home.html
Sponsors "Eating Disorders Awareness Week" each February with a network of state coordinators and educational info. Sponsors conference and publishes newsletter, and develops educational and prevention programs.

Healing Connections, Inc.
212-585-3450
FAX: (212) 585-3452
Nonprofit organization raising funds to help to defray costs of treatment for individuals and families who cannot otherwise afford care.

Christy Henrich Foundation
P.O. Box 414287
Kansas City, MO 64141-4287
816-395-2611
Nonprofit organization dedicated to fighting the battle against eating disorders, founded in memory of Christy Henrich, an elite gymnast who lost her battle with anorexia on July 26, 1994.

IAEDP: International Association of Eating Disorders Professionals
427 Wooping Loop #1819
Altamonte Springs, FL 32701
800-800-8126
FAX: 407-832-2661
http://www.iaedp.com
Membership organization for professionals: provides certification, education, local chapters, a newsletter, and an annual symposium.

MEDA: Massachusetts Eating Disorders Association, Inc.
92 Pearl Street
Newton, MA 02158
617-558-1881
http://www.medainc.org
Provides newsletter, referral network, local support groups, educational seminars, and conference.

NAAFA: National Association to Advance Fat Acceptance, Inc.
P.O. Box 188620
Sacramento, CA 95818
916-558-6880
http://www.naafa.org
Advocacy group: provides newsletter, educational materials, regional chapters, annual convention, and pen-pal program.

NEDO: National Eating Disorders Organization
Affiliated with Laureate Eating Disorders Program; administrative office for ANRED
See also ANRED
6655 S. Yale Ave.
Tulsa, OK 74136
918-481-4044

http://www.laureate.com/nedointro.html
Focuses on prevention, education, research, and treatment referrals; distributes information and newsletter; conference.

NEDSP: The National Eating Disorders Screening Program
A program of the National Mental Health Illness Screening Project, Inc.
One Washington Street, Suite 304
Wellesley Hills, MA 02181
781-239-0071
http://www.nmisp.org
Free anonymous public outreach and education program: offers information, written self-tests, one-on-one meetings with health professionals, and referrals for further evaluation if necessary.

OA: Overeaters Anonymous Headquarters
P.O. Box 44020
Rio Rancho, NM 87174-4020
505-891-2664
http://www.overeatersanonymous.org
12-step self-help fellowship; free local meetings listed in the telephone white pages under "Overeaters Anonymous."

Vitality, Inc. Promoting Wellness and Respect for All Shapes & Sizes
91 S. Main St.
West Hartford, CT 06107
860-521-2515
http://www.tiac.net/users/vtlty
Diet industry watchdog group: information packet on diet laws, three newsletters, and articles on non-dieting approach, $10.

Videos on Eating Disorders and Weight-Related Issues

The following videos (listed alphabetically by title) are available directly from the producers or distributors listed below. The prices, which are subject to change, illustrate a wide range of charges. For example, films that run about 30 minutes can cost as little as $19.95 or as much as $299, with many prices in between. Also, some distributors offer rental or preview rates while others do not. Contact information for the production companies/distributors follows the listing of videos.

Afraid to Eat: Eating Disorders and the Student Athlete—17 min. $14.95
Karol Media; developed by the NCAA

An Anorexic's Tale: The Brief Life of Catherine—80 min. $159
Films for the Humanities and Sciences

Anorexia and Bulimia—19 min. $89.95
   Films for the Humanities and Sciences

Anorexia Nervosa: The Covert Rebellion—26 min.
$149.95
   Aims Media

Beyond the Looking Glass: Body Image and Self-Esteem—$189
   Hourglass Productions, Inc.

Body Trust: Undieting Your Way to Health and Happiness—60 min. $24.95
   Production West

Bulimia: Out-of-Control Eating—23 min.
$149.95
   Aims Media

Bulimia: The Binge-Purge Obsession—25 min.
$150
   Baxley Media Group

Bulimia: The Binge Purge Syndrome—28 min.
$99.95
   Aims Media

Dark Secrets, Bright Victory: One Woman's Recovery from Bulimia—13 min. $60
   Hazelden Foundation

The Discovery of Dawn: Body Image and Eating Disorders—30 min. $195
   NEWIST/CESA 7

Dying to be Thin—25 min. $250
   Baxley Media Group

Dying to be Thin—28 min. $149
   Films for the Humanities and Sciences

Eating: Out of Control—30 min. $79.95
   Karol Media

Eating Disorders—26 min. $89.95
   Films for the Humanities and Sciences

Eating Disorders. From the American College of Physicians—25 min. $20
   Karol Media

Eating Disorders. From the Teen Health Series—30 min. $39.93
   Karol Media

Eating Disorders: Myths vs. Realities—27 min.
$145
   Therapeutic Education Inc.

Eating Disorders: The Hunger Within—48 min
$129
   Films for the Humanities and Sciences

Eating Disorders: The Slender Trap—21 min.
$149.95
   Aims Media

Eating Disorders: What Can You Do?—15 min.
$14.95
   Karol Media

The Enigma of Anorexia Nervosa—58 min. 3 parts $250 each, or $695 total
   Baxley Media Group

Faces of Recovery: Kathy Rigby on Eating Disorders—35 min. $29.95
   Increase Video

The Famine Within—55, 90, 118 min. versions.
Call for prices.
   Direct Cinema Limited

Fat Chance: The Big Prejudice—72 min. $29.95
   Bullfrog Films

Feeling Good About Me—15 min. $95
   Sunburst

Foodfright—30 min. Call for price.
   Direct Cinema Limited

Healthy Woman 2000: Women and Eating Disorders—20 min. $19.95
   ITV

Heavy Load—36 min. $99
   Baxley Media Group

In Our Own Words: Personal Accounts of Eating Disorders—30 min. $39.95
   Gürze Books

It's Not About Food—3 videos, 2@ 50min, 1 @ 1hr. 15min. $85 ea, $225 set.
   Alternatives

Killing Us Softly—29 min. $299
   Cambridge Documentary Films Inc.

Mirror, Mirror—14 min. $150
   UCSB Student Health Service

The Myth of the Perfect Body: Accepting Your Physical Self—21 min. $89
   Karol Media

Out of Balance: Nutrition and Eating Disorders—16 min. $14.95
   Karol Media; developed by the NCAA

The Perfect Body—14 min. $150
   UCSB

Pregnancy and Eating Disorders—28 min.
$89.95
   Aims Media

The Problem with Food—27 min. $19.95
   Karol Media

Real People: Coping with Eating Disorders—27 min. $169
   Sunburst

A Season in Hell—59 min. $199
 New Day Films

Recovering Bodies: Overcoming Eating Disorders—34 min. $175
 Media Education Foundation

The Secret Life of Mary-Margaret: Portrait of a Bulimic—30 min. $69.95
 Aims Media

Self-Image and Eating Disorders: A Mirror for the Heart—24 min. $89.95
 Films for the Humanities and Sciences

Shaping the Future: Freedom from Eating Disorders—6 @15min. each $179 total
 NCES

The Silent Hunger: Anorexia and Bulimia—46 min $149
 Films for the Humanities and Sciences

Skin Deep—26 min. $199
 Disney Educational Productions

Slim Hopes: Advertising & the Obsession with Thinness—30 min. $250
 Media Education Foundation

Still Killing Us Softly—32 min. $299
 Cambridge Documentary Films Inc.

Teen Health Series: Eating Disorders—30 min $39.95
 Total Marketing Services

Thea's Mirror: A Guide to Helping Teens with Eating Disorders—25 min. $95
 Karol Media

Thin Dreams—21 min. $99
 Baxley Media Group

Wasting Away—25 min. $180
 Agency for Instructional Technology

When Food is an Obsession: Overcoming Eating Disorders—$189
 Hourglass Productions

When Food Is Love—3 one hr. videos—$30 ea. or $75 for all 3
 Breaking Free

VIDEO DISTRIBUTORS AND PRODUCERS

Agency for Instructional Technology
Box A
Bloomington, IN 47402
812-339-2203

Aims Media
9710 DeSota Ave.
Chatsworth, CA 91311
800-367-2467

Alternatives
217 State St., #306
Santa Barbara, CA 93101
805-899-1970

Baxley Media Group
110 W. Main St.
Urbana, IL 61801-2700
800-421-6999

Breaking Free
PO Box 2852
Santa Cruz, CA 95063
408-685-8601

Bullfrog Films
Box 149
Oley, PA 19547
610-779-8226; 800-543-3764

Cambridge Documentary Films, Inc.
PO Box 385
Cambridge, MA 02139
617-484-3993

Direct Cinema Limited
PO Box 10003
Santa Monica, CA 90410
310-396-4774

Disney Educational Productions
105 Terry Dr., Ste 120
Newton, PA 18940
800-295-5010

Films for the Humanities and Sciences
PO Box 2053
Princeton, NJ 08543
206-382-3587

Gürze Books
PO Box 2238
Carlsbad, CA 92018
760-434-7533

Hazelden Foundation
PO Box 176, 1525 Pleasant Valley Rd.
Center City, MN 55012-0176
800-328-9000 ext 4073

Hourglass Productions, Inc.
277 Old Army Rd.
Scarsdale, NY 10583
914-723-3065

Increase Video
6860 Canby Ave., #118
Reseda, CA 91335
818-707-0300

ITV
1 Park Place
621 NW 53rd St., #350
Boca Raton, FL 33487
800-INFO ITV (407-997-5433)

Karol Media
350 N. Pennsylvania Ave., Box 7600
Wilkes-Barre, PA 18773-7600
800-526-4773

Media Education Foundation
26 Center St.

Northampton, MA 01060
413-586-4170; 800-897-0089

NCES
1904 E. 123rd St.
Olathe, KS 66061
888-545-5653

New Day Films
22-D Hollywood Ave.
Hohokus, NJ 07423
201-652-6590

NEWIST/CESA 7
Studio B, IS 1040, UW Green Bay
Green Bay, WI 54311
800-633-7445

Production West
2110 Overland Ave., Suite 120
Billings, MT 59102
406-656-9417

Sunburst
39 Washington Ave.
Pleasantville, NY 10570
800-431-1934

Therapeutic Education Inc.
514 S. Livingston Ave.
Livingston, NJ 07039
201-740-9085

Total Marketing Services
Dept 59293, 400 Morris Ave.
Long Branch, NJ 07740
800-888-school4u

UCSB Student Health Service
Health Education Department
Santa Barbara, CA 93106

Internet Sites on Eating Disorders

Anyone who has searched the World Wide Web for information on eating disorders knows that it can be a frustrating task. A recent Internet search for "eating disorders" found more than 150,000 sites—hardly a practical method to find anything useful. Additionally new Web pages appear every day, and addresses are often quickly obsolete.

The best way to find information about eating disorders on the Internet is to visit an established, well-maintained site that provides general information as well as links to other eating-disorders sites. The first three sites listed below are excellent resources for eating-disorders information and contain numerous links to additional information as well. These sites have been in service for several years and are regularly updated.

The remaining entries in the first list (listed alphabetically) include a variety of sites specifically about eating disorders. The second list contains additional addresses for various health organizations. More Web sites may also be found in entries in the sections on "Nonprofit Eating Disorders Organizations" and "Treatment Facilities", (pages xxx–xxx).

COMPREHENSIVE RESOURCES FOR EATING-DISORDERS INFORMATION

Eating-Disorders Resource Catalog
http://www.bulimia.com
Contains a list of more than 125 books and a comprehensive list of videos on eating-disorders, links to many national eating-disorders organizations, links to many of the eating disorders sites listed below, and an index of *Eating Disorders Review* articles.

Mirror-Mirror
http://www.mirror-mirror.org/eatdis.htm
Contains definitions, signs and symptoms, information on physical dangers of eating disorders, specific information on athletes, men, and children with eating disorders, relapse warning signs, and much more; also has links to many personal Web sites of individuals who have had or have recovered from eating disorders.

The Something Fishy Website on Eating Disorders
http://www.something-fishy.com/
Includes information on signs and symptoms, physical dangers of eating disorders, definitions,

words from victims, a family and friends bulletin board, and information on treatments. Also includes a memorial page dedicated to those who have died of eating disorders, links to other sites, and much more.

OTHER GENERAL RESOURCES FOR EATING-DISORDERS INFORMATION

Aliveness Experience for Healing Emotional Eating & Related Disorders

http://www.aliveness.net/index.htm
Created by Jane E. Latimer, a writer of books on food issues, contains information on healing emotional eating and free workbook pages, an online newsletter, and ongoing programs.

American Society of Bariatric Physicians

http://www.sni.net/bariatrics/
Presents information on obesity and treatment options from a professional association of physicians who specialize in the medical treatment of obesity.

Anorexia-Information and Guidance for Patients, Family and Friends

http://users.neca.com/cwildes/
A comprehensive and personal site by Cheryl A. Wildes, includes pages on special interest areas (males, older victims, children, etc.), links to other pages, and online support.

Ask Noah About: Eating Disorders: Anorexia and Bulimia Nervosa

http://www.noah.cuny.edu/wellconn/
eatdisorders.html
Lists questions and brief, but complete, answers on a variety of topics; includes an updated bibliography of journal articles and various links to other eating-disorders sites.

Eating Disorders Recovery Online

http://www.edrecovery.com
Provides online treatment consultations (fee required) and message boards, along with basic information.

Eating Disorders Support & Information

http://www.geocities.com/HotSprings/5395/
Contains facts, personal testimonies, stories and poetry, links to other pages, book reviews, and online support.

Healthy Weight Network

http://www.healthyWeightNetwork.com/
Produced by the publishers of the *Healthy Weight Journal,* contains scientific information on weight and eating issues and reports on controversial topics.

HUGS International

http://www.hugs.com

Maintained by advocates of not dieting, contains information on International No-Dieting Day, teen programs, and adult nondieting programs.

Information On Weight Control/Obesity and Eating Disorders

http://www.weight.com/
With up-to-date information that is particularly thorough on obesity and weight control, contains general information on various eating disorders and related medical conditions, such as diabetes, cholesterol, and hypertension.

Males and Eating Disorders

http://www.primenet.com/~danslos/males.html
Includes lists of articles on males and eating disorders, Dan's story, and numerous links.

Mental Health Net: Eating Disorders

http://eatingdisorders.cmhc.com/
Includes information on eating-disorders symptoms and treatments, lists of eating disorders organizations and online resources. Also includes a support group.

New Realities Eating Disorders Recovery Centre

http://www.newrealitiescan.com/
Toronto treatment center which contains basic information about eating-disorders, a self-assessment questionnaire, a free newsletter, and links to other sites.

Optimal Eating

http://www.healthyeating.com/
Contains information for therapists, information on professional workshops, and eating-disorders articles.

Overcoming Overeating Home Page

http://www.overcomingovereating.com/
Originated by Jane Hirschmann and Carol Munter, authors of books on recovery from compulsive eating and body acceptance, includes their campaign for women to end body hatred and dieting, personal stories, and links to more information.

Lucy Serpell

http://www.iop.bpmf.ac.uk/home/depts/psychiat/
edu/eat.htm
One of the Web's most comprehensive eating-disorders sites (based in the UK), lists eating-disorder information, resources, links, and much more.

OTHER SELECTED GENERAL HEALTH SITES

American Academy for Child and Adolescent Psychiatry

http://www.aacap.org/web/aacap

American Diabetes Association
   http://www.diabetes.org

American Diabetic Association
   http://www.eatright.org

Center for Disease Control and Prevention
   http://www.cdc.gov

FDA Center for Food Safety & Applied Nutrition
   http://www.vm.cfsan.fda.gov/index.html

Healthgate's Medline
   http://www.healthgate.com

National Institutes of Health
   http://www.nih.gov

National Library of Medicine
   http://www.nlm.nih.gov

Physicians Online
   http://www.po.com/Welcome.html

World Health Organization
   http://www.who.ch

INDEX

Index

by Francine Cronshaw